Guide to Neuropsychiatric Therapeutics

Guide to Neuropsychiatric Therapeutics

C. Edward Coffey, MD, FANPA

Kathleen and Earl Ward Chair of Psychiatry,
Vice President, Behavioral Health Services,
Henry Ford Health System;
Professor of Psychiatry and of Neurology,
Wayne State University, Henry Ford Campus,
Detroit, Michigan

Thomas W. McAllister, MD, FANPA

Professor of Psychiatry, Director, Neuropsychiatry,
Dartmouth-Hitchcock Medical Center,
Lebanon, New Hampshire

Jonathan M. Silver, MD, FANPA

Clinical Professor of Psychiatry, New York
University School of Medicine, New York, New York

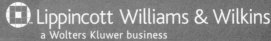 Lippincott Williams & Wilkins
a Wolters Kluwer business
Philadelphia · Baltimore · New York · London
Buenos Aires · Hong Kong · Sydney · Tokyo

Acquisitions Editor: Charles W. Mitchell
Managing Editor: Lisa Kairis
Project Manager: Bridgett Dougherty
Associate Director of Marketing: Adam Glazer
Design Coordinator: Doug Smock
Production Services: Laserwords Private Limited, Chennai, India
Printer: R.R. Donnelley, Crawfordsville

530 Walnut Street
Philadelphia, PA 19106 USA
LWW.com

Printed in the USA

Library of Congress Cataloging-in-Publication Data
Guide to neuropsychiatric therapeutics / [edited by] C. Edward Coffey,
    Thomas W. McAllister, Jonathan Silver.
    p. ; cm.
Includes bibliographical references and index.
ISBN 13: 978-0-7817-9935-5
ISBN 10: 0-7817-9935-X
    1. Neuropsychiatry. 2. Neurobehavioral disorders.   I. Coffey, C.
Edward, 1952- . II. McAllister, Thomas W. III. Silver, Jonathan M.,
1953- .
    [DNLM: 1. Neurologic Manifestations. 2. Mental Disorders—physio-
pathology. 3. Mental Disorders—therapy. 4. Nervous System Diseases
—physiopathology. 5. Nervous System Diseases—therapy. 6. Neuropsychology—methods.   WL 340 G946 2007]
RC341.G852 2007
616.89—dc22
                                                    2006028360

Care has been taken to confirm the accuracy of the information presented and to describe generally accepted practices. However, the authors, editors, and publisher are not responsible for errors or omissions or for any consequences from application of the information in this book and make no warranty, expressed or implied, with respect to the currency, completeness, or accuracy of the contents of the publication. Application of this information in a particular situation remains the professional responsibility of the practitioner.

The authors, editors, and publisher have exerted every effort to ensure that drug selection and dosage set forth in this text are in accordance with current recommendations and practice at the time of publication. However, in view of ongoing research, changes in government regulations, and the constant flow of information relating to drug therapy and drug reactions, the reader is urged to check the package insert for each drug for any change in indications and dosage and for added warnings and precautions. This is particularly important when the recommended agent is a new or infrequently employed drug.

Some drugs and medical devices presented in this publication have Food and Drug Administration (FDA) clearance for limited use in restricted research settings. It is the responsibility of the health care provider to ascertain the FDA status of each drug or device planned for use in their clinical practice.

To purchase additional copies of this book, call our customer service department at (800) 638-3030 or fax orders to (301) 223-2320. International customers should call (301) 223-2300.

Visit Lippincott Williams & Wilkins on the Internet: at LWW.com. Lippincott Williams & Wilkins customer service representatives are available from 8:30 am to 6 pm, EST.

10 9 8 7 6 5 4 3 2 1

*To our patients, whose lives we are dedicated
to improving through excellence in the science
and art of health care and healing*

Contents

Contributors

Karen E. Anderson, MD
*Assistant Professor of Psychiatry
and Neurology, Division of Psychiatry
and Neurosciences, University
of Maryland Medical Center,
Baltimore, Maryland*

David B. Arciniegas, MD
*Director, Neurobehavioral Disorders
Program, Associate Professor of Psychiatry
and Neurology, University of Colorado
School of Medicine, Denver, Colorado;
Co-Medical Director, Brain Injury
Rehabilitation Unit, HealthONE Spalding
Rehabilitation Hospital,
Aurora, Colorado*

Sheldon Benjamin, MD
*Professor, Department of Psychiatry and
Neurology, University of Massachusetts
Medical School; Director of Psychiatric
Education and Training, Director
of Neuropsychiatry, Department
of Psychiatry, UMass Memorial
Healthcare, Inc.,
Worcester, Massachusetts*

Kevin J. Black, MD
*Associate Professor, Department
of Psychiatry, Neurology, Radiology,
and Neurobiology, Washington University
School of Medicine; Attending
Psychiatrist, Department of Psychiatry,
Barnes-Jewish Hospital,
St. Louis, Missouri*

Nash N. Boutros, MD
*Professor, Department of Psychiatry
and Behavioral Neurosciences
and Neurology, Wayne State University,
School of Medicine,
Detroit, Michigan*

C. Edward Coffey, MD
*Kathleen and Earl Ward Chair
of Psychiatry, Vice President, Behavioral
Health Services, Henry Ford Health
System; Professor of Psychiatry and
of Neurology, Wayne State University,
Henry Ford Campus,
Detroit, Michigan*

John J. Campbell, MD
*Medical Director of Hospital Psychiatric
Services, Maine Medical Center; Clinical
Associate Professor of Psychiatry,
University of Vermont
College of Medicine,
Portland, Maine*

Jeffrey L. Cummings, MD
*Professor of Neurology and Psychiatry,
Department of Neurology, University
of California, Los Angeles,
Los Angeles, California*

James D. Duffy, MD, FANPA
*Professor of Psychiatry in Public Health,
Weill Medical College of Cornell
University; Director, Institute
for Palliative Medicine,
The Methodist Hospital,
Houston, Texas*

Jess G. Fiedorowicz, MD
*Fellow Associate, Department
of Psychiatry, The University of Iowa;
Fellow Associate, Department
of Psychiatry, The University of Iowa
Hospitals and Clinics,
Iowa City, Iowa*

Laura A. Flashman, PhD, ABPP-Cn
*Associate Professor, Department
of Psychiatry, Dartmouth Medical School,
Dartmouth-Hitchcock Medical Center,
Lebanon, New Hampshire; Co-Director,
Neuropsychology Program,
Dartmouth-Hitchcock Medical Center
and New Hampshire Hospital,
Concord, New Hampshire*

Robin A. Hurley, MD, FANPA
*Associate Chief of Staff, Mental Health &
Behavioral Sciences; Co-Director for
Education, Veterans Integrated Service
Network 6 Mental Illness Research,
Education, and Clinical Center, Salisbury
Veterans Affairs Medical Center,
Salisbury, North Carolina; Associate
Professor, Department of Psychiatry
and Radiology, Wake Forest University
School of Medicine, Winston-Salem, North
Carolina; Clinical Associate Professor,
Department of Psychiatry,
Baylor College of Medicine,
Houston, Texas*

Daniel I. Kaufer, MD
*Associate Professor, Director, Memory
and Cognitive Disorders, Department
of Neurology, The University of North
Carolina at Chapel Hill,
Chapel Hill, North Carolina*

Walter Knysz, III, MD
*Director, Consultation-Liaison Psychiatry,
Assistant Director, Brain Stimulation
Service, Department of Behavioral Health,
Henry Ford Health System,
Detroit, Michigan*

**Edward C. Lauterbach, MD, FANPA,
DFAPA**
*Chief, Division of Adult and Geriatric
Psychiatry, Department of Psychiatry
and Behavioral Sciences, Mercer
University School of Medicine; Medical
Staff, Department of Psychiatry, The
Medical Center of Central Georgia,
Macon, Georgia*

Po H. Lu, PsyD
*Assistant Clinical Professor, Department
of Neurology, University of California
at Los Angeles,
Los Angeles, California*

Thomas W. McAllister, MD, FANPA
*Professor of Psychiatry,
Director, Neuropsychiatry
Dartmouth-Hitchcock Medical Center,
Lebanon, New Hampshire*

**James R. Merikangas, MD, FACP,
FANPA**
*Clinical Professor of Psychiatry
and Behavioral Neuroscience, Department
of Psychiatry, George Washington
University, Washington, DC; Attending
in Psychiatry and Neurology, Department
of Psychiatry, Suburban Hospital,
Bethesda, Maryland*

Fred Ovsiew, MD
*Professor, Department of Psychiatry,
University of Chicago; Medical Director,
Adult Inpatient Psychiatry; Chief, Clinical
Neuropsychiatry, Department
of Psychiatry, University of
Chicago Hospitals,
Chicago, Illinois*

Alya Reeve, MD
*Associate Professor, Department
of Psychiatry and Neurology,
The University of New Mexico;
Co-Investigator, Continuum
of Care Project, University
of New Mexico,
Albuquerque, New Mexico*

Robert G. Robinson, MD
*Professor and Head, Department
of Psychiatry, Carver College of Medicine,
The University of Iowa; Head, Department
of Psychiatry, The University of Iowa
Hospitals and Clinics,
Iowa City, Iowa*

Steven A. Rogers, PhD
*Assistant Professor, Department
of Psychology, Westmont College,
Santa Barbara, California*

Jonathan M. Silver, MD
*Clinical Professor of Psychiatry, New York
University School of Medicine,
New York, New York*

Katherine H. Taber, PhD
*Adjunct Associate Professor, Department
of Physical Medicine and Rehabilitation,
Baylor College of Medicine, Houston,
Texas; Assistant Co-Director
for Education, Mental Illness Research,
Education and Clinical Center, Salisbury
Veterans Affairs Medical Center,
Salisbury, North Carolina*

Stuart C. Yudofsky, MD
*D.C. and Irene Ellwood Menninger
Professor and Chairman, Department
of Psychiatry and Behavioral Sciences
of Baylor College of Medicine; Chief
of Psychiatry Service,
The Methodist Hospital,
Houston, Texas*

Preface

Neuropsychiatry is a rapidly evolving clinical specialty that is devoted to the diagnosis and treatment of psychiatric or behavioral disorders in persons with disturbances of brain function. Brain dysfunction in the form of a stroke for example, may produce depression (a psychiatric disorder traditionally addressed by "neuropsychiatrists") or an aphasia (a "deficit" syndrome traditionally addressed by "neurobehaviorists" or "behavioral neurologists"). Both approaches—neuropsychiatry and behavioral neurology—are essential to the care of persons with brain dysfunction.

The growth of neuropsychiatry is fueled by the remarkable advances in the neurosciences (and particularly our understanding of brain-behavior relations), as well as by the development of new and powerful clinical tools (e.g., structural and functional brain imaging) and treatments (e.g., safe and effective psychotherapies, medications, and brain stimulation therapies) to improve the care of persons with disturbed brain-behavior relations.

The purpose of this volume—*The Manual of Neuropsychiatric Therapeutics*—is to build upon these advances in clinical and basic neuroscience in order to clearly and concisely provide a rational and evidence-based approach to the diagnosis and biopsychosocial treatment of the neuropsychiatric disorders commonly encountered by practitioners, house officers, and students of brain-behavior relations. For each of these disorders we describe the syndrome and what is known about its pathophysiology, and then provide evidenced-based guidelines for assessment and treatment. While there may be more than one legitimate clinical approach for a given neuropsychiatric disorder, the approaches to care described herein reflect the current practices of the Fellows of the American Neuropsychiatric Association, all of whom are senior clinicians or clinical scientists and noted experts in the care of persons with brain dysfunction.

We are confident this text will enable practitioners to provide state-of-the-art care to their patients with brain dysfunction, and at the same time stimulate consideration of fundamental brain-behavior relations.

C. Edward Coffey, MD
Thomas W. McAllister, MD
Jonathan M. Silver, MD

Chapter 1

APATHY AND RELATED DISORDERS OF DIMINISHED MOTIVATION

James D. Duffy

BACKGROUND

Historical Context

During the eighteenth and nineteenth centuries, disorders of motivation represented the theoretical foundation for most psychiatric classifications. The Swiss psychiatrist André Matthey wrote in 1816 that psychiatric illness was a manifestation of "perversions of the will and the natural inclinations without obvious impairment of the intellectual functions." Matthey distinguished between a behavioral disturbance caused by a physical etiology (délire) and a behavioral disorder produced by a disturbance of the individual's free will (fureur sans délire). According to Matthey's nosology, behaviors such as kleptomania, ennui, melancholia, and tigridoanie (an irresistible urge to spill blood) were all considered "disorders of the will." Matthey's seminal writings became the foundation for the development of nineteenth-century neuropsychiatry and a clinical approach that placed disorders of will as the primary derangement in pathologic behaviors.

The German neuropsychiatrist Heinroth (1818) rejected earlier explanations for mental illness such as "bile or worms or a hundred other irritations" and suggested, "there are many involuntary movements, but not a single involuntary action, for action cannot be imagined without willing." Heinroth went on to write that pathologic behaviors occurred when "the will separates itself from reason and is no longer determined by feeling or intellect." By distinguishing intellect from emotion and motivation, Heinroth laid the foundation for the triad approach of Mood, Cognition, and Conation that became the basis for psychiatric classification for the most part of the nineteenth century. The term abulia appeared in psychiatric literature as early as 1847 and was defined in medical dictionaries as "absence of will, a type of insanity in which this symptom is dominant." Ribot described abulia as a "pure disease of will" in which the individual's ability to act was abolished and he or she was reduced to an individual of "pure intellect." Although most neuropsychiatrists at the end of the nineteenth century agreed on the concept of abulia, there was considerable disagreement on whether the disorder was caused by a deficit in cognition or was a consequence of a dysfunction in a specific motivational system within the brain.

By the beginning of the twentieth century, *abulia* had become a household word and parents were even urged to "combat the evil of abulia amongst students." Despite this, the neuropsychiatric concept of disorders of will fell quickly into decline and by the end of World War I they had essentially disappeared from psychiatric nosology. The reasons for this shift include (i) the rise of behaviorism that posited a simple reflex response that did not require an intervening variable; (ii) psychiatry's preoccupation with psychoanalysis and its emphasis of psychodynamic predeterminism; (iii) the burgeoning field of neurology with its emphasis on somatosensory disorders; (iv) the emergence of postmodernism and its emphasis on individuality and self-determinism (v) the reassignment of disorders of free will to diagnostic concepts such as "negative symptoms" and "executive cognition."

Definitions of Motivation

A universal definition of the term *motivation* remains elusive. This single issue represents the most important barrier to our scientific attempts to understand the neural basis of goal-directed behavior and clinical disorders of motivation.

From a theoretical perspective, *motivation is the heuristic construct that describes the amalgam of forces acting within an organism to initiate and direct behavior. Motivation serves to influence the activation, persistence, and direction of an organism's behavioral response across different levels of behavioral complexity.*

From a *neuropsychiatric* perspective, motivation describes the neurologically mediated variables that energize and direct an individual's response to the environment. These variables include the following:

1. The emotional response to a stimulus
2. The motor reactivity to the stimulus
3. The level of arousal elicited by the stimulus
4. The cognitive interpretation of a stimulus

This approach provides a simple framework for assessing the character and etiology of behaviors that are characterized by a decrease in the expected response to a particular stimulus. It also provides a heuristic framework that is inclusive of and consistent with each of the different approaches to motivation described in the preceding text and does not fall prey to Cartesian models that attempt to separate mind-driven behaviors (i.e., free will) from homeostatic drive theories and instinctual reflex behavior patterns.

Definition of Apathy

Apathy may be either a symptom or a syndrome. As a syndrome, Marin has proposed Diagnostic and Statistical Manual of Mental Disorders (DSM)-like criteria (see subsequent text). Although not yet formally accepted, these criteria do provide the framework for the clinical assessment of apathy.

As per Marin's proposed criteria, apathy is defined as "A lack of motivation, relative to the patient's previous level of functioning or the standards of his/her age and culture as evidenced by all three of the following":

1. Diminished goal-directed overt behavior, as indicated by the following:
   a. Lack of productivity
   b. Lack of effort
   c. Lack of time spent in activities of interest
   d. Lack of initiative or perseverance
   e. Behavioral compliance or dependency on others
   f. Diminished socialization or recreation
2. Diminished goal-directed cognition as indicated by the following:
   a. Lack of interests
   b. Lack of concern about one's personal, health, or functional problems
   c. Diminished importance or value attributed to such goal-related domains as socialization, recreation, productivity, initiative, curiosity
3. Diminished emotional concomitants of goal-directed behavior as indicated by the following:
   a. Unchanging affect
   b. Lack of emotional responsiveness
   c. Euphoria or flat affect
   d. Absence of excitement or emotional intensity

Classification of Apathy and Disorders of Motivation

Apathy and the Diagnostic and Statistical Manual of Mental Disorders text revision (DSM-IV-TR)— The DSM glossary does not include the term apathy, but related symptoms such as indifference, emotional unresponsiveness, lack of symptoms, and lack of concern are included in the diagnostic criteria and symptoms of several disorders. Further examples of related symptoms in DSM-IV-TR include the following:

Major depressive disorder: "Diminished interest or pleasure in all, or almost all, activities"

Post-traumatic stress disorder: "Markedly diminished interest or participation in significant activities"

Schizophrenia: Catatonic behavior characterized by "decrease in reactivity to the environment;" negative symptoms include avolition, alogia, and affective flattening

Apathy is explicitly included as a diagnostic criterion in only the following four disorders:

Inhalant intoxication (criterion B—"maladaptive changes e.g., apathy")
Opioid intoxication (criterion B—"euphoria followed by apathy")

Apathetic type of personality change due to a general medical condition (i.e., predominant feature is apathy or indifference)

Postconcussional disorder (criterion C—"apathy or lack of spontaneity")

Epidemiology of Apathy and Disordered Motivation

No data are currently available on apathy as a primary disorder. However, a considerable amount of research indicates that apathy is perhaps the most common behavioral syndrome associated with neurologic disease. A recent analysis of prevalence data revealed that neurologic diseases involving the cerebral cortex are associated with a point prevalence of apathy of approximately 60%, whereas disorders primarily involving subcortical structures are associated with a 40% prevalence of apathy.

Alzheimer disease: At least six studies have examined the prevalence of apathy in Alzheimer disease (AD) with a reported prevalence ranging from 37% to 86.4% (composite prevalence 55.5%). Apathy has also been reported to be the most common behavioral symptom in mild cognitive impairment (MCI) with a point prevalence of 39%. It is important to recognize that apathy may be a herald symptom in MCI and AD that antedates the onset of observable cognitive decline. The prevalence of apathy in AD appears to be higher in community-dwelling AD patients and may be the most important determining factor for patients' families seeking medical evaluation.

Traumatic brain injury: Several studies have reported the prevalence of apathy in traumatic brain injury (TBI) to range from 46% to 71% with a composite average of 61%. One study reported that apathy occurred in only 13.8% of patients following a TBI.

Vascular dementia: Two studies have reported a combined prevalence of 33.8% in a sample of patients with vascular dementia.

Poststroke: The prevalence of apathy in a heterogeneous group of patients following cerebrovascular accidents ranges from 22.5% to 56.7%. Apathy appears to be most frequent following a lesion involving the posterior limb of the internal capsule and is slightly higher in patients with right hemisphere lesions.

Anoxic encephalopathy: A study including 14 subjects reported a prevalence of 78.6% in patients with postanoxic encephalopathy.

Parkinson Disease: Using self report or informant-based measures, several studies have reported that between 16.5% and 42% of patients with Parkinson disease (PD) exhibit apathy. Low serum testosterone has been found to be an independent variable predicting the presence of apathy in PD.

Huntington disease: One study reported that 38% of patients with Huntington disease exhibit apathy and depression, with 7% exhibiting apathy alone. Apathy was found to be a powerful predictor of activities of daily living (ADL) ability.

Multiple sclerosis: Apathy has been reported to occur in 20.5% of patients with multiple sclerosis (MS); however, 53.3% of MS patients with depression are apathetic.

Human immunodeficiency virus: Three studies in patients with human immunodeficiency virus (HIV) report a prevalence ranging from 29.8% to 50%.

Interestingly, the presence of apathy does not appear to correlate with absolute CD4 count.

Nursing home residents: Probably as a consequence of the additive effect of severity of disease and impoverished social environment, nursing home residents have an extremely high prevalence of apathy. This finding has important implications for patient compliance and undoubtedly negative impacts on disease progression, morbidity, and mortality.

Although no data is available, given their pathophysiology, it is reasonable to assume that normal pressure hydrocephalus, sleep apnea, amyotrophic lateral sclerosis, Lyme disease, and thyroid disease are associated with atrophy.

Negative symptoms of schizophrenia: The overlap between apathy and the negative symptoms of schizophrenia is discussed elsewhere in this text.

Prescription medications: Although no data is available on prevalence, anecdotal reports indicate that apathy may occur as a side-effect of selective serotonin reuptake inhibitors (SSRIs), neuroleptics, metaclopramide, and felbamate.

Prognosis

Several studies have reported significant morbidity associated with the presence of apathy. Four studies in patients with Alzheimer dementia that utilized standardized assessment tools for the diagnosis of apathy, have reported an association between the presence of apathy and diminished performance on *activities of daily living* (independent of the presence of depression). Patients who are apathetic following a stroke have been reported to be more functionally impaired, with the comorbidity of apathy and depression having the greatest impact on functional capacity. A study of geriatric patients admitted to a nursing home found apathy to be an important predictor of functional capacity at discharge, independent of admission diagnosis.

Apathy appears to be associated with *more rapid cognitive and functional decline* in patients with AD. Apathy has also been reported to be an important predictor of poor prognosis in patients with major depressive disorders.

Apathy appears to be an important predictor of medication compliance in patients with schizophrenia, and in identifying those patients who are less likely to benefit from social skills training.

Although there is no data available to support the hypothesis, it is reasonable to suggest that apathy may contribute to *patient medication and treatment noncompliance*, thereby indirectly increasing the morbidity and mortality of comorbid disorders (such as diabetes, hypertension etc.) that may themselves produce apathy. Patients and caregivers often interpret the patient's apathetic behavior as volitional and label the patient as lazy, passive aggressive, or ungrateful. This inevitably results in resentment or hostility toward the patient, thereby perpetuating a downward spiral of diminishing functional capacity and diminishing social supports. In this regard, apathy has been reported to be significantly correlated with caregiver distress in AD, thereby being an important determinant of nursing home placement.

The *longitudinal clinical course* of apathy remains unclear. One study in AD has reported that apathy is likely to persist and worsen over the course of the disease.

THE NEURAL SUBSTRATES OF MOTIVATION

Since the construct of motivation describes the neurologically mediated variables that energize and direct an individual's response to the environment, a discussion of the neural substrates of goal-directed behavior could conceivably include a description of the entire brain. However, understanding the neural substrates that serve the different components of goal-directed behavior does provide the clinician with a framework that is helpful in developing clinical hypotheses and effective treatment plans.

Subcircuit No. 1—Motivational working memory

Components: The ventral tegmental area (VTA)—nucleus accumbens (NA) and the ventral pallidum (VP).
Function: Provides "the neural template for motivational working memory" that allows the prioritization of motivational valencies across the temporal domain.

Subcircuit No. 2—Cognitive coordination

Components: VP, mediodorsal (MD) nucleus of thalamus, prefrontal cortex (PFC), NA, and VTA.
Function: Provides the cognitive coordination of motivational response.

Subcircuit No. 3

Components: VP, pedunculopontine nucleus (PPN), VTA.
Functions: Integration of arousal into motivational response.

Subcircuit No. 4

Components: The ventral tegmentum, amygdala, and the NA.
Function: Integration of reward memory into motivation.

Neurochemical Aspects of Motivation

Although dopamine (DA) and glutamine appear to be the primary modulators of motivation, the neurochemical foundations of motivation are extremely complex and have not been fully elucidated. However, substantial experimental data indicates a pivotal role for DA and glutamate as the key modulators of goal-directed behavior.

In simple terms, one can state that DA is necessary for modulating relative motivational valency (i.e., the direction of behavior) while glutamate is primarily involved in the enactment of the behavioral response (the intensity of behavior).

The cholinergic system exerts a modulatory influence on motivational response through projections from the PPN (located in the mesencephalic locomotor region) to widespread targets that include the limbic system, extrapyramidal system, thalamic nuclei, and tectal and cortical regions. These ascending cholinergic projections influence locomotor goal-directed behavior through their stimulatory influence on DA efflux.

The serotinergic system appears to exert an inhibitory effect upon motivational response through its 5-HT$_{1b}$ modulatory activity of glutamate pathways in the NA and an inhibitory effect on DA release through 5-HT$_2$ activation.

Clinical Implications of This Circuitry

The neural circuitry described in the preceding text provides the theoretical framework for a reasoned clinical approach to the assessment and treatment of disorders of diminished motivation. Dysfunction within particular subcircuits produces a predictable and specific disorder of diminished goal-directed behavior (Table 1.1). This approach suggests that rather than representing a single syndrome, the disorders of diminished motivation include at least four distinct behavioral syndromes. Each of these syndromes requires a treatment approach based on the particular characteristics of each syndrome.

Diagnosis

It is important to be aware of other conditions and syndromes, the clinical presentation of which may overlap or mimic apathy and disorders of motivation.

Differential Diagnosis of Apathy

DEPRESSION

Although apathy may occur as a symptom of depression, several studies have demonstrated apathy to be a disorder distinct from depression. Although patients suffering from a depressive disorder often exhibit diminished goal-directed behavior, the hallmark of depression is the presence of depressed mood and neurovegetative symptoms. While apathetic patients fail to verbalize any subjective distress, depressed patients are usually characterized by negativism and despair. The depressed person typically and purposively avoids interpersonal contacts. In contrast, the apathetic patient is passive and will engage in interpersonal behaviors only if others initiate and facilitate the social engagement.

DELIRIUM

Lethargy, impersistence, distractibility, and diminished goal-directed behavior are all components of delirium. When these features dominate the delirious patient's clinical picture the patient is described as suffering from "apathetic delirium." Apathy, however, is not associated with the disorder of attention and arousal that represents the hallmark of delirium. In addition, while apathy is associated with diffuse background frequency slowing on electroencephalogram (EEG), apathy is not associated with any particular EEG abnormality.

AGNOSIAS

Patients with specific agnosias may exhibit a diminished behavioral response to a specific sensory or categorical stimulus. In particular, anosagnosic patients manifest a "laissez-faire" attitude to their illness and its social and personal implications (in this respect, it is probably better defined as apathy, cognitive subtype).

AKINESIA

Patients who are exhibiting akinetic mutism manifest no goal-directed motor behavior in the absence of any motor deficit or abnormal motor movements. In this regard, rather than a motor disorder, akinetic mutism may be regarded as apathy, motor type.

TABLE 1.1 Components and Functions of Motivational Circuitry

	Circuit No. 1	Circuit No. 2	Circuit No. 3	Circuit No. 4
Neuroanatomic components	VT-NA-VP	VP-MD-PFC-NA-VTA	VP-PPN-VTA	VTA-Amygdala-NA
Function	Provides the neural template for "motivational working memory" that allows the prioritization of motivational valencies across the temporal domain	Provides cognitive framework for response coordination	Integrates autonomic state into motivational readiness	Integrates the incentive value (reward memory) into motivational response
Clinical syndrome associated with lesion in circuit	Diminished motivational flexibility and increased threshold of behavioral response to stimulus	Diminished cognitive planning	Diminished arousal in response to motivationally relevant stimulus.	Diminished stimulus discrimination
Clinical syndrome	Motor apathy	Cognitive apathy	Arousal apathy	Emotional apathy

VT-NA-VP, ventral tegmental-nucleus accumbens-ventral pallidum; VP-MD-PFC-NA-VTA, ventral pallidum-mediodorsal-prefrontal cortex-nucleus accumbens-ventral tegmental area; VP-PPN-VTA, ventral pallidum-pedunculopontine nucleus-ventral tegmental area; VTA-Amygdala-NA, ventral tegmental area-Amygdala-nucleus accumbens.

FATIGUE

Pathologic fatigue is increasingly recognized as an important determinant of diminished goal-directed behavior. Unlike apathy, fatigue is an ego-dystonic experience with the patient typically frustrated by the inability to function at his/her usual level.

DESPAIR AND DEMORALIZATION

These occur in response to experienced helplessness in the context of an apparently overwhelming stress. Unlike apathy, these are experienced as painful psychological states. Demoralized individuals will exhibit a negative emotional orientation regarding their future while apathetic patients will exhibit very little concern.

SUBSTANCE ABUSE

Although there is no data available, anecdotal experience suggests that the chronic abuse of marijuana and possibly amphetamines may produce a chronic behavioral state characterized by apathy.

HISTORY

Obtain a thorough history from the patient *and* his/her family or caregivers. Because apathetic patients will not be motivated to participate in the interview process, it is important to obtain historical data from both the patient and his/her family and/or social supports. Typically, apathetic patients will underestimate their lack of motivation and its social consequences. *Neuropsychiatric treatment is therefore typically sought by family members and/or caregivers and not by the identified patient.*

When obtaining the history, it is important to assess not only the content, but also the patient's response style. Apathetic patients typically initiate very few spontaneous statements. The interviewer typically needs to drive the interview and provide increased motivational relevance by either being more persistent or raising the volume of the interaction. Make sure that the patient's caregiver/family member does not compensate for the patient's apathy by assuming a more active role in the conversation. Also, while attempting to obtain historical information, carefully assess the patient's level of arousal and monitor for evidence of distractibility, impersistence, or perseveration (all signs of delirium that can mimic apathy).

When obtaining the history, particular attention should be given to the following:

1. Changes in goal-directed activities from premorbid level (it is important to realize that goal-directed behaviors usually diminish with advancing age)
2. Previous and current functional capacity (i.e., occupational status, recreational pursuits)
3. Overt evidence for cognitive slippage (i.e., has the patient exhibited memory loss, diminished organizational skills, or diminished work performance?)
4. The patient's insight regarding his/her diminished goal-directed behavior and the amount of concern the patient exhibits about this decline
5. History of increased irritability and/or aggressive behaviors
6. Changes in gait, posture, falls, tremor, urinary incontinence
7. Neurovegetative signs and symptoms of depression
8. Past or present substance abuse

9. The patient's living environment and its motivational implications (i.e., patients living in an impoverished environment such as nursing facilities will experience fewer motivationally relevant stimuli)
10. Current and past medical history with particular reference to a previous history of TBI due to neurologic disease
11. Any recent or past history of substance abuse (particularly marijuana, solvents, N-methyl-D-aspartate [NMDA], and designer drugs)
12. Consider administering a clinical assessment tool such as the Apathy Evaluation Scale (AES) (patient-rated and observer-rated versions) or neuropsychiatric inventory (NPI)

Perform a Thorough Neurologic Examination

Patients exhibiting diminished goal-directed behavior should undergo a full physical and neurologic examination. The general physical examination should make particular reference to clinical signs of thyroid disease and cerebrovascular disease, and other conditions that result in general asthenia. In patients exhibiting features of delirium, it is important to recognize that delirium may be the manifestation of a medical emergency. In addition to detailed neurologic examination, the examiner should evaluate the patient for any evidence of frontal release signs.

Perform a Cognitive Examination

As stated above, it is important to assess the patient for any behavioral features of delirium. In patients exhibiting altered arousal, distractibility, impersistence, and/or perseveration, it is important to immediately perform a formal assessment of the patient's attentional status (i.e., digit span, reverse serial days and months). In addition to assessing quantifiable cognitive functions such as memory, language, math and so on, it is also important to formally assess the patient's executive functioning (open and closed set word generation, insight, and abstraction). The cognitive examination typically provides important information regarding the etiology of the patient's apathy. Formal neuropsychological assessment can be helpful in providing more sensitive and specific assessments of cognitive functioning.

Perform a Psychosocial Assessment

Apathy will inevitably produce very significant social dysfunction. It is important to evaluate the patient's current functional capacity and determine any evidence for deteriorating work performance. Although patients may be able to continue in their premorbid work capacity, close questioning regarding performance evaluations will usually uncover evidence for employer discontent with the patient's productivity.

Since family members will typically compensate for changes in the patient's behavior, it is important to perform a detailed family assessment. In this regard, the approach of a system to family assessment that includes a review of the different domains of family functioning is particularly useful (i.e., role assignment, instrumental problem solving, affective problem solving, discipline, finances). This assessment is particularly helpful in developing an effective treatment plan.

Clinical Instruments for Assessing Apathy

Although there is no universal definition of apathy, several assessment tools are available. These instruments were developed to support research in disorders of motivation but they do, however, have clinical utility. In particular, they provide clinicians with a method for quantifying the patient's level of motivation and monitoring the patient's clinical course over time.

The AES (as well as its shortened version, the Apathy Scale) is the most widely used scale and has demonstrated specificity for distinguishing apathy from depression (see Table 1.1). There are three versions of the AES for use by the patient, i.e., self (AES-S), by an informant such as a family member (AES-I), or by a clinician (AES-C). They are essentially the same, with only the pronoun referring to the subject changed. However, the AES-C has patient and clinician/caregiver versions, with at least one study reporting that families may be more reliable in accurately reporting the identified patients' goal-directed behavior. One major challenge when using the AES is to recognize that the cutoff score for a diagnosis of apathy is arbitrary and is not sensitive to premorbid functional capacity and/or age. In this regard, the AES is most helpful as a tool for assessing treatment response and disease progression.

The NPI includes several behavioral domains including apathy. As an observer rating scale, the NPI is simple to administer and has been utilized in several neuropsychiatric conditions. The scale, however, is not clear on the appropriate cutoff score for the presence of apathy.

Laboratory Investigations

1. EEG provides important diagnostic information in patients who exhibit attentional deficits suggestive of delirium.
2. Magnetic resonance imaging provides important information regarding subcortical and white matter disease.
3. Neuropsychological assessment provides useful quantitative data in different domains and may be particularly helpful in patients with a presumptive diagnosis of MCI.
4. Perform tests for thyroid function and serum testosterone on all patients. Other tests should be performed depending upon the patient's clinical picture.
5. Consider a formal sleep study in patients with a history of body habitus (i.e., overweight, bull necked, etc.) consistent with sleep apnea.
6. Perform urine toxicology screen.

MANAGEMENT

Effective treatment should include both psychopharmacological and psychosocial interventions. The efficacy of therapeutic interventions can be assessed utilizing ongoing clinical assessment tools such as the AES. When developing a treatment plan, it is important to appreciate that most apathetic patients are, by definition, not bothered by their behavior. Treatment goals should therefore be established on the basis of the needs of the patient and family and not on the basis of the clinician's agenda.

When developing a treatment plan it is important to characterize the nature of the patient's apathy syndrome and its etiology. Patients with apathy characterized by diminished cognitive planning are likely to respond to medications only if their PFC is intact (i.e., they have an intact end organ). For example, (i) a patient who has sustained prefrontal trauma will not benefit from DA agonist therapy whilst a patient with a ventral tegmental lesion will likely exhibit marked improvement at high doses of DA agonist, (ii) patients with motor apathy (e.g., parkinsonism) will benefit from strategies intended to enhance motor responsivity, that is, DA agonists, and (iii) patients with emotional apathy may benefit from a nonserotoninergic antidepressant—however, patients with lesions involving the medial temporal structures are unlikely to benefit from this approach.

PSYCHOPHARMACOLOGICAL APPROACHES
The following principles should be observed when treating a patient with apathy:

1. Optimize physical status.
2. Evaluate and modify psychosocial modifiers (see subsequent text).
3. Optimize endocrine status.
4. Optimize treatment of comorbid psychiatric conditions.
5. Discontinue medications that may produce diminished motivation, that is, metaclopramide, paroxetine (and possibly other SSRIs), felbamate, and neuroleptics.
6. In patients with AD, acetylcholinesterase inhibitors represent the first-line treatment for apathy. A meta-analysis of randomized clinical trials (RCT) demonstrated a significant benefit of metrifonate for treating apathy in AD. An RCT has also demonstrated positive response with tacrine and donezepil. An open study of rivastigmine reported benefit in a small sample of patients with Lewy body dementia. The author's preference is to begin donezepil 5 mg daily PO. Intolerance to side effects limits the use of other psychostimulants in patients with AD—however, patients may tolerate and benefit from low doses starting with methylphenidate 2.5 mg at breakfast and lunchtime. Patients who will benefit from psychostimulant therapy are likely to do so quickly and at these low doses.
7. There are no RCTs to guide the treatment of apathy in other disease populations. Pharmacologic approaches are therefore largely anecdotal and dictated by the side effect profile and close monitoring of the response. In one open trial with bromocriptine (doses 10 to 120 mg daily) patients post-TBI reported increased motivation. Although there are no published data to support their use, the newer DA agonists (pergolide, pramipexole, selegiline) should theoretically have a therapeutic benefit in the treatment of apathy. Pramipexole, with its selectivity for limbic D3 receptors, may have some theoretical advantage. The author's preference is to begin with bromocriptine starting at 5 mg and titrate dosage upward against the patient's response and tolerance. Patients may require very high doses to drive their motivational responsivity.
8. Anecdotal case studies have reported benefit from amantadine (50 to 200 mg per day) in TBI patients. One study reported that nursing home patients who were taking amantadine for viral prophylaxis demonstrated increased social interaction, personal care, caloric intake and weight gain.

9. Although there are no RCTs, several case reports suggest that methyl-phenidate (doses up to 1 mg/day/kg body weight) and D-amphetamine have clinical utility as a treatment for apathy in patients with TBI.
10. There is considerable evidence to support the efficacy of novel antipsy-chotics in reducing the negative symptoms in schizophrenia. Their utility in improving motivation in other neuropsychiatric disorders has not been ascertained.

PSYCHOSOCIAL APPROACHES TO TREATING APATHY

It is probably true to state that at this time, psychosocial treatment approaches offer more benefit than medications in treating apathy. Unfortunately, the impact of these psychosocial interventions is frequently underestimated or completely ignored.

It is critical to engage family members and/or caretakers in all psychoso-cial interventions. In particular, they should be empowered to assume a very active role in shaping the patient's behavior and supporting adaptive behav-iors. It is important to clarify from the outset that the patient's apathy is not intentional but a manifestation of neurologic disease. This simple interpreta-tion typically frees family members from the vicious cycle of accusations and misattribution.

Apathetic patients are typically incapable of generating and sustaining novel behavioral repertoires. They therefore benefit from a repetitive structured daily schedule. Because apathy is frequently associated with irritability, they also benefit from a low expressed emotion environment. Unfortunately, family and caregivers have to walk a tightrope—supporting positive goal-directed behaviors while also avoiding overt frustration. It is important that caregivers recognize their own needs and identify other resources that will lower their caregiving burden, that is, daycare, volunteers, other family members, and inpatient respite. Failure to address the needs of the patient's caregivers will inevitably result in their becoming demoralized, exhausted, angry, and being likely to relinquish their critical role in supporting the patient. It is important to realize that psychosocial treatment will inevitably be a long-term regular endeavor.

CONCLUSION

Apathy is not formally recognized as a distinct symptom or syndrome in current psychiatric nosology. The clinician should, however, remain alert to recognizing that disorders of diminished motivation are a common and potentially treatable cause of profound psychosocial disability. Utilizing targeted psychopharmacologic and sustained psychosocial interventions can significantly improve the quality of life for both patients and their caregivers.

Selected Readings

Marin RS. Apathy: A neuropsychiatric syndrome [Review]. *J Neuropsychiatry Clin Neurosci.* 1991;3(3):243–254.

Marin RS. Apathy: Concept, syndrome, neural mechanisms, and treatment. *Semin Clin Neuropsychiatry.* 1996;1(4):304–314.

Van Reekum R, Stuss DT, Ostrander L. Apathy: Why care? [Review]. *J Neuropsy-chiatry Clin Neurosci.* 2005;17(1):7–19.

Chapter 2

DELIRIUM

Walter Knysz, III, C. Edward Coffey

I. BACKGROUND

A. **Definitions**
1. *Delirium* refers to a clinical syndrome characterized by a disturbance of arousal, attention, perception, and other cognitive domains, which tends to have a fluctuating course. Onset is usually (but not always) acute. Numerous disorders may cause delirium (see subsequent text).
2. Diagnostic and Statistical Manual of Mental Disorders, 4th edition (DSM-IV) criteria for delirium:
   a. Disturbance of consciousness with a reduced ability to focus, sustain, or shift attention
      (1) We prefer to think of this as a disturbance in arousal that can range from the hypoaroused (drowsy, lethargic, obtunded) to hyperaroused (agitated and hypervigilant).
   b. A change in cognition (such as memory deficit, disorientation, or language disturbance) or the development of a perceptual disturbance that is not better accounted for by a preexisting, established, or evolving dementia.
   c. The disturbance developing over a short period of time (usually hours to days) and tending to fluctuate during the course of the day.
3. The term "delirium" is generally considered synonymous with the term *encephalopathy*. Other terms found in the literature include organic brain syndrome, confusional state, acute brain failure, acute dementia, reversible dementia, cerebral insufficiency, toxic psychosis, posttraumatic amnesia, and "ICU psychosis" among others.

B. **Classification of delirium**
1. The DSM-IV differentiates delirium by etiology:
   a. Delirium due to a general medical condition
   b. Substance-induced delirium
   c. Delirium due to multiple etiologies
   d. Delirium not otherwise specified

2. Some authors propose two other subtypes of delirium not in the DSM-IV.
   - *Hyperkinetic* or *hyperactive* delirium is characterized by hyperarousal, hypervigilance, elevated psychomotor activity, fast or loud speech, restlessness, irritability, anger, euphoria, laughter, delusions, hallucinations, distractibility, or tangentiality. Patients suffering from hyperkinetic delirium are more likely to generate psychiatric consultation (the squeaky wheel gets the oil) for assistance in managing behavior or psychosis, or possibly the capacity to sign out of the hospital against medical advice.
   - *Hypokinetic*, or *hypoactive*, delirium is characterized by decreased arousal and psychomotor activity, lethargy, apathy, and slow or decreased speech. These patients are less likely to generate a psychiatric consultation and often when they do, it is to assess for depression. The presence of delirium in these patients tends to be underappreciated, which can result in morbidities including dehydration, medication noncompliance, pressure ulcers, and aspiration pneumonia. It is thought that approximately half the patients with delirium will experience features of both subtypes over the course of the delirium.

      Additionally, some authors describe two subtypes of delirium, namely, "acute confusional states" and "acute agitated delirium"

   As noted in the preceding text, there are several classifications of delirium. Each has its usefulness with certain clinicians in certain clinical situations. Use of the DSM-IV classification is apt to be the most clear when communicating with other clinicians.

C. **Presentation.** The clinical syndrome of delirium typically has an acute onset (hours to days) and is manifest by a disturbance of consciousness (arousal → remember hyperkinetic/hypokinetic) with reduced ability to focus, sustain, or shift attention; a change in cognition (such as disorientation, problems with memory, or a language disturbance); or the development of a perceptual disturbance (not better accounted for by a dementing process) with an overall fluctuating course.

   Keep in mind that delirium can present with a wide range of signs and symptoms including disturbances in the following:
   - Level of arousal
   - Speech and language
   - Mood (dysphoria/euphoria)
   - Affect (crying, laughing, yelling, labile, constricted, etc.)
   - Thought process (tangential, circumstantial, disorganized)
   - Thought content (paranoia, delusions)
   - Perception (illusions; hallucinations visual more than auditory, tactile, and other domains)
   - Insight and judgment
   - All domains of cognition (especially attention, orientation and memory)

Some patients may also display neurologic signs such as myoclonus, nystagmus, or asterixis.

D. Epidemiology. The incidence and prevalence of delirium depend on the definitions being used and the populations being studied. The prevalence of delirium in hospitalized patients ranges from 10% to 30%. The prevalence is higher in elderly hospitalized patients (up to 40%) and in postoperative patients (as high as 50%). Patients who have undergone a cardiotomy, hip surgery, or organ transplant are at a particularly increased risk. The prevalence of delirium in terminally ill patients who are near death has been reported to be as high as 80%.

E. Potential etiologies. There are numerous potential etiologies of delirium. It is quite common for the etiology to be multifactorial. However, on occasion, no clear etiology is identified. It is imperative to remember that just because an etiology has not been identified it does not mean the diagnosis is no longer correct. Common etiologies include substance intoxication and/or withdrawal states, polypharmacy, metabolic derangements, and infection. Table 2.1 provides a more complete (yet partial) list of etiologies.

F. Prognosis. Generally, patients with delirium whose etiology is identified and treated in a timely manner will recover without observable sequelae. Full recovery is less likely in the elderly patient population. If untreated, delirium may progress to stupor, coma, seizures, or death, depending upon its etiology. It has been reported that there is a 25% mortality rate at 6 months associated with patients suffering from delirium. It is possible that these data may be skewed by the high prevalence of delirium in terminally ill patients.

The patient with delirium may experience morbidity from decubitus ulcers, aspiration pneumonia, and increased cardiovascular stress. When delirium is associated with cognitive impairment, patients may have difficulty relating a reliable medical history, thereby making diagnosis and treatment more difficult, possibly prolonging hospitalization. Patients suffering from delirium are also at risk for posthospital institutionalization (skilled nursing facility, rehab, nursing home).

G. Risk factors. Common risk factors for delirium include the following:
- Advancing age
- Polypharmacy

TABLE 2.1   Potential Causes of Delirium (Partial Listing)

Medication side effect	Metabolic derangements	Infections
Medication/drug intoxication	Head trauma	Fever
Withdrawal syndromes	Neoplasm	Epilepsy
Postoperative states	Central nervous system, space-occupying lesions	Vascular disorders
Hypoxia or hypercapnia	Malnutrition	Sleep and sensory deprivation

- Multiple medical problems (certainly, the more unstable those medical problems are the higher the risk)
- Preexisting central nervous system (CNS) pathology or cognitive impairment
- Substance abuse/dependence
- Human immunodeficiency virus (HIV)/acquired immunodeficiency syndrome (AIDS)
- Infection
- Metabolic derangements
- Severe burns
- Visual and auditory impairment
- Fever
- Thiamine deficiency
- Low serum albumin (protein-bound medication)

H. **Differential diagnosis**
   1. *Dementia* is probably the most difficult diagnosis to distinguish from delirium. An adequate history is essential. Unlike delirium that typically has an abrupt onset and a fluctuating course, and is reversible, dementias often have an insidious onset, gradual and progressive decline without fluctuation and are irreversible. However, Lewy body dementia is the exception to this rule and can be easily confused with delirium as it too has a fluctuating course. In addition, some patients can have an acute onset of symptoms and an initial period of delirium after a stroke.
   2. In addition, some patients' presentation may mimic *primary psychiatric disorders*. For instance, a patient who is hyperaroused may appear manic; a hypoaroused and dysphoric patient may appear to be suffering from depression; a patient who is hallucinating and/or suffering from a disturbance in thought content (paranoia/delusions) and/or thought process (tangential or disorganized) may appear to be suffering from a primary psychotic disorder. Again, the key to making the diagnosis is history, history, history (focusing on the timeline of onset and course of symptoms) and cognitive examination.

II. NEUROBIOLOGY AND PATHOPHYSIOLOGY OF DELIRIUM

The neurobiology of delirium is not fully understood. Delirium may be the result of a transient disruption of normal neuronal activity in certain brain regions (likely the prefrontal cortex, thalamus, right basal ganglia, and right temporoparietal cortex) and neurotransmitter systems (decreased cholinergic and increased dopaminergic activity and possibly γ-aminobutyric acid (GABA), glutamine, serotonin, histamine systems, and others as well). This neuronal dysfunction may result from metabolic disturbances (e.g., hypoxia, infection, trauma, etc.) or toxins (e.g., medications, substance use or abuse, hepatic encephalopathy, etc.). Certain neurons are more vulnerable to a mismatch between energy supply and demand (which is caused by these toxic and metabolic disturbances). Specifically, neurons with a higher surface area to volume ratio (such as neurons with long, thin axons) are considered to be more vulnerable. Neuroanatomically, this vulnerability correlates to those brain regions and neurotransmitter systems noted in the preceding text (particularly neurons originating in the brainstem traveling to the hippocampus, frontal cortex, and other neocortical regions). As the energy supply–demand discrepancy increases, there is a predictable progression of neuronal dysfunction from more susceptible neurons to more resilient neurons.

III. MANAGEMENT

The management of delirium is focused on identifying and treating the underlying etiology, and on managing the symptoms until the etiology is resolved. In general, the management of delirium should follow the American Psychiatric Association Practice Guidelines for patients with delirium.

A. Perform a diagnostic evaluation

1. Obtain a thorough history including history from collateral sources (family, friends, nursing staff, or others who are familiar with the patient). Careful review of the medical record should be done including the emergency medical services (EMS) run sheet, emergency department documentation, any operative and anesthesia records, all multidisciplinary documents, and diagnostic and laboratory results. Special attention should be paid to the time course of mental status changes (acute onset and fluctuating course versus insidious onset with progressive and gradual decline) as well as the history of recent medication changes and the possibility of substance abuse. Longitudinal history is the key to distinguishing between delirium and dementia. A thorough medical review of systems should be performed to identify clues to an underlying etiology.

2. A physical examination should include particular attention to vital signs and the evaluation of cardiac, pulmonary, and neurologic systems. A thorough examination of the mental status is essential, and the assessment of attention is important, as attentional deficits are a defining feature of delirium. Attention can be assessed in a number of ways such as having the patient recite the months of the year in reverse or performing serial subtraction. Short-term memory can be assessed by encoding three words and asking the patient to recall them after 5 minutes of distraction. An additional task that can be quite helpful is asking the patient to draw the face of a clock which requires sustained attention, planning, and spatial orientation.

3. Laboratory testing is done to confirm an etiology suspected on the basis of history or examination. Table 2.2 provides a list of diagnostic tests to be considered. We specifically recommend obtaining a urinalysis in all elderly patients and patients with significant premorbid cognitive impairment, who have acute changes in mental status or behavior. These patients are far more sensitive to even the smallest infection because of their lack of cognitive reserve. We recommend

TABLE 2.2   Laboratory Tests for Patients with Delirium

Basic laboratory tests (consider for all patients with delirium):
- Complete blood count (with differential and platelet count)
- Serum chemistries (electrolytes, glucose, blood urea and nitrogen, creatinine, albumin, serum glutamic oxaloacetic transaminase, serum glutamic pyruvic transaminase, bilirubin, calcium, magnesium, phosphorus, alkaline phosphatase)
- B_{12}, folate, sedimentation rate
- Thyroid-stimulating hormone, free thyroxine
- Urinalysis and culture
- Electrocardiogram
- Chest x-ray
- Oxygen saturation and arterial blood gas
- Urine drug screen

Additional laboratory tests (ordered as indicated by clinical status and results of work-up to date):
- Blood tests (serum levels of medications, Venereal Disease Research Laboratory test, heavy metal screen, lupus erythematosus preparation, antinuclear antibody, urinary porphyrins, ammonia, human immunodeficiency virus)
- Blood cultures
- Lumbar puncture
- Neuroimaging (computed tomography scan of the head; magnetic resonance imaging of the brain)
- Electroencephalogram

a low threshold for treating urinary tract infections in these populations.

If a specific CNS disease process is suspected, then neuroimaging, lumbar puncture, and an electroencephalogram (EEG) should be considered. An EEG is particularly useful if seizure activity (particularly nonconvulsive status epilepticus, complex partial status epilepticus and toxic ictal psychosis) is suspected. Diffuse slowing is the most common EEG finding in patients with delirium. However, false-negative results can occur particularly if a patient's dominant posterior rhythm slows down relative to their baseline rhythm but does not reach the theta range (the EEG thereby being read as normal despite a relative slowing). In addition, alcohol withdrawal or benzodiazepine intoxication may show low-voltage fast activity.

B. **Nonpharmacologic management**
1. Any suspicion of an active disease process found through the history and physical examination should trigger an appropriate medical workup and appropriate medical management. The patient's vital signs, hydration status, and oxygenation should be monitored. As diagnostic tests reveal further abnormalities, these should be addressed promptly.
2. Evaluate the *safety* of the patient and others. Patients with delirium are at an elevated risk of self-harm, both unintentional and

suicidal. They are also at an elevated risk of injuring the staff and other patients. Patients should be monitored for behavioral and cognitive disturbances that may endanger themselves, the staff, or other patients. These behaviors may include being agitated; wandering; falling; pulling out IVs, central lines or catheters; and committing suicide. The nature of delirium is to wax and wane, and this can happen rapidly. Therefore, careful monitoring of the patient's mental status is required. It is often helpful to enlist the assistance of the patient's family. If the family is not available then a one-to-one observer may at times be necessary.

3. It is important to determine and continually evaluate the *treatment setting* (intensive care unit [ICU], general medical floor, rehab setting) based on the patient's clinical status. In addition, simple environmental changes such as minimizing environmental stimulation (a quiet, dimly lit [not dark] room is optimal) can be quite helpful in decreasing agitation. Furthermore, patients should be provided with corrective lenses and hearing aids if they normally wear them. It should be no surprise that a confused patient, who does not know or understand where he or she is or why, becomes agitated, particularly when strangers are approaching him or her with needles and several tubes. Remember the fight or flight response. When the staff come in contact with the patient they should introduce themselves, reorient the patient to time, place, and context and explain any actions toward the patient beforehand (blood draws, IVs, placement of a catheter, monitoring of vital signs). Family and friends should be instructed similarly about environmental stimulation and encouraged to frequently reorient the patient and provide reassurance. *Treatment adherence* can often be improved with the assistance of family members. A clock and calendar should be visible to the patient. Familiar objects from home such as pictures may also provide comfort. The use of mechanical restraints should be used judiciously (not out of convenience) and should be in compliance with Joint Council of Accreditation of Healthcare Organizations (JCAHO) standards.

4. *Coordinate the care* with other clinicians. Delirium is frequently a medical emergency, with the patients being managed in a hospital *treatment setting* often with several consulting services. Appropriate management of the delirious patient begins with seeking and treating the underlying cause and relieving the symptoms. Coordination between the primary and consulting services (including psychiatry, neurology, and other specialty services) is necessary to ensure appropriate evaluation and safe and effective management. It is also important to ensure that nurses, case management teams, and ancillary services are informed so that the patient's behavioral, cognitive, or emotional disturbances are monitored and not misconstrued.

5. Medications that are nonessential should be minimized or eliminated. The use of opiates, benzodiazepines (unless being used

to treat the underlying cause such as a withdrawal state), other sedative-hypnotics, and anticholinergic medications should also be minimized when possible. Of course, there may be times when medications with delirogenic effects are required to treat a significant medical condition. If alternate medications are available they should be considered. If not, then a risk–benefit analysis must be made.

6. Provide *education and support to patient and family*. Patients' families may have fears that the patient is suffering from a major mental illness with life-long implications (and all the stigma that goes along with it). Explaining the nature, etiology, and course of delirium can be very reassuring and prevent unnecessary and persisting concerns about a patient's psychiatric stability. The patient's memory of events during a delirium is variable. Some patients are completely amnesic while others have vivid and detailed recollection of events that can be quite disturbing. Upon resolution of the delirium, it is helpful to educate the patient (as with the patient's family) about the transient nature of the change in mental status and its etiology. It is important to reassure the patient that the recent change in mental status is not an indication of permanent mental illness.

C. **Pharmacologic management strategies**

1. A quietly confused patient can generally be managed with the nonpharmacologic interventions and strategies mentioned in the preceding text.

2. Antipsychotic medication is considered the medication of choice for managing many of the symptoms of delirium. For patients who are agitated, hallucinating, frightened, or otherwise suffering, the use of a neuroleptic agent is widely accepted. Some clinicians and researchers have proposed that the use of dopamine-blocking agents may also have a neuroprotective effect when used in delirious patients and therefore encourage their use. Contraindications would include a history of allergic reaction and significantly prolonged QTc (see subsequent text).

   a. Haloperidol—a high-potency dopamine-blocking agent, is generally considered first. It has the advantage of minimal anticholinergic side effects (if any), minimal cardiovascular side effects, and no active metabolites. In addition, there is the option of intravenous injection, which, in many situations is desirable (emergency setting or lack of oral access). One must monitor for side effects including extrapyramidal effects (less severe when given intravenously), neuroleptic malignant syndrome, excess sedation, and lowering of the seizure threshold. It should be noted that haloperidol may prolong the QTc interval that can lead to *torsades de pointes*. Therefore, it is recommended to check a baseline electrocardiogram (ECG) and monitor for the prolonging of the QTc interval. A QTc of >450 msec or an increase >25% from previous ECGs may warrant telemetry, cardiac consultation, reduction in dose, or discontinuation. We also recommend monitoring potassium and magnesium levels in critically ill patients, especially those with a baseline QTc of 440 msec or longer, those with electrolyte derangements, and those receiving other medications that can prolong the QTc.

(1) Dosing is individualized and can vary greatly, depending on the clinical situation. Intravenous haloperidol is twice as potent as when taken orally. A common dose range is 1 to 2 mg every 2 to 4 hours as needed. However, dosing can be as low as 0.25 to 0.5 mg every 4 hours as needed (particularly in the elderly population). At times, a simple, low bedtime dose may be enough to regulate a patient's sleep–wake cycle and ease mild agitation. In other instances, as in a severely agitated ICU patient, titration to much higher doses, such as repeating a 5 to 10 mg bolus every 15 to 20 minutes, may be needed until the desired effect is achieved (doses between 50 and 500 mg in 24 hours have been reported to have been used with minimal side effects). The use of continuous infusion in severe cases may also be helpful. When higher doses are used it is often helpful to supplement the antipsychotic with a benzodiazepine as the two together can have an additive effect and you may be able to get adequate sedation using smaller doses of each compared with using only a single agent. In cases involving more significant agitation where more rapid sedation is desired, we recommend starting with haloperidol 3 to 5 mg and lorazepam 0.5 to 1 mg, repeating every 20 to 30 minutes as needed. As mentioned in the preceding text, the patient should be monitored for excess sedation, extrapyramidal symptoms, neuroleptic malignant syndrome, prolonged QTc, and lowering of the seizure threshold.

b. Atypical antipsychotics—Although haloperidol is generally accepted as the first choice, there is growing experience with the use of atypical antipsychotics such as risperidone (0.25 to 2 mg), olanzapine (2.5 to 10 mg) and quetiapine (12.5 to 50 mg). Although these agents theoretically have less of a risk for extrapyramidal side effects, the option of administering them intravenously is not available. There have been recent reports and warnings of cerebrovascular events in elderly patients being treated with antipsychotic medication. The clinical significance of these reports is not clear as it pertains to using antipsychotic medication generally at low doses in a transient manner when managing delirium in the elderly. A risk–benefit analysis must be made and clinical judgment used. By using the lowest possible dose for the shortest period of time any cerebrovascular risk will be minimized, especially in the context of the benefit gained.

3. Benzodiazepines—In general, benzodiazepines should be minimized in delirious patients, with the following exceptions:
   a. When benzodiazepines are the treatment of choice for an underlying etiology such as in alcohol or benzodiazepine withdrawal. A common mistake is to use a benzodiazepine to treat alcohol withdrawal successfully only to abruptly discontinue the benzodiazepine, leading to a second withdrawal syndrome.
   b. When a patient is significantly agitated. In these patients using a benzodiazepine in conjunction with a neuroleptic can be quite helpful in controlling the patient's behavior (see preceding text).
   c. When seizure threshold is a concern.
   d. When akathisia is treated.

The preferred benzodiazepine is lorazepam because it is relatively short acting with no active metabolites. Dosing should be titrated to effect (0.25 to 2 mg), where the most common starting doses are between 0.5 and 1 mg. Higher doses are sometimes required when treating alcohol or benzodiazepine withdrawal (with severe cases requiring a lorazepam drip of several milligrams an hour). Clearly, benzodiazepines are associated with sedation and doses should be held in the setting of excess sedation. Other associated effects to be mindful of include respiratory depression, ataxia, behavioral disinhibition, delirium, and withdrawal syndromes. Should a patient require daily benzodiazepines for more than 2 continuous weeks (such as in an ICU setting), or if benzodiazepines are being used to treat alcohol or benzodiazepine withdrawal, then a gradual discontinuation (10% to 15% per day) is required.

Chapter 3

COGNITIVE IMPAIRMENT

David B. Arciniegas,
Thomas W. McAllister, Daniel I. Kaufer

I. BACKGROUND

A. **Definitions**

1. **Arousal**—refers to a state of wakefulness that underlies the capacity to respond appropriately to environmental stimuli. Arousal is a continuum of function, with *coma* at the severely deficient end of that continuum and *hyperarousal* (as manifested in some delirious, manic, psychotic, or anxious individuals) at the other end of that continuum.

2. **Speed of processing** refers to the rate at which an individual is able to process and respond to a stimulus. Information processing speed is most often described clinically in terms of *reaction time* or *response latency* (latency between stimulus presentation and a behavioral response).

3. **Attention**—refers to the capacity to detect, select, and focus on a stimulus (external or internal). Several component processes of attention include: (a) Multimodal filtering of sensory and cognitive information to select a stimulus for processing (*sensory gating* and *selective attention*, respectively); (b) maintaining focus on a stimulus over time (*sustained attention*); and (c) simultaneously attending to two or more stimuli (*divided attention*).

4. **Memory** refers to the ability to learn, store, and retrieve information. There are several different but overlapping types and ways of categorizing memory based on the type of information learned (e.g., spatial vs. verbal) and the temporal interval between learning and retrieving (immediate vs. short term vs. long term). *Working memory* describes the process of keeping information in mind or "on-line" for short-term use in processing additional information, and overlaps both conceptually and nosologically with *registration* and also *immediate memory*.

Declarative memory (also known as explicit memory) refers to the ability to learn and store (or *encode*) and to retrieve factual information. Declarative memory is generally divided into two subcategories: *Semantic memory*, or memory for general knowledge ("who, what, where"), and *episodic memory*, or memory for personal experiences that are tied to particular times and places. Declarative memory also encompasses *spatial memory*, the learning, storage, and retrieval of visual-spatial information, and *verbal memory*, the learning, storage, and retrieval of verbally encoded information. *Procedural memory* (also known as *implicit memory*) denotes the ability to learn, store, and retrieve how to do things; conceptually and clinically, procedural memory overlaps considerably with praxis (defined in the subsequent text). *Short-term memory* refers to the ability to retain information for a period of several minutes to a few days, and *long-term memory* refers to retention of information over a period of days of longer.

5. **Language** refers to the communication of thought using symbolic (verbal or written) means. Language is generally divided into four domains: (a) *Fluency*, the ability to produce syntactically normal phrase lengths of six or more words without undue word-finding pauses; (b) *repetition*, the ability to reproduce phrases without error; (c) *comprehension*, the ability to recognize written or spoken symbols across multiple sensory domains and to attach linguistic meaning to them; and (d) *naming*, the ability to identify actions and objects across multiple sensory domains accurately. Language is distinct from *speech*, the motor capacity for producing verbal output (impairment of which is described as *dysarthria*), and from *voice*, the laryngeal function required for phonation (impairment of which is described as *dysphonia*).

6. **Prosody** refers to the affective import and *kinesics* (gestural elements) of language. Prosodic modulation permits communication of the emotion associated with spoken (or written or signed) language. Changes in prosody also permit emphasis on particular words in a sentence so as to change the meaning of that sentence.

7. **Recognition**—refers to the ability to integrate sensory information at a cortical level regarding objects, people, sounds, shapes, or smells (cortically based perception) and to attach meaning to those percepts (association).

8. **Praxis**—refers to the ability to execute skilled purposeful movements on demand given normal comprehension of the request and the elementary motor abilities to execute it. Praxis is most often classified into three types: *Limb-kinetic, ideomotor,* and *ideational. Limb-kinetic praxis* describes the ability to make finely graded, precise, individual finger movements on demand. *Ideomotor praxis* refers to the ability to perform a single previously learned skilled movement on demand. *Ideational praxis* refers to the ability to carry out a specific sequence of tasks on demand.

9. **Visuospatial function** refers to the ability to assess spatial relationships between objects in the environment and also between the environment and oneself. This function is also involved in spatial attention, working memory, and short-term memory.

10. **Executive function**—refers to a variety of cognitive processes that contribute to selection, planning, and execution of adaptive behavior. These include: *Volition* (conceptualize what one wants), *planning* (outline and sequence a set of behaviors to achieve a desired end), *purposive action* (initiation and maintenance of behaviors that increase the likelihood of a desired end), and *monitoring* (assess progress of previously decided sequence of behavior in the furtherance of the goal). *"Mental flexibility"* (integrate feedback and consider alternative actions), *insight* (the ability to realistically appraise one's capacities and deficits, and to recognize and accurately attribute aberrant behaviors to illness), and *judgment* (the capacity to assess current situation, potential future action options, assign outcome probabilities to those options and pursue the one that best fits the short- and long-term goals) are other examples of executive cognitive functions.

II. NEUROANATOMY AND NEUROCHEMISTRY OF COGNITION

A. **Arousal**
1. Arousal is the most fundamental cognitive function, and is supported by a set of selective distributed reticulothalamic, thalamocortical, and reticulocortical networks.
2. The reticulothalamic portion of the arousal system consists of cholinergic projections arising from the pendunculopontine and laterodorsal tegmental nuclei. These projections terminate in the body of the thalamus as well as the reticular nucleus of the thalamus, the balance of activity between which appears to modulate the degree of thalamic activity.
3. Thalamocortical projections, which are predominantly glutamatergic, also contribute to arousal by activating cortex and preparing it for information processing.
4. Cortical readiness to engage in information processing is modulated by the reticulocortical portion of the arousal system. This portion of the arousal system consists of dopaminergic projections arising from the ventral tegmental area of the midbrain, noradrenergic projections arising from the locus ceruleus, serotonergic projections arising from the median and dorsal raphe nuclei, and cholinergic projections arising from the medial septal nucleus and vertical limb of the diagonal band of Broca (to medial temporal structures) and also from the nucleus basalis of Meynert (to neocortical, and especially frontal, parietal, and lateral temporal areas). The balance between and reciprocal influences of the reticulothalamic and reticulocortical systems on the diencephalic and cortical targets to which they project influence level of arousal.

5.   Injury to or dysfunction of any of these elements of the arousal system may impair this most basic cognitive function.

B.   Attention and processing speed

1.   Attentional processes are mediated by several large-scale, selective distributed neural networks. These networks include those involved in arousal described in the preceding text. Additionally, primary and secondary sensory cortices, heteromodal parietal cortical areas, medial temporal (i.e., hippocampal and entorhinal) areas, the striatum and pallidum, several prefrontal (i.e., cingulate, inferolateral, and dorsolateral) cortices, and the axonal connections between them are components of these distributed attentional networks.

2.   Electrophysiologic and functional neuroimaging studies suggest that the neurobiological bases of sensory gating, selective attention, and sustained attention differ from one another. Sensory gating appears most strongly related to the function of a cholinergically dependent hippocampal inhibitory circuit, and is a prerequisite for the development of selective attention within sensory cortical-hippocampal-thalamo-frontal networks. Sustained attention is most strongly related to the function of inferolateral frontal-subcortical and dorsolateral prefrontal-subcortical circuits.

3.   The function of attentional networks is dependent on a complex set of interactions between the major neurotransmitter systems, including those regulating the availability and function of cortical dopamine, norepinephrine, serotonin, acetylcholine, glutamate, and γ-aminobutyric acid (GABA).

4.   Acute or chronic structural and neurochemical dysfunction within the several networks serving attention contribute to impairments in this cognitive domain. Impairments in attention may also contribute to problems with the speed of information processing.

C.   Declarative memory

1.   Declarative memory is a hippocampally dependent process.

2.   Highly processed multimodal sensory information is transmitted from the inferior parietal (heteromodal) association cortices to the entorhinal-hippocampal complex. When that information produces a sufficiently robust signal in the hippocampus (a process that is, at least in part, predicated on assignment of motivational, emotional, or other "survival-related" significance by amygdala–hippocampal interactions), the process of *long-term potentiation (LTP)* is initiated and that information is encoded for later recall.

3.   Output from the hippocampus travels to several target sites. Most hippocampal output travels through the fornix to the mamillary bodies and anterior thalamus; this pathway is generally regarded as that through which the hippocampus participates most strongly in the process of declarative memory. A smaller portion of hippocampal efferents in the fornix split off anterior to the anterior commissure as the precommissural

fornix, from where they continue to their targets in the septal and preoptic areas, orbital cortex, and anterior cingulate cortex. Although these areas may also be important to the development of declarative memory, their function appears to be more closely tied to homeostatic processes mediated by the limbic system.

4. After information is communicated through the hippocampal-forniceal-mamillo-thalamic pathway, it is further distributed to frontal areas involved in the process of memory development (*consolidation*). The time required for consolidation is variable, ranging from only a few minutes to many months.

5. Following consolidation of memories, retrieving declarative information requires prefrontal structures to activate the selective distributed networks where that information was originally encoded.

6. By virtue of the distributed nature of the networks involved in encoding of declarative information, declarative memory is highly associative: Memories may be retrieved by reactivation of nearly any part of the network involved in the original encoding of that information or by activation of other networks whose constituent elements are shared by the network involved in the original encoding of that information.

7. Although the neurochemistry of declarative memory is complex, glutamate and acetylcholine appear to be particularly important. The action of glutamate at N-methyl-D-aspartate (NMDA) receptors is involved in the process of LTP. Acetylcholine appears to facilitate this process, possibly through its establishment of pre- and postsynaptic excitatory potentials in the neurons involved in the process of LTP.

8. Acute or chronic structural and neurochemical dysfunction within the several networks serving declarative memory may contribute to impairments in this cognitive domain.

D. **Procedural memory**

1. Procedural memory is predicated on the development and fine-tuning of the sensorimotor-frontal-subcortical-cerebellar networks that are required for learning and efficiently retrieving complex sensorimotor routines.

2. Procedural memory is not hippocampally dependent and its function and dysfunction are dissociable from declarative memory.

3. Procedural memory is not associative, but is instead dedicated: It is inflexibly limited to the context (i.e., the specific sensorimotor processes) in which it is acquired.

4. Normal performance in this domain is dependent on many of the same neurotransmitters required by the frontal-subcortical circuits involved in retrieval of declarative information.

5. Acute or chronic structural and neurochemical dysfunction within the several networks serving procedural memory may contribute to impairments in this cognitive domain.

E. **Language**

1. Language refers to the symbolic means of representing and communicating thought, and is in most cases a function of the dominant cerebral hemisphere.

2. *Fluency* is predicated on a network of frontal structures, including dorsolateral prefrontal motor association, and anterior insular cortices, white matter, and subcortical structures through which these areas are connected, and the frontal opercular (Broca) area. Output from this network of structures requires intact connections between primary motor cortex and the parts of the body used to communicate verbally or by writing. Communication impairments related to disturbances in elementary motor function are generally distinguishable from true language disturbances (*aphasias*).

3. *Comprehension* is predicated on a network of temporoparietal structures, including at least the superior temporal language association cortex (Wernicke area), inferior parietal heteromodal association cortex, and the white matter structures connecting them. Comprehension depends on the integrity of peripheral sensory structures, their connections to primary sensory cortices, and the connection of these areas to sensory association systems. Communication disturbances due to impairments in peripheral sensory organs, primary sensory cortices, and also the connections between them, are distinguishable from aphasias.

4. The neural networks serving fluency and comprehension are distinct and dissociable, resulting in the distinct patterns of language impairments referable to dysfunction in each of these networks.

5. *Repetition* is served by a distinct network composed of Wernicke area, a phonologic output area at the anterior border of Wernicke area, Broca area, and the arcuate fasciculus that connects the posterior and anterior language areas. Disruption in any of these areas results in impairment of repetition.

6. *Naming* is subserved by widely distributed neural networks that overlap substantially with those upon which fluency, comprehension, and repetition are predicated. Consequently, impairment of naming (anomia) usually accompanies impairments in these other areas of language.

7. The neurochemistry of language impairment is understood less fully than is the neurochemistry of arousal, attention, and memory impairment. Reports of the pharmacotherapy of aphasia suggest a role for augmentation of dopamine and acetylcholine in the treatment of language disturbances in individuals with stroke, traumatic brain injury (TBI), and other neurologic conditions.

8. Acute or chronic structural and neurochemical dysfunction within the several networks serving language may contribute to impairments in this cognitive domain.

F. **Prosody**
    1. Prosody demonstrates a pattern of nondominant hemispheric specialization. The nondominant hemisphere structures and networks serving prosody are simplistically understood as roughly homologous with those in the dominant hemisphere serving the syntactic and semantic aspects of language.
    2. Impaired function of the nondominant frontal structures involved in prosody may produce disturbances in the affective and kinesic aspects of language production, resulting in flat or monotonous expression that fails to communicate effectively its emotional relevance and nuance.
    3. Impaired function of the nondominant temporoparietal structures involved in prosody results in disturbances in the appreciation of the affective and kinesic aspects of the communications of others.
    4. At present, little is known about the neurochemistry of prosody.
G. **Praxis**
    1. Praxis displays a pattern of dominant hemisphere specialization.
    2. The dominant hemisphere neural networks subserving praxis are anatomically colocated, and may overlap, with those serving language. Consequently, the *apraxias* tend to be associated with the aphasias, and particularly the nonfluent aphasias.
    3. The neurochemistry of praxis is not well established, but striatal dopaminergic function appears to play an important role in this cognitive function.
    4. Acute or chronic structural and neurochemical dysfunction within the several networks serving praxis may contribute to impairments in this cognitive domain.
H. **Visuospatial function**
    1. Visuospatial function displays a pattern of nondominant hemisphere specialization.
    2. The nondominant hemisphere networks subserving visuospatial function (including spatial attention, spatial working memory, and spatial orientation) includes elements of the reticular system, thalamus, superior colliculus, striatum, posterior parietal cortex, frontal eye fields, and parietal cortex.
    3. Most of the major neurotransmitter systems (i.e., glutamate, GABA, acetylcholine, and dopamine, among others) are involved in visuospatial function. Cortical noradrenergic projections, which have a right-hemisphere predilection, and cortical dopaminergic pathways, which are frontally predominant, may be particularly important for spatial attention.
    4. Acute or chronic structural and neurochemical dysfunction within the several networks serving visuospatial function may contribute to impairments in this cognitive domain.
I. **Executive function**
    1. Executive function is mediated primarily by the dorsolateral prefrontal-subcortical circuit, which integrates the processing, interaction, and output of other cognitive processes (i.e., language, memory) carried out elsewhere in the brain.

2. Although the role of the dorsolateral prefrontal-subcortical circuit is essential for executive function, there is evidence suggesting that the anterior cingulate and also the lateral orbitofrontal-subcortical circuits participate in the development of executive function as well.

3. The function of these circuits is dependent on a host of neurotransmitters including glutamate (serving as the primary excitatory neurotransmitter), acetylcholine, dopamine, norepinephrine, serotonin (serving various modulatory functions), and GABA (serving as the primary inhibitory neurotransmitter), among others.

4. Executive dysfunction may arise as a direct effect of injury to any element (cortical, subcortical, or axonal) of this circuit, the neurochemical systems that modulate function within this circuit, and/or the connections between the "basic" cognitive processing networks and this circuit.

III. CLASSIFICATION OF COGNITIVE IMPAIRMENT

A. The Diagnostic and Statistical Manual of Mental Disorders, 4th edition (DSM-IV) (1) describes several disorders where cognitive impairment is the defining feature. These include delirium, the dementias, amnestic disorders, developmental disorders, and cognitive disorder not otherwise specified (NOS).

B. *Delirium* (see Chapter ??) is characterized by an alteration in attention, perceptual disturbances (i.e., hallucinations), and consciousness (altered and/or fluctuating). Other terms often used to describe delirium include acute confusional state and encephalopathy.

C. *Amnestic disorders* are characterized by deficits in memory in the absence of, or out of proportion to, deficits in other cognitive domains. The DSM-based classification system specifies three general categories of amnestic disorders: Amnestic disorder due to a general medical condition, substance-induced persisting amnestic disorder, and amnestic disorder NOS (i.e., amnesia due to any other cause). To meet criteria for an amnestic disorder, the memory impairment must represent a decline from a previous level of ability and be sufficiently severe to impair functioning in one or more important domains of activity (i.e., social, occupational, etc.). The DSM-based diagnosis of an amnestic disorder also requires that the impairment is not better accounted for by delirium, dementia, substance use or withdrawal, or another psychiatric disorder.

D. In the DSM-based classification system, *dementia* (see Chapter 4) is characterized by prominent impairments of memory and at least one other cognitive domain (e.g., attention, language, praxis, recognition, and/or "complex cognition" [executive function]). Additionally, the cognitive impairments must impair social, occupational, or other important daily functions. Although there is an explicit relationship between cognitive impairment and functional disability in this definition of dementia, recent evidence suggests that cognitive impairments contribute to, but do not entirely account for, functional disability; other neuropsychiatric impairments (e.g., emotion, behavior, and/or elementary sensorimotor impairments) are likely contributors to functional disturbances as well. Dementias may be reversible (e.g., dementia due to hypothyroidism, and nutritional deficiencies), static (e.g., dementia due to TBI), or progressive (e.g., Alzheimer dementia).

E. The diagnosis of *cognitive disorder NOS* is used when the patient presents with functionally significant cognitive impairments that do not meet criteria for any of the other cognitive disorders listed in the DSM. For example, this diagnosis might be applied to a patient with isolated impairments of language (*aphasia*), praxis (*apraxia*), recognition (*agnosia*), visuospatial function, or executive function, particularly when such impairments occur in the absence of memory impairment (absent which they fail to meet DSM criteria for dementia). Although the DSM-IV-TR mentions "mild neurocognitive disorder" and "postconcussional disorder" as examples of cognitive disorder NOS, the criteria provided for these diagnoses are for research purposes only and should not be used in clinical practice.

F. Although not included presently in the DSM-based classification of disorders, *mild cognitive impairment* (MCI) is an emerging term that has been applied as a descriptor for impairment in any of the major domains of cognition (e.g., "mild memory loss," or "mild problems with attention"). More recently, MCI has been used to describe a syndrome characterized by complaints of memory difficulty and (1) minimal or no functional impairment of usual activities of daily living, (2) normal general cognitive function, (3) abnormal memory test performance relative to age norms and the individual's baseline memory function, and (4) does not meet criteria for clinical diagnosis of dementia.

G. Cognitive impairment may be a feature of other conditions where non-cognitive symptoms are the defining feature of the illness. For example, individuals with depression have measurable decrements in attention and memory, and individuals with schizophrenia frequently demonstrate impairments in visual and auditory information processing, sustained attention, working memory, verbal episodic memory, and executive function.

IV. TREATMENT OF COGNITIVE IMPAIRMENT

A. **General issues**
  1. **Epidemiology.** Cognitive complaints are common among individuals with neurologic and neuropsychiatric disorders (e.g., TBI, stroke, Parkinson disease, multiple sclerosis, or HIV/AIDS, etc.). In some cases, for example, the dementias, cognitive impairment, and associated impairments in day-to-day function are the defining features of the clinical presentation and are therefore present among all individuals with such conditions. In other settings, for example, TBI, HIV/AIDS, and multiple sclerosis, cognitive impairments are a common but not

invariant element of a multidimensional set of neuropsychiatric problems. Across all of these conditions, the frequency and severity of cognitive complaints or impairments varies with a host of premorbid (e.g., age, or education), condition-specific (e.g., degenerative, traumatic, or demyelinating), and associated psychiatric, medical, and psychosocial factors. Despite the influence of these factors on clinical presentation, however, two points are clear: (1) Cognitive complaints and deficits can be the presenting symptom in all of these disorders, and (2) cognitive complaints and deficits are an important source of distress and disability in all of these disorders.

2. **Prognosis**

   a. Treatment of cognitive deficits is directed at three broad groups. The first includes individuals with progressive neurodegenerative or neurologic disorders (e.g., Alzheimer disease and other neurodegenerative dementias—see Chapter 4). The second includes individuals with delirium or dementing disorders that are reversible with appropriate treatment (e.g., dementia due to depression, endocrine or nutritional disorders, and/or infectious encephalopathies). The third consists of individuals with static brain insults that affect cognitive function (e.g., individuals with TBI, focal vascular events, radio- or chemotherapy-induced brain injury, neurodevelopmental disorders, etc.).

   b. The prognosis and goals of treatment vary considerably with the cause and severity of such impairments. From a therapeutic standpoint, treatment for cognitive deficits may fall into the category of *disease altering* (correction of the underlying disorder), or *symptomatic* (treatment of the cognitive deficits that are causing excess disability).

   c. There are at present no disease-altering treatments for individuals with progressive neurodegenerative disorders. Accordingly, the long-term prognosis for cognitive function in these populations is universally poor. Appropriate goals of treatment are to augment current cognitive functions to the greatest extent possible, to delay progression of symptoms when possible, and to improve quality of life despite persistence and/or progression of symptoms.

   d. Among individuals with delirium or "reversible" dementia syndromes, the prognosis is generally favorable provided proper diagnosis is made and appropriate treatment provided. With prompt and effective treatment of the underlying medical/neurologic condition, the goal of treatment is to effect a "cure" of cognitive impairments resulting from that condition.

   e. Among individuals with static neurologic disorders affecting cognitive function (e.g., TBI, stroke, or hypoxic-ischemic brain injury), the prognosis for recovery of cognitive function typically varies as a function of the nature, severity, and chronicity (i.e., time since onset) of the disorder. Facilitating cognitive recovery to the greatest extent possible and improving quality of life despite persistent disability are appropriate treatment goals.

3. **General management principles**

   a. **Diagnosis**

     (1) **History**—The diagnosis of cognitive impairment in neuropsychiatric disorders should follow a logical process. It is important to ask about the following areas:

       (a) **Complaints or deficits**—Determine first whether the problem is subjective (cognitive complaints), objective (cognitive impairment), or both. This requires a careful history regarding premorbid factors (and especially the highest level of cognitive function obtained before symptom onset), the types of cognitive impairments experienced, their severity, and their functional consequences. Collateral history from reliable informants (e.g., observers, data describing prior function, etc.) is essential.

       (b) **Time course**—Carefully outline the time course of the problem. Did the problem develop acutely or insidiously? Has the decline shown a continuous or interrupted trajectory? Answers to these questions help inform whether one is dealing with a static or progressive problem, and may yield important clues regarding the etiology of the problem.

       (c) **Relationship to other neurologic symptoms and events**—Clarify whether the cognitive problems are an isolated symptom/syndrome, manifestations of an identifiable neurologic disorder, or associated features of a primary psychiatric disorder (e.g., depression, or anxiety). Identifying and interpreting cognitive complaints with respect to each of these possibilities is essential for developing a refined differential diagnosis for the patient's clinical presentation and formulating appropriate treatment goals.

       (d) **Profile of symptoms and signs** Define the spectrum of symptoms and signs that are the target behaviors. Clarify whether the problems fall primarily within the domain of attention, memory, language, praxis, recognition, visuospatial function, executive function, or some combination of these. This assessment sheds light on the likely underlying etiology and will also help inform initial treatment. This process requires a careful history, "bedside" cognitive testing, and often additional assessments (see subsequent text).

(2) **Diagnostic assessment**—Diagnostic assessments generally fall into two broad categories. The first involves characterizing the profile of cognitive complaints and capacities, and the second involves identifying the cause of these problems.

   (a) **Profile of cognitive deficits** Initial office or "bedside" assessment of cognition is the first step in characterizing whether one is dealing with cognitive complaints, cognitive deficits, or both. There are a variety of bedside assessments of cognition, the most commonly used of which include the Mini-Mental State Examination (MMSE), the Clock Drawing Test (including the CLOX), the EXIT25 (a measure of executive function), and the Frontal Assessment Battery (FAB). Each of these and similar measures have their individual strengths and weaknesses.

   Normative databases describing age- and education-adjusted performance expectations are available for many of these measures. Given the strong influence of age and education on performance on such measures, comparison of an individual patient's score on these measures is strongly recommended over use of "cutoff" scores. Because the latter does not account for the influence of such variables on cognitive performance, some individuals with "normal" cognitive function will be misclassified as impaired, and *vice versa*, when cutoff scores are used.

   When screening assessments fail to identify impairments in the cognitive domains suggested by patient complaints or history, referral for formal cognitive assessments (neuropsychological testing) and performance of additional diagnostic testing (see subsequent text) is recommended. Formal neuropsychological testing should include indicators of psychiatric/psychological processes known to adversely affect performance on cognitive assessment measures, particularly anxiety, and depression.

   (b) **Physical examination**—A general medical and neuropsychiatric examination is required on all patients.

   (c) **Additional diagnostic assessments**—The selection of additional diagnostic assessments varies with the clinical context. Serum laboratory assessments for common reversible causes of cognitive impairment (i.e., vitamin B_{12} and thyroid stimulating hormone) is recommended; when justified by the clinical history, other serum (e.g., HIV, rapid plasma reagin [RPR], antinuclear antibodies [ANA], liver function tests, electrolytes, and complete blood count, etc.) and urine (e.g., urinalysis, and urine toxicology) assessments may be appropriate. When epilepsy or delirium is suspected, electroencephalography (EEG) may inform the diagnostic assessment. Structural brain imaging is strongly recommended in the evaluation of all patients with cognitive impairment, and particularly among those in whom the clinical examination suggests existence of structural brain disease.

b. **General treatment considerations**

(1) **Development of a therapeutic alliance and promotion of treatment adherence**—Many individuals with cognitive impairments may have limited awareness of the nature, severity, or functional consequences of their deficits. This can make developing a therapeutic alliance challenging. Patient "resistance" may reflect psychological denial (not wanting to be labeled as "brain damaged" or "demented"), a deficit in self-monitoring and awareness of illness (*anosognosia*), or both. Nonetheless, establishing such an alliance with these patients and, when relevant, their caregivers is essential for developing a realistic and effective treatment plan.

(2) **Treat comorbid conditions**—A variety of conditions can produce or exacerbate cognitive impairments; among the most common are depression, anxiety, substance use disorders, sleep disorders, and physical discomfort or pain. Side effects from medications used to treat many medical, neurologic, and psychiatric conditions are also common causes of cognitive impairment. A thorough assessment of these issues is imperative before prescribing medications or nonpharmacologic treatments specifically for cognition. Optimizing treatment of comorbid conditions and reducing or eliminating medications with potentially adverse effects on cognition are important steps before treating cognition specifically.

(3) **Cognitive remediation or rehabilitation** Nonpharmacologic interventions may be effective for the treatment of cognitive impairments, particularly among individuals with static brain disorders (e.g., TBI, stroke, hypoxic-ischemic brain injury, and possibly schizophrenia). Such interventions for domain-specific cognitive impairments are described in the following sections of this chapter. Successful cognitive remediation or rehabilitation interventions generally include a

mix of stimulus modalities, complexity, and response demands, and active involvement of the therapist in terms of performance monitoring, feedback, and skills/strategy training. These interventions are "successful" to the extent that they generalize beyond the context of treatment—in other words, these interventions should be designed in such a way that they improve not only performance on the office-based tasks (e.g., attention training on a computerized test) involved but are applicable to everyday function (e.g., attentional processing in real-world settings).

(4) **Environmental strategies and approaches**—Several strategies can be effective in minimizing the functional consequences of cognitive impairments.

    (a) **Time for performance**—One of the core deficits associated with many neurologic disorders is reduced speed of information processing. "Absolute" function or task-accuracy may be reasonably normal if the patient is afforded sufficient time to perform. Simple interventions such as waiting longer for verbal responses (i.e., teaching others not to respond or perform immediately for the individual) and allowing longer intervals to accomplish tasks, whether in the context of activities of daily living, educational endeavors, or in vocational settings, may permit the individuals to maximize their "real-world" functional performance.

    (b) **Cognitive prosthetics** Encouraging the use of memory notebooks, timers with alarms and messages, tasks lists, and provision by others of verbal or nonverbal cues may permit the individuals to compensate for cognitive deficits and maximize their functional independence. The use of cognitive prosthetics may reduce affective responses (i.e., anxiety, anger/agitation) that may otherwise result from real or perceived cognitive failures.

    (c) **Technology**—Assistive technologies may permit compensation for more severe cognitive impairments, and particularly language impairments. Consultation with speech and occupational therapists experienced in the selection and use of such technologies is recommended.

    (d) **Environmental accommodation** Stimulating environments may tax the ability of individuals to select and sustain attention appropriately, to process information at the speed demanded by the environment, and to develop flexible and adaptive responses to environmental demands. As suggested in the preceding text, overtaxing environments may produce cognitive failures and precipitate otherwise avoidable and unwanted affective and behavioral responses. Identifying environmental antecedents to cognitive failures and the affective–behavioral problems they produce may facilitate improvements in functional cognition, reduce disability, and alleviate patient and caregiver distress.

(e) **Tailor demands to peak capacity** Individuals with cognitive impairment and neurologic disorders often struggle with physical and cognitive fatigue. Performance of tasks otherwise within the functional abilities of such individuals may decline significantly as they fatigue. It is helpful to outline daily events and challenges and schedule them to coincide with periods when the individual is well rested and refreshed.

(5) **Pharmacotherapy** Pharmacologic interventions for cognitive impairments are most usefully regarded as adjuncts to nonpharmacologic therapies. The individual response to treatment is highly variable, both with respect to specific agents and also doses. Although a "start-low, go-slow" approach is prudent when prescribing neuroactive agents to individuals with neurologic disorders, standard doses of such agents are often required. Because there are no U.S. Food and Drug Administration (FDA)-approved medications for the treatment of these cognitive impairments described in this chapter, individual treatment remains a matter of clinical judgment and empiric trial.

(6) **Integrate treatment from multiple clinicians** Patients with cognitive impairments receive treatment from multiple clinicians. Communication between clinicians is needed to ensure that treatments offered are not working at cross-purposes.

(7) **Document treatment effects** Serial assessment of cognition, whether by bedside or formal neuropsychological assessments, allows accurate recording of the degree of response (or lack thereof) to a given intervention, whether nonpharmacologic or pharmacologic, and avoids repeat administration of previously unsuccessful treatments.

V. DISORDERS OF AROUSAL

A. **Clinical background**
   1. **Occurrence and prevalence.** Disturbances of arousal may fall on the continuum from states of hyperarousal, as seen among individuals with mania, anxiety disorders, and some forms of delirium, to hypoarousal of varying degrees of severity. The former are considered elsewhere in this volume. Here

we consider impairments of arousal including *coma, vegetative states* (VS), including *persistent vegetative states* (PVS), and the *minimally conscious state* (MCS). TBI, hypoxic-ischemic brain injury, cerebrovascular events (especially subarachnoid hemorrhage), metabolic disturbances due to conditions such as hyper- or hypoglycemia, hepatic or renal failure, endocrine disorders (e.g., severe hypothyroidism), medication intoxications (both accidental and intentional), cerebral neoplasms, and congenital/developmental disorders are among the most common causes of impaired arousal. The frequency of coma and other states of impaired arousal (consciousness) varies with the type and severity of the underlying conditions.

2. **Phenomenology**
   a. Coma represents a complete failure of the arousal system: Patients in coma appear unconscious, demonstrate no spontaneous eye opening, and are unable to be awakened by application of vigorous sensory stimulation. Patients in coma do not demonstrate evidence of sleep–wake cycles.
   b. VS describes a condition in which "core" consciousness (simple arousal) is relatively preserved but "higher" consciousness (i.e., self- and environmental awareness) is completely absent. However, patients in VS may retain capacity for spontaneous or stimulus-induced arousal, and may demonstrate sleep–wake cycles. When such impairment lasts for more than a few weeks, the term PVS is used to describe the condition.
   c. MCS is characterized by inconsistent but clearly discernable behavioral evidence of consciousness such as following simple commands, gestural or verbal yes/no responses (regardless of accuracy), intelligible verbalization, and purposeful behavior. The latter include movements or affective behaviors that occur in response to an understandable environmental stimulus and are not better attributable to reflexive behavior.

3. **Course and prognosis.** The course and prognosis impaired arousal varies with the type and severity of underlying illness as well as the depth and duration of the state of impaired arousal.
   a. Emergence from coma within the first day after onset is generally associated with a more favorable prognosis. Conversely, persistence of impaired consciousness beyond the first 24 hours after onset, and certainly beyond the first week thereafter, is usually associated with a poor prognosis for recovery.
   b. The transition from coma to VS is marked by fading of decerebrate reactions (when present initially), development of sleep–wake cycles, and the emergence of spontaneous or stimulus-induced arousal.
   c. Patients with coma or PVS may progress to MCS; for some of these patients, MCS is a transient state during the process

of continued recovery, although for others MCS may become a permanent condition. The distinction between MCS and higher states of consciousness is somewhat arbitrary, but the development of functional interactive communication, functional use of at least two different objects (suggesting a capacity for object discrimination), or both is generally regarded as evidence supporting emergence from MCS. In a minority of individuals with severe congenital cerebral disorders, MCS may be a permanent outcome. MCS may also be a late feature of neurodegenerative disorders.

B. **Neuropathogenesis.** Coma and other states of impaired arousal reflect impairment of the brainstem, diencephalic, and cortical structural and neurochemical networks serving this basic domain of cognition. Impairment of the deeper (i.e., reticular, reticulothalamic, reticulocortical) elements of these systems is generally associated with more severe impairments of arousal such as coma and VS/PVS. Disruption of the thalamocortical elements of these networks is more often associated with VS/PVS and MCS.

C. **Diagnosis.** Although impaired arousal is usually evident on basic clinical examinations, the distinction between coma, VS/PVS, and MCS is challenging. Giacino et al.[1] recommend the following steps be taken to establish an accurate diagnosis:

1. Provide adequate stimulation to ensure that arousal is maximized.
2. Reduce factors that may impair arousal (e.g., sedating medications, or seizures, etc.).
3. Avoid verbal or other stimuli that provoke reflexive responses.
4. Design command-follow trials that are within the patient's motor abilities.
5. Assess a broad range of behavioral responses using a broad range of eliciting stimuli.
6. Conduct examinations in an environment free of potentially distracting stimuli.
7. Perform serial reassessments using systematic observations and reliable measurement strategies to confirm findings from initial assessments.
8. Observe interactions between the patient and others; this may be useful for the purpose of data collection and for the development of assessment procedures tailored to the condition and capabilities of the patient.

Structural neuroimaging of individuals with impaired arousal using computed tomography and/or magnetic resonance imaging (MRI) of the brain is strongly recommended as it may elucidate the neurologic basis of the patient's condition and guide prognostication. Functional neuroimaging is not sufficiently developed to recommend its routine use in this context. Electrodiagnostic testing, including EEG and evoked potentials (especially somatosensory evoked potentials) may also help identify the cause (e.g., seizure) and inform the prognosis of states of impaired arousal.[2,3] Laboratory assessment for metabolic, endocrine, toxic, and other medical conditions is also essential.

D. **Treatment**

1. **Optimize the physical health.** In light of the many and varied causes of states of impaired arousal, identification and treatment of the underlying cause is the first and most important intervention. Use of supportive measures and prevention of medical complications is essential.

2. **Optimize the patient's environment.** Manage the patient's environment to provide cues that may facilitate adaptive engagement while minimizing the potential for overstimulation and attendant behavioral disturbances. For example, it may be useful to structure the environment such that sleep–wake and feeding cues are provided in a manner that may entrain circadian rhythms. Avoiding unnecessary procedures and minimizing pain may also be useful. Although such interventions are intuitively appealing, the evidence supporting their effectiveness is lacking.

3. **Nonpharmacologic interventions.** The term "coma stimulation" refers to structured sensory stimulation in the service of promoting recovery of sensory awareness, and hence recovery from coma. Although three randomized controlled trials of such programs suggest a possible benefit of coma stimulation, a recent review of these and other studies concluded that the data is insufficient to definitively support or refute the effectiveness of such programs.[4] However, the safety of this treatment is not a subject of controversy. Because it is unlikely to cause harm, we recommend use of a time-limited trial of coma stimulation in the treatment of individuals in coma, VS, PVS, and MCS.

4. **Pharmacotherapy.** There are no FDA-approved treatments for coma, VS, PVS, or MCS. The neurochemical bases of arousal predict that augmentation of cerebral catecholaminergic, glutamatergic, and/or cholinergic function might improve impaired arousal. The clinical literature most strongly supports the use of agents that directly or indirectly augment catecholaminergic function for this purpose. We recommend amantadine as a first-line agent for coma, VS, PVS, and MCS, based on its safety and demonstrated efficacy in two randomized, double-blind, placebo-controlled studies.[5,6]

Amantadine is generally started at a dose of 50 mg twice daily, and is usually increased every week by 100 mg/day for either symptomatic improvement is achieved or medication intolerance develops. Amantadine 100 mg twice daily is often sufficient to improve these symptoms without undue side effects. The maximum dosage of amantadine should not exceed 400 mg daily. Common side effects include headache, nausea, diarrhea, constipation, anorexia, dizziness, lightheadedness, and orthostatic hypotension. Anxiety, irritability, depression, and hallucinations may also develop during treatment with this agent, but are relatively uncommon. At higher doses, psychosis and confusion may occur. Abrupt withdrawal of this agent has been associated (rarely) with neuroleptic malignant syndrome. Additionally, coadministration of triamterene/hydrochlorothiazide may decrease renal excretion of amantadine, resulting in medication intolerance at doses that would ordinarily be regarded as within the usual therapeutic range. Amantadine also potentiates the effects of agents with anticholinergic properties. Adverse reactions to amantadine appear to occur more often in elderly patients than in younger patients. Amantadine may lower seizure threshold, and clinicians are advised to be vigilant for the development or worsening of seizures when using this agent.

References

1. Giacino JT, Ashwal S, Childs N, et al. The minimally conscious state: Definition and diagnostic criteria. *Neurology*. 2002;58(3): 349–353.
2. Brenner RP. The interpretation of EEG in stupor and coma. *Neurologist*. 2005;11(5):271–284.
3. Carter BG, Butt W. Are somatosensory evoked potentials the best predictor of outcome after severe brain injury? A systematic review. *Intensive Care Med*. 2005;31(6):765–775.
4. Lombardi F, Taricco M, De Tanti A, et al. Sensory stimulation for brain injured individuals in coma or vegetative state. *Cochrane Database Syst Rev*. 2002;(2)CD001427.
5. Meythaler JM, Brunner RC, Johnson A, et al. Amantadine to improve neurorecovery in traumatic brain injury-associated diffuse axonal injury: A pilot double-blind randomized trial. *J Head Trauma Rehabil*. 2002;17(4):300–313.
6. Whyte J, Katz D, Long D, et al. Predictors of outcome in prolonged posttraumatic disorders of consciousness and assessment of medication effects: A multicenter study. *Arch Phys Med Rehabil*. 2005;86(3):453–462.

VI. IMPAIRMENTS OF ATTENTION AND PROCESSING SPEED

A. **Clinical background**
   1. **Occurrence and prevalence.** Impairments of attention and processing speed are common cognitive manifestations of many neurologic and neuropsychiatric conditions. However, firm estimates of the prevalence of such impairments both within and across these disorders is lacking. Impairment of attention is the cardinal feature of attention deficit hyperactive disorder (ADHD) and also delirium. The Centers for Disease Control and Prevention (www.cdc.gov/ncbddd/adhd/) estimate that, 4.4 million youth, ages 4 to 17, were diagnosed with ADHD during 2003.
   2. **Phenomenology.** Attention is best understood as a category of cognitive function with several components; selective, sustained, and divided attention are the domains where clinical impairments are most often identified. Impairments of selective attention (including sensory gating) manifest as difficulties directing robust attention to even a single environmental or cognitive target. By contrast, impairments of sustained attention

(concentration) manifest as difficulty with continued attention to a target after its selection (distractibility). Impaired speed of processing generally manifests as delayed response or reaction times to stimuli or tasks, delayed completion times, and a general "slowing" of cognitive processing. The boundaries of these processes overlap with many other aspects of cognition, including arousal, perception, recognition, memory, and executive function. Accordingly, attention disturbances may exacerbate impairments in these other domains of cognition.

   3. **Course and prognosis.** Impairments of attention and processing speed may be transient and reversible manifestations of some neurologic conditions (e.g., TBI, medication, other intoxication or withdrawal states, etc.), static problems in other conditions (e.g., ADHD), or progressive impairments in others (e.g., multiple sclerosis, neurodegenerative dementias such as diffuse Lewy body disease, Parkinson disease, etc.). Accordingly, the course and prognosis of such impairments vary with the underlying condition on which they are predicated.

B. **Neuropathogenesis.** Because attention is predicated on several large-scale selective distributed neural networks, dysfunction of the cortical, subcortical, brainstem, or axonal elements of these networks may produce impairments in attention. Electrophysiologic and functional neuroimaging studies suggest that the neurobiologic bases of sensory gating, selective attention, and sustained attention differ from one another.[1] Sensory gating appears most strongly related to the function of a cholinergically dependent hippocampal inhibitory circuit, and is a prerequisite for the development of selective attention within sensory cortical-hippocampal-thalamo-frontal networks. Sustained attention is most strongly related to the function of inferolateral frontal-subcortical and dorsolateral prefrontal-subcortical circuits. The function of these circuits is dependent on a complex set of interactions between the major neurotransmitter systems, including those regulating the availability and function of cortical dopamine, norepinephrine, serotonin, acetylcholine, glutamate, and GABA. Although the neuropathologic bases of impaired processing speed overlap substantially with those producing attention impairments, reduced speed of processing is most commonly attributed to disturbances in structure or function of the cerebral white matter.

C. **Diagnosis.** Identification of impaired attention and/or processing speed involves clinical interview of the patient and/or other reliable informants and also objective testing. In the DSM-based classification system, a diagnosis of ADHD requires not only subjective report of attention problems but also evidence of functional disturbances resulting from such problems in at least two important domains of daily activity (e.g., school, work, or interpersonal relationships, etc.). Most commonly used bedside measures of cognition are inadequate for the assessment of impairments in attention and processing speed. The use of continuous performance tasks such as the Paced Auditory Serial Addition Test, or other quantitative measures of accuracy and reaction time, are recommended for the diagnosis and monitoring of impairments in attention and processing speed.

D.   **Treatment**

1.   **Optimize the physical health.** As with the treatment of any cognitive impairment, maximizing treatment of underlying neurologic, psychiatric, medical, or substance conditions is a prerequisite to the prescription of treatments (nonpharmacologic and somatic) for impairments in attention and processing speed.

2.   **Optimize the patient's environment and lifestyle.** It is important to address environmental factors that exacerbate or maintain problems with attention and processing speed. For example, identifying and minimizing potential sources of overstimulation and distraction may permit patients with such problems to make the most effective use of their innate attention abilities. Providing adequate time for completion of required tasks may allow an individual to perform more accurately and effectively on such tasks. Encouraging adequate rest and recovery after periods of intense or sustained mental effort may permit patients to maximize their functional abilities.

3.   **Nonpharmacologic interventions.** The use of attention training exercises is a common component of cognitive rehabilitation programs, although the data regarding these interventions suggests that they are more effective during the late (rather than the acute) period after injury or stroke.[2,3] Although other reviews of attention training are less favorable,[4,5] our experience suggests that these interventions may be useful in highly-motivated patients with relatively mild impairments, particularly when tailored to generalize from the office to real-world contexts, and when conducted by a therapist with experience in their selection and administration. Pairing attention retraining with pharmacotherapy may maximize the benefit afforded by both interventions.[6] We recommend this type of combined treatment of attention and processing speed impairments.

Although there are reports describing possible benefits of biofeedback (or "neurofeedback") on attention and speed of processing, the cost–benefit ratio of such treatments precludes recommending their use presently.

4.   **Pharmacotherapy.** There are several FDA-approved treatments for attentional impairments among individuals with ADHD;[7,8] however, there are no FDA-approved treatments for impaired attention due to other neuropsychiatric or neurologic conditions. The neurochemistry of attention predicts that augmentation of cerebral catecholaminergic and cholinergic function may be useful targets for the treatment of attention and speed of processing impairments. Consistent with that hypothesis, several small-scale, randomized, double blind, placebo-controlled studies of methylphenidate[9] and donepezil[10] suggest that these agents are effective and safe for the treatment of impaired attention following TBI. A single-site, open-label study suggests that donepezil

may be similarly effective for the treatment of impaired attention due to multiple sclerosis.[11] There remains insufficient evidence on which to predicate the use of these agents for impairment attention in other conditions, but they are often used for this purpose nonetheless.

In clinical practice, we generally begin pharmacotherapy of attention and processing speed impairments with methylphenidate. Treatment with methylphenidate generally begins with doses of 5 mg twice daily and is gradually increased in increments of 5 mg twice daily until either beneficial effect or medication intolerance is achieved. Most studies suggest that optimal doses of methylphenidate are in the range of 20 to 40 mg twice daily (i.e., 0.15–0.3 mg/kg/twice daily). This medication generally takes effect quickly (within 0.5 to 1 hour following administration), although this effect may wane after only a few hours. Therefore, the first issue in the administration of this agent is determining optimal dose and dosing frequency. Individuals requiring relatively high and frequent doses of methylphenidate may benefit from use of longer-acting preparations of this medication.

Mild increases in heart rate or blood pressure may occur during treatment with methylphenidate, although these tend to occur relatively infrequently in patients without other cardiac or vascular problems and are only rarely of sufficient magnitude to require treatment discontinuation. Serious adverse reactions to these medications are most often related to increases in central dopamine, and to a lesser extent central norepinephrine activity; when these occur, they may include paranoia, dysphoria, anxiety, agitation, and irritability. However, these adverse effects are in practice very uncommon at doses typically used to treat attention and speed of processing impairments. Although lowering seizure threshold is often cited as a risk associated with the use of these agents, this risk appears to be minimal, even among individuals with epilepsy. Clinicians are advised to become familiar with prescribing information regarding other side effects, drug interactions, and contraindications before using methylphenidate or related agents.

Subjective reports of improvement in the absence of improvement on objective measures of cogniton should prompt reevaluation of the etiology of those impairments. Because stimulants may improve mood, increase motivation, or lessen fatigue, discrepancy between subjective and objective measures of improvements may suggest that the primary problem lies in depression, apathy, fatigue, or some combination of these noncognitive problems.

When methylphenidate fails to improve attention, or does so incompletely, use of a cholinesterase inhibitor is recommended. Donepezil is prescribed most commonly when a cholinesterase inhibitor is used; treatment with this agent begins with 5 mg daily. If this dose is tolerated but does not produce improvements in attention after approximately 4 weeks of treatment, titration to 10 mg daily is generally undertaken. Slower dose titration may limit the development of treatment-emergent side effects, which are gastrointestinal in nature. Rivastigmine and galantamine have shorter half-lives, and require twice daily dosing. Rivastigmine is generally started at 1.5 mg b.i.d. and increased in 1.5 mg b.i.d. increments every 4 weeks until maximal benefits are attained or treatment intolerance develops. Galantamine is generally started at 4 mg b.i.d. and increased in 4 mg b.i.d. increments until maximal benefits are attained or treatment intolerance develops. An extended-release once-daily preparation of galantamine is also available; treatment with this agent is generally started at 8 mg daily and increased to 16 mg daily after 4 weeks. A further increase to 24 mg daily after 4 weeks at 16 mg daily may be considered if maximal benefits are not achieved at the lower dose.

All of these agents produce, with variable frequency, headache, nausea, diarrhea, vomiting, fatigue, insomnia, muscle cramping, pain, and abnormal dreams. These side effects are frequently a consequence of overly rapid dose escalation, although they will occur in a minority of patients during treatment with standard dosing strategies. When intolerable side effects develop and/or persist during treatment with any of these agents, dose reduction is prudent. Such reductions may reduce adverse effects and permit patients to continue treatment. Clinicians are advised to familiarize themselves with prescribing information regarding other side effects, drug interactions, and contraindications before using these agents for any purpose. Todate, there are no reports suggesting that the use of these agents in individuals with neurologic disorders is associated with altered seizure frequency. Nonetheless, remaining vigilant for the development of seizures and/or changes in seizure frequency is recommended.

If this strategy produces improvements, we taper the first medication (methylphenidate) to determine whether the benefit is best attributed to the combination of medications or instead to the cholinesterase inhibitor alone. Some patients will respond to stimulants alone, some to cholinesterase inhibitors alone, some to either or both classes of medication, and some to neither. In all cases, treatment of attention and processing speed impairments remains a matter of empiric trial.

References

1. Arciniegas DB, Topkoff JL. Applications of the P50 evoked response to the evaluation of cognitive impairments after traumatic brain injury. *Phys Med Rehabil Clin N Am.* 2004;15(1): 177–203.
2. Cicerone KD, Dahlberg C, Kalmar K, et al. Evidence-based cognitive rehabilitation: Recommendations for clinical practice. *Arch Phys Med Rehabil.* 2000;81(12):1596–1615.
3. Cicerone KD, Dahlberg C, Malec JF, et al. Evidence-based cognitive rehabilitation: Updated review of the literature from 1998 through 2002. *Arch Phys Med Rehabil.* 2005;86(8):1681–1692.
4. Lincoln NB, Majid MJ, Weyman N. Cognitive rehabilitation for attention deficits following stroke. *Cochrane Database Syst Rev.* 2000;4:CD002842.

5. Riccio CA, French CL. The status of empirical support for treatments of attention deficits. *Clin Neuropsychol.* 2004;18(4): 528–558.
6. Michel JA, Mateer CA. Attention rehabilitation following stroke and traumatic brain injury. A review. *Eura Medicophys.* 2006;[Epub ahead of print].
7. Biederman J, Spencer T, Wilens T. Evidence-based pharmacotherapy for attention-deficit hyperactivity disorder. *Int J Neuropsychopharmacol.* 2004;7(1):77–97.
8. Jadad AR, Boyble M, Cunningham C, et al. Treatment of attention-deficit/hyperactivity disorder. *Evid Rep Technol Assess (Summ).* 1999;11:i–viii, 1–341.
9. Whyte J, Vaccaro M, Grieb-Neff P, et al. Psychostimulant use in the rehabilitation of individuals with traumatic brain injury. *J Head Trauma Rehabil.* 2002;17(4):284–299.
10. Arciniegas DB, Silver JM. Pharmacotherapy of posttraumatic cognitive impairments. *Behav Neurol.* 2006;17(1,2):76–119.
11. Greene YM, Tariot PN, Wishart H, et al. A 12-week, open trial of donepezil hydrochloride in patients with multiple sclerosis and associated cognitive impairments. *J Clin Psychopharmacol.* 2000;20(3):350–356.

VII. MEMORY IMPAIRMENT

A. **Clinical background**

1. **Occurrence and prevalence.** Impairments of working, declarative, and procedural memory are common cognitive manifestations of many neurologic and neuropsychiatric conditions. Declarative memory impairment is, among these, the most common reason for neuropsychiatric evaluation and treatment. In most cases, this and other memory impairments are comorbid with other cognitive and neurobehavioral problems. Alcohol amnestic disorder (also known as *Korsakoff syndrome* or *Korsakoff psychosis*), transient global amnesia (TGA), and MCI are the most common causes of isolated impairment of declarative memory. Memory impairment may develop as a complication of electroconvulsive therapy (ECT). Amnesia may also be a feature of some seizures (i.e., complex partial or generalized seizures), severe alcohol intoxication ("alcoholic blackouts"), and a consequence of a variety of nutritional, metabolic, endocrine, and toxic conditions.

2. **Phenomenology.** In clinical practice, impairment of declarative memory is the most commonly recognized form of memory dysfunction. As described earlier, declarative memory refers to new learning (encoding) and retrieval of both semantic (conceptual) and episodic (autobiographic or event-related) information. Working memory describes the process of keeping information in mind or "on-line" for short-term use in processing additional information, and overlaps with immediate memory and sustained attention. When present, impaired working memory may contribute to impairment in new learning and retrieval.

Impaired learning reflects an inability to encode new information. In some contexts, and particularly in the setting of traumatic and hypoxic-ischemic brain injuries, this form of memory impairment is described as *anterograde amnesia*. Patients with severe "pure" forms of this problem are unable to learn new information subsequent to the onset of their condition (e.g., memory stimuli, facts about their injuries, current time, and location, etc.), but are able to retrieve previously learned information (e.g., name, date of birth, or major life events, etc.). Individuals with severe anterograde amnesia sometimes demonstrate *confabulation*, the unconscious filling of gaps in their memory that is accepted by the individual as fact. Confabulated information is usually not stable over time (often a period as short as a few minutes). The variable nature of confabulations distinguishes them from *delusions*, which denote fixed (i.e., sustained and unchanging) false beliefs. More commonly, patients with anterograde amnesia demonstrate partial impairment of their ability to learn new information; some items are learned, some are not. Information with higher emotional valence tend to be preferentially encoded for later retrieval.

Retrograde amnesia denotes impaired ability to retrieve previously learned information. Patients with isolated retrograde amnesia are unable to retrieve previously learned information, often including autobiographic data, but retain the ability to learn new information. Although there are a small number of case reports describing isolated retrograde amnesia in the setting of traumatic and vascular brain injuries, this is a rare occurrence. When isolated retrograde amnesia occurs, it generally involves loss of the ability to retrieve specific autobiographic (episodic) rather than conceptual (semantic) information. Isolated retrograde amnesia is a relatively common manifestation of conversion (psychogenic) memory disorders and psychogenic fugue states. In clinical practice, retrograde amnesia is usually accompanied by anterograde amnesia, with the latter generally being more severe than the former.

Impairments of procedural memory manifest as difficulty learning new perceptual-motor tasks and performing those tasks once learned. Procedural memory impairments may be difficult to distinguish from apraxia; formal neuropsychologic assessment is often needed to make this distinction.

It is important to note that declarative memory and procedural memory are distinct and dissociable. Many patients with impaired declarative memory retain relatively normal procedural memory; the preservation of the latter carries implications for rehabilitation efforts designed to help patients compensate for impaired declarative learning and retrieval.

3. **Course and prognosis.** Memory impairments may be transient and reversible manifestations of some conditions (e.g., mild TBI, TGA, alcoholic blackouts, or ECT), static problems in

other conditions (e.g., severe traumatic or hypoxic-ischemic brain injuries), or progressive impairments in still others (e.g., MCI, or Alzheimer disease, etc.). Accordingly, the course and prognosis of such impairments varies with the underlying condition. It is important to note, however, that the development of anterograde amnesia precludes the formation of declarative memories during the time in which the condition is present. As such, patients with anterograde amnesia following traumatic, hypoxic-ischemic, alcoholic, or other acute neurologic events should not expect to fully recover memory for information presented during the period of anterograde amnesia. Offering patients an explanation of this phenomenon may alleviate the anxiety that awareness of a gap in memory may produce in some of these individuals.

B. **Neuropathogenesis.** Memory impairment may result from injury to or degeneration of the cortical, subcortical, and white matter elements of the networks that serve the various aspects of memory. The specific location of injury gives information on the type of memory impairment it produces. For example, injury to the entorhinal-hippocampal formation, fornix, mamillary bodies, and anterior/dorsomedial thalamus produces impairments in new learning. Although susceptible to damage from a large number of conditions, these structures are particularly susceptible to the effects of hypoxic-ischemic, hypoglycemic, or metabolic injury (i.e., CA1 region of the hippocampus), increased glucose metabolism in the setting of thiamine deficiency (i.e., mamillary bodies and thalamus), trauma (i.e., hippocampus and fornix), and Alzheimer disease (i.e., entorhinal-hippocampal formation). By contrast, injury to the frontal-subcortical systems is more often associated with difficulty retrieving recently learned information. Consistent with this anatomy, TBI, cerebrovascular disease, multiple sclerosis, HIV/AIDS, and other conditions that impair the structure or function of frontal-subcortical circuits are among the more common causes of impaired memory retrieval. Conditions with a predilection for damaging subcortical structures involved in perceptual-motor processing (e.g., Parkinson disease, or Huntington disease) are among the more common causes of impaired procedural memory.

Acute excesses of glutamate produce a series of excitotoxic events (i.e., increases in intracellular calcium and activation of second messenger systems) that damage entorhinal and hippocampal areas involved in memory. Such excesses are common in the setting of traumatic, vascular, and hypoxic-ischemic brain injuries. Excitotoxic injury thereby contributes to the development of declarative memory impairments in these conditions. Persistent neurochemical dysfunction in these and other structures required for declarative memory, including alterations in glutamatergic function and cholinergic function, also contribute to declarative memory impairments. Deficits in cholinergic function are particularly common contributors to such problems, and are believed to contribute to the declarative memory impairments observed among individuals with Alzheimer disease, vascular dementia, TBI, and possibly alcohol amnestic disorder. Deficient or excessive catecholaminergic function in frontal-subcortical systems may also contribute to impairments in the frontally mediated aspects of memory, including working memory, retrieval of declarative information, and procedural memory.

C. **Diagnosis.** Diagnosis requires first a careful description of the symptom of concern. Some individuals and their caregivers will use the phrase "memory problems" to describe impairments that are more accurately understood as difficulties with attention, language (i.e., word-finding problems or semantic impairments), recognition (agnosia), praxis, visuospatial function (i.e., "getting lost" due to visuospatially mediated difficulties navigating in their environment), and executive function. Thereafter, history should seek to identify the onset, course, and possible etiology of the memory impairment.

Physician evaluations of memory generally make use of one or more bedside assessments. The MMSE is particularly useful for such evaluations given the relatively high number of items that assess memory (three for registration, three for recall, five for temporal orientation, and five for geographic location). Screening for memory impairment with this measure is best made using the prompt for new learning originally described:[1] "I am going to test your memory. Please repeat these three items (e.g., apple, table, or penny)." Note that the patient is *not* prompted to remember the items for later recall; instead, recall after a short delay (no more than 5 minutes) without cued rehearsal is assessed. If patients are unable to remember the items, then semantic or recognition cues may be provided to determine whether recall can be facilitated. Inability to recall items even with cues suggests impairment in new learning; facilitation of recall by cues suggests a retrieval deficit. Although only non-cued recall contributes to MMSE score, performance on new learning and retrieval tasks may help the clinician understand the anatomy of the patient's memory impairments and develop an appropriate differential diagnosis. When this screening assessment is insufficient for the identification and characterization of the patient's memory difficulties, formal neuropsychological testing is recommended. Following the other diagnostic principles described in the preceding section of this chapter is also important.

D. **Treatment**
   1. **Optimize the physical health.** Maximizing treatment of underlying neurologic, psychiatric, medical, or substance conditions is a prerequisite to the prescription of treatments (nonpharmacologic and somatic) for memory impairments.
   2. **Optimize the patient's environment and lifestyle.** Addressing environmental factors that exacerbate or maintain memory problems is essential. Identifying and minimizing potential sources of overstimulation and/or distraction may permit patients with such problems to make the most effective use of their abilities. Providing adequate time for completion of required tasks may allow individuals whose "memory" problems actually reflect impairments of processing speed to perform more accurately

and effectively on such tasks. Because such problems may reflect aberrant (excessive) allocation of processing resources in the service of normal or near-normal performance, individuals with impairments of working memory may fatigue quickly after sustained mental effort.[2] Encouraging rehearsal of new information and also providing environmental cues, whether written or verbal, to facilitate retrieval of information may limit the functional consequences of memory impairments. Encouraging adequate rest and recovery after periods of intense or sustained mental effort may permit patients to maximize their functional abilities.

3. **Nonpharmacologic interventions.** The use of nonpharmacologic interventions is a required component of the treatment of memory impairment. Use of memory books, other memory prosthetics, and technologies that assist with cued retrieval of information may be useful.[3,4] Two systematic reviews of the cognitive rehabilitation literature suggest that mild memory impairments experienced by individuals with traumatic brain injuries and stroke may be amenable to treatment with strategy-training exercises. Although other reviews reach more equivocal conclusions regarding the use of such interventions,[5] our experience suggests that these interventions may be useful in highly-motivated patients with relatively mild impairments, particularly when tailored to generalize from the office to real-world contexts. We recommend use of individually tailored and functionally adaptive memory training and compensatory strategies, and usually refer patients with memory impairments to a therapist with experience in their selection and administration.

4. **Pharmacotherapy.** There are no FDA-approved treatments for memory impairments. Although several agents (i.e., donepezil, rivastigmine, galantamine, memantine) are indicated for the treatment of dementia due to Alzheimer disease, the FDA indications for the use of these agents does not extend to memory specifically. The neurochemistry of memory predicts that augmentation of cholinergic, stabilization of glutamatergic, and possibly augmentation of catecholaminergic function may be useful targets for the treatment of memory impairments. Multiple case reports, open-label trials, and small-scale, double-blind, placebo-controlled trials of cholinesterase inhibitors suggest that these agents may be safe and effective for the treatment of impairments in new learning and retrieval across many neurologic conditions.[6]

When working memory impairments are the focus of clinical concern, catecholaminergic augmentation may improve working memory impairments.[2,7] Methylphenidate is the most commonly prescribed agent for this purpose; recommendations for the use of this agent are described in the section on the pharmacologic treatment of attention and processing speed impairments (see preceding text).

We recommend donepezil as a first-line agent for the treatment of declarative memory impairment due to a neurologic condition. This agent may also be useful for the treatment of working memory impairments.[7] Donepezil increases the availability of cerebral acetylcholine by inhibiting the enzyme (acetylcholinesterase) that metabolizes this neurotransmitter. Treatment with this agent begins with 5 mg daily. If this dose is tolerated but does not produce improvements in memory after approximately 4 weeks of treatment, titration to 10 mg daily is generally undertaken. Slower dose titration may limit the development of treatment-emergent side effects that are gastrointestinal in nature.

We regard rivastigmine and galantamine as second-line agents for the treatment of memory impairments due to a neurologic condition. These agents have shorter half-lives and require twice daily dosing. Rivastigmine is generally started at 1.5 mg b.i.d. and increased in 1.5 mg b.i.d. increments every 4 weeks until maximal benefits are attained or treatment intolerance develops. Galantamine is generally started at 4 mg b.i.d. and increased in 4 mg b.i.d. increments until maximal benefits are attained or treatment intolerance develops; if the extended-release form of galantamine is used, treatment begins with 8 mg daily and is titrated in 8 mg daily increments until maximal benefits are attained or treatment intolerance develops. The side effects and cautions regarding the use of this class of medication are as described for the treatment of attention and processing speed impairments (see preceding text).

When cholinesterase inhibitors confer only a partial or no treatment response, we generally attempt to augment these agents using memantine. When cholinesterase inhibitors are not tolerated or contraindicated, we recommend an empiric trial of memantine alone. Memantine is an uncompetitive NMDA receptor antagonist that may secondarily improve dopaminergic function in frontal-subcortical circuits. Treatment with memantine begins with 5 mg daily, and is increased by 5 mg daily at intervals of 1 week until a dose of 10 mg twice daily is reached or treatment intolerance emerges. Memantine is generally well tolerated, although confusion may develop during treatment initiation or dose titration. Temporary dose reduction may mitigate this adverse effect of treatment. Drug–drug interactions are few, but vigilance for their development is recommended.

Among patients who are unwilling to use any of these agents, some may use and benefit from CDP-choline up to 1 mg orally per day.[8] Because the FDA does not regulate the manufacturing of CDP-choline, and because the safety profile of this agent is incompletely characterized, we do not recommend use of this agent. Nonetheless, CDP-choline remains a treatment option among individuals for whom no other pharmacologic interventions for memory impairment are useful or tolerated.

References

1. Folstein MD, Folstein SE, McHugh PR. "Mini-mental state." A practical method for grading the cognitive state of patients for the clinician. *J Psychiatr Res*. 1975;12(3):189–198.

2. McAllister TW, Flashman LA, Sparling MB, et al. Working memory deficits after traumatic brain injury: Catecholaminergic mechanisms and prospects for treatment—a review. *Brain Inj.* 2004;18(4):331–350.
3. Cicerone KD, Dahlberg C, Kalmar K, et al. Evidence-based cognitive rehabilitation: Recommendations for clinical practice. *Arch Phys Med Rehabil.* 2000;81(12):1596–1615.
4. Cicerone KD, Dahlberg C, Malec JF, et al. Evidence-based cognitive rehabilitation: Updated review of the literature from 1998 through 2002. *Arch Phys Med Rehabil.* 2005;86(8):1681–1692.
5. Majid MJ, Lincoln NB, Weyman N. Cognitive rehabilitation for memory deficits following stroke. *Cochrane Database Syst Rev.* 2000;3:CD002293.
6. Devi G, Silver J. Approaches to memory loss in neuropsychiatric disorders. *Semin Clin Neuropsychiatry.* 2000;5(4):259–265.
7. Barch DM. Pharmacologic manipulation of human working memory. *Psychopharmacology (Berl).* 2004;174(1):126–135.
8. Fioravanti M, Yanagi M. Cytidinediphosphocholine (CDP-choline) for cognitive and behavioural disturbances associated with chronic cerebral disorders in the elderly. *Cochrane Database Syst Rev.* 2005;2:CD000269.

VIII. LANGUAGE IMPAIRMENTS

A. **Clinical background**
   1. **Occurrence and prevalence.** *Aphasia* (from Greek, *a*- "without" + *phasis* "utterance") is seen in conditions that produce dysfunction in the neural networks of the dominant (in most cases) hemisphere serving language. *Aprosodia* (from Latin, *a*- "without" + *pros*- "to" + *oide* "song, poem") is seen in conditions that produce dysfunction within the neural networks of the nondominant (in most cases) hemisphere serving language. Although the frequency of aphasia is not well established, approximately one in three stroke survivors will develop aphasia.[1,2] The frequency of aprosodia in this and other contexts is less well established. Subtle functional communication impairments, including mild word-finding and naming problems, are also manifestations of many neuropsychiatric disorders.
   2. **Phenomenology.** Disturbances of the syntax and semantics of language are described as *aphasias*, and may involve impairment in any of the four primary domains of language (fluency, repetition, comprehension, and naming). The clinical features and classification of the aphasias are described in Table 3.1.

   Impairment of cortically based, sensory domain-specific stimulus recognition (*agnosia*) is distinguished from naming impairment (*anomia*) by demonstrating that presentation of the stimulus in a different sensory modality permits naming of that stimulus. Individuals with anomia fail to name the stimulus regardless of the sensory modality in which it is presented.

   The development of nonfluent aphasia is often associated with depression. Whether depression in this context is a psychological reaction to impaired communication ability, a reflection of a

TABLE 3.1   Classification of Aphasias

Aphasia	Fluency	Repetition	Comprehension	Naming
Global	−	−	−	−
Broca	−	−	+	−
Transcortical motor	−	+	+	−
Conduction	+	−	+	−
Wernicke	+	−	−	−
Transcortical sensory	+	+	−	−
Mixed transcortical	−	+	−	−
Anomic	+	+	+	−

+ indicates that the function is relatively intact; − indicates that the function is impaired, although the degree of impairment may vary from mild (as in the transcortical and anomic aphasias) to severe (as in Broca and Wernicke aphasia).

shared neurobiologic underpinning (i.e., left frontal stroke), or both, is a matter of controversy.

Nonfluent aphasias (and particularly Wernicke aphasia) are sometimes associated with paranoia or frank psychosis. Again, the relative contributions of psychological reaction to impaired understanding of the environment, neuroanatomic areas associated with psychosis in other conditions (i.e., planum temporale), or both, remains uncertain.

Impairments of the affective and kinesic aspects of language production are described as *nonfluent aprosodias*, and manifest as flat or monotonous expressions that fail to communicate emotional relevance and subtlety. Impairments of the ability to appreciate the affective and kinesic aspects of the communications of others are described as *prosodic comprehension impairments*. Inability to repeat phrases using the same affective and kinesic import with which they are expressed describes *conduction aprosodia*.

Although nonfluent aphasia is associated with depression, nonfluent aprosodia may be confused with depression: The relative paucity of affective import and gesturing during communication may be mistaken for the monotonous speech and psychomotor deficits of depression.

3. **Course and prognosis.** The course and prognosis of aphasia is highly variable, and appears to be influenced strongly by lesion type and location, age, education, and handedness, among other variables.[3] In general, patients with aphasia due to cortical injuries tend to recover less fully than patients with aphasia following white matter or subcortical injuries. Advanced age, lower premorbid educational levels, strongly lateralized language function, and associated neurologic comorbidities (e.g., hemiplegia, or visual field defects) appear to negatively influence recovery from aphasia.

Spontaneous recovery from aphasia tends to be greatest during the first 3 months after onset, with most additional spontaneous recovery occurring over the next 3 months. Without treatment, the prognosis for spontaneous recovery of aphasia thereafter is poor. The functional consequences of aphasia are considerable, and persistent language dysfunction contributes substantially to reduced quality of life.[4]

The course and prognosis for recovery from aprosodia is not well defined.

B. **Neuropathogenesis.** In most individuals, including left-handed individuals, the syntax and semantics of language are functions of the dominant hemisphere. By contrast, prosody is, in most individuals, a function of the nondominant hemisphere. Aphasia and aprosodia reflect injury to or dysfunction of the cortical, white matter, or subcortical elements (alone or in combination) of the networks serving language. Vascular injury (e.g., stroke in any of its forms) is by far the most common cause of aphasia and aprosodia, although traumatic, neoplastic, infectious (and especially type I herpes simplex virus), and other causes are described.

The neurochemistry of language has not been described fully. However, pharmacologic interventions studies (see subsequent text) suggest that catecholaminergic and cholinergic systems are likely to play a critical role in this domain of cognition.

C. **Diagnosis.** The assessment of individuals with aphasia entails testing of each of the major domains of language (fluency, repetition, comprehension, and naming). This assessment should include testing of both verbal and written (reading and writing) communication. Among individuals whose primary means of communication is International Sign Language or Braille, assessment of communication by these means is essential. Additionally, assessment of motor (i.e., limb, and buccofacial) and sensory (i.e., visual, auditory, and tactile) function must discriminate between aphasia and *aphemia* (impaired motor output required for speech usually manifest as *mutism* without other evidence of aphasia); *verbal (speech) apraxia*, impaired sequencing of motor output required for verbal communication; *agraphia*, impaired writing ability without impaired verbal ability; *dysarthria*, weakness of the muscles required for speech; *dysphonia*, weakness of the laryngeal muscles required for phonation; *pure-word deafness*, an auditory agnosia for words in the setting of normal hearing and comprehension of non-language sounds; *visual agnosia for words*, an impaired ability to recognize written words (often accompanied by agnosia for faces) despite intact verbal comprehension; *alexia*, inability to read without impaired verbal comprehension; and other motor and sensory impairments that may interfere with communication.

The MMSE is often used as a screening assessment for aphasia. It contains several items assessing language, including repetition ("no ifs, ands, or buts"), naming ("pen," "watch"), and comprehension (3-step command). The latter item is understood more accurately as an assessment for ideational praxis; failure to perform correctly the 3-step item on the MMSE requires the clinician to "dissect" this problem to determine whether it reflects an impairment of ideational praxis, ideomotor apraxia for one of the elements of this task, language comprehension difficulties, impairments of working memory or attention, or other sensorimotor impairments.

A more careful bedside assessment of language among individuals suspected of suffering from aphasia is recommended. This assessment should include: Fluency, including phrase length, word finding, grammatical structure; repetition of agrammatical, simple, and complex statements; comprehension of yes/no, true/false, and short-story questions; and naming of objects and parts of objects. Evaluation by a speech-language pathologist or neuropsychologist is often helpful for this purpose, and may assist in the characterization of the type and severity of aphasia and also in the development of a language rehabilitation plan.

Assessment of prosody parallels the assessment of aphasia: Prosodic fluency, repetition, and comprehension is required. For this purpose, we often use variations of the phrase "He is going to sing." For example, "*He* is going to sing?" communicates surprise that it is this individual, among others, who will be singing; "He is *going* to sing?" communicates surprise that this individual will be singing in the future; and "He is going to *sing*?" communicates surprise that what this individual will be doing is singing (as opposed to speaking, for example). We usually begin by asking the patient to repeat each variation of the phrase used so as to reproduce exactly the manner in which it is stated by the examiner. The patient is then asked to interpret the meaning of each variation of the phrase as stated by the examiner. Finally, the examiner asks the patient to state each phrase so as to communicate the meaning specified by the examiner. Referral to a speech-language pathologist or neuropsychologist for more detailed and formal assessment of aprosodia may be of diagnostic value and also useful for treatment planning.

D. **Treatment**
   1. **Optimize the physical health.** Maximizing treatment of underlying neurologic, psychiatric, or general medical conditions is a prerequisite to the prescription of treatments (nonpharmacologic and somatic) for language impairments.
   2. **Optimize the patient's environment and lifestyle.** As described earlier in this chapter, addressing environmental factors that exacerbate or maintain language problems is essential. Identifying and minimizing potential sources of overstimulation and distraction may permit patients with such problems to make the most effective use of their abilities. Providing adequate time for completion of required tasks may allow individuals with word-finding difficulties to communicate more accurately and independently. Interacting with an individual with aphasia should allow the patient to attempt to communicate independently to the greatest extent possible; this approach, sometimes structured as a "constraint-induced" therapy for aphasia, may

facilitate recovery of functional language abilities and reduce the aphasic patient's feelings of frustration and inadequacy.[5] Using direct, simple, and concrete communication with the patient, and encouraging the same of the patient, may also facilitate functional adaptation despite persistent aphasia. Augmenting verbal communication with pointing (whether to real objects, pictures, or items on a communication board) may also be useful. Encouraging both the patient and individuals interacting with the patient to state their intended meaning (rather than using prosody to create meaning and nuance in those communications) may allow patients to understand others and to be understood by others correctly despite persistent aprosodia. Encouraging adequate rest and recovery after periods of intense or sustained mental effort also permits patients to maximize their functional abilities.

3. **Nonpharmacologic interventions.** The use of nonpharmacologic interventions is a requisite component of the treatment of language impairments. Cicerone et al.,[6,7] based on two systematic reviews of the cognitive rehabilitation literature, strongly recommend the use of nonpharmacologic interventions for the treatment of aphasia, aprosodia, and non-aphasic functional communication impairments experienced by individuals with traumatic brain injuries and stroke. We concur with this recommendation, and routinely refer patients to a speech therapist with experience in their selection and administration.

    Cognitive rehabilitation of aphasia combined with administration of piracetam[8] or bromocriptine[9] improves aphasia outcome, even in the late period after onset, when compared with cognitive rehabilitation combined with placebo. Although piracetam is not available in the United States, we often combine speech-language therapies with other pharmacologic interventions (described in the subsequent text). Although our experience can only be regarded as anecdotal, we have observed similar superiority to this combined-treatment approach during the acute rehabilitation of individuals with aphasia due to stroke or TBI. Accordingly, we recommend use of a combined cognitive rehabilitation-pharmacotherapy approach.

    There is emerging evidence that slow frequency (1 Hz) repetitive transcranial magnetic stimulation applied to the nondominant posterior pars triangularis (a portion of the nondominant homolog of Broca area) may improve nonfluent aphasia.[10] Although it is premature to recommend the use of this treatment in routine clinical practice, we strongly encourage clinicians to remain apprised of the evidence regarding this intervention and to consider its use pending the availability of additional information describing its safety and efficacy.

4. **Pharmacotherapy.** There are no FDA-approved treatments for aphasia, and the literature describing pharmacotherapy for aphasia is limited to several small-scale, open-label studies describing various dopaminergic augmentation or donepezil.[1] The *a priori*

rationale for the use of these agents is limited, but includes: (a) The possibility that pharmacologically mediated improvements in motor function, attention, speed of processing, and memory may facilitate recovery of language skills; and (b) laboratory and clinical evidence suggesting that such agents may partially restore metabolic function in the areas damaged by stroke, trauma, and other conditions that produce aphasia. However, clinicians are encouraged to remain mindful of the fact that the efficacy and safety of pharmacologic treatments of aphasia are not well established.

In light of evidence that methylphenidate may also facilitate recovery of motor impairments and emotional disturbances following a stroke,[11] this agent is our first-line choice when a pharmacologic treatment of aphasia (alone or in combination with cognitive rehabilitation) is undertaken. Treatment is generally initiated at 5 mg twice daily, a titrated to a target dose of 0.15-0.3 mg/kg b.i.d. in 5 mg b.i.d. increments every 3 to 5 days. When this agent fails to afford improvements in aphasia at maximally tolerated doses, we generally augment methylphenidate with or switch entirely to treatment with donepezil 5 mg daily. If tolerated but not fully effective after 2 to 4 weeks of treatment, the dose of donepezil is increased to 10 mg daily. As suggested in the preceding text, these agents are best provided as adjuncts to cognitive rehabilitation interventions.

It has been suggested that dopaminergic dysfunction may contribute to aprosodia. At present, there is only one report describing improvement in poststroke aprosodia during treatment with the dopamine agonist bromocriptine.[12] Although interesting and encouraging, we recommend the use of nonpharmacologic interventions alone pending additional evidence demonstrating effectiveness of medications for the treatment of aprosodia.

References
1. Berthier ML. Poststroke aphasia: Epidemiology, pathophysiology and treatment. *Drugs Aging.* 2005;22(2):163–182.
2. Bakheit AM. Drug treatment of poststroke aphasia. *Expert Rev Neurother.* 2004;4(2):211–217.
3. Aichner F, Adelwohrer C, Haring HP. Rehabilitation approaches to stroke. *J Neural Transm Suppl.* 2002;63:59–73.
4. Bays CL. Quality of life of stroke survivors: A research synthesis. *J Neurosci Nurs.* 2001;22(6):310–316.
5. Pulvermuller F, Neininger B, Elbert T, et al. Constraint-induced therapy of chronic aphasia after. *Stroke.* 2001;32(7):1621–1626.
6. Cicerone KD, Dahlberg C, Kalmar K, et al. Evidence-based cognitive rehabilitation: Recommendations for clinical practice. *Arch Phys Med Rehabil.* 2000;81(12):1596–1615.
7. Cicerone KD, Dahlberg C, Malec JF, et al. Evidence-based cognitive rehabilitation: Updated review of the literature from 1998 through 2002. *Arch Phys Med Rehabil.* 2005;86(8):1681–1692.
8. Greener J, Enderby P, Whurr R. Pharmacological treatment for aphasia following stroke. *Cochrane Database Syst Rev.* 2001;4: CD000424.

9. Bragoni M, Altieri M, Di Piero V, et al. Bromocriptine and speech therapy in non-fluent chronic aphasia after stroke. *Neurol Sci.* 2000;21(1):19–22.
10. Martin PI, Naeser MA, Theoret H, et al. Transcranial magnetic stimulation as a complementary treatment for aphasia. *Semin Speech Lang.* 2004;25(2):181–191.
11. Grade C, Redford B, Chrostowski J, et al. Methylphenidate in early poststroke recovery: A double-blind, placebo-controlled study. *Arch Phys Med Rehabil.* 1998;79(9):1047–1050.
12. Raymer AM, Bandy D, Adair JC, et al. Effects of bromocriptine in a patient with crossed nonfluent aphasia: A case report. *Arch Phys Med Rehabil.* 2001;82(1):139–144.

IX. AGNOSIA

A. **Clinical background**

1. **Occurrence and prevalence.** The development of agnosia (from Greek, *a-* "without" + *gnosis-* "knowledge") as an isolated cognitive deficit is relatively rare, and is most often a consequence of a stroke. Agnosia is more commonly seen as a feature of dementing illnesses such as Alzheimer disease, dementia with Lewy bodies, frontotemporal dementia, and vascular dementia.

2. **Phenomenology.** Agnosia is characterized by an inability to integrate sensory information at a cortical level regarding objects, people, sounds, shapes, or smells (cortically based perception) and to attach meaning to those percepts (association). *Visual agnosia* is the most common type of agnosia. Individuals with *visual apperceptive agnosia* are unable to recognize the features of visual stimuli. This results in an impaired ability to recognize, discriminate between, and copy visual stimuli. Individuals with *visual associative agnosia* perceive the constituent elements of visual stimuli but are unable to recognize them; in contrast to individuals with visual apperceptive agnosia, they are able to copy visual stimuli. Common forms of visual agnosia include *object agnosia*, an inability to identify objects (that may involve some, but not all, object categories); *form agnosia*, an inability to recognize the whole object due to impaired recognition of one or more of its parts; *shape agnosia*, an inability to recognize the shape of the object despite recognition of its other features (e.g., color, size, etc.); *finger agnosia*, an inability to recognize figures on the hand—sometimes seen in the setting of *Gerstmann syndrome* that also includes *agraphia* (inability to write), *acalculia* (inability to calculate), and *left–right disorientation; mirror agnosia*, an inability to recognize objects or activity in either the left or right field of view; *"pure alexia"* or *alexia without agraphia*, an inability to read despite preserved perception of letters, words, and/or sentences (evidenced by ability to copy the text that they cannot "read"); *color agnosia*, an inability to recognize colors despite the ability to distinguish between colors—this deficit is distinct from *central achromatopsia*, which refers to a cortically based impairment of color perception; *simultanagnosia*, the inability

to synthesize multiple elements in a simultaneously displayed visual presentation into a cohesive whole despite recognition of its constituent elements; and *prosopagnosia*, an inability to recognize familiar faces (sometimes including the patient's own face).

Visual agnosia features prominently in *Bálint syndrome*, an acquired disturbance in the ability to perceive the visual field as a whole resulting from the combination of simultanagnosia, *optic ataxia* (an impairment of visually guided reaching), and *oculomotor apraxia* (an impairment of saccadic initiation). Deficits in face recognition may also contribute to *Capgras syndrome*, a delusional misidentification syndrome where the patient believes that a familiar person has been replaced by an impostor or exact double despite recognition of the familiarity of that person's appearance and behavior.[1] Deficits in face recognition may also be related to impaired social development among patients with Asperger syndrome.[1]

The auditory agnosias involve an inability to recognize auditory stimuli, and include *auditory agnosia*, an inability to recognize environmental sounds (e.g., a dog's bark, a car engine, etc.); *auditory/verbal information agnosia*, also known as *pure-word deafness*, an inability to recognize verbal stimuli in the absence of impaired language comprehension; and *receptive amusia*, an inability to recognize music. Auditory agnosia is distinct from *cortical deafness*, a condition where there is a cortically based failure to perceive auditory stimuli despite intact peripheral hearing.

Tactile agnosia refers to an inability to recognize somatosensory stimuli. Common forms of tactile agnosia include *astereognosia*, an inability to recognize objects by touch; and *agraphesthesia*, an inability to recognize a number or letter written on the skin (usually the palm or first finger).

Olfactory agnosia refers to an inability to recognize stimuli by smell. *Gustatory agnosia* refers to an inability to identify stimuli by taste.

Anosognosia refers to an inability to recognize disease in oneself (from Greek *a-* "without," *nosos-* "disease" and *gnosis-* "knowledge"). Although sometimes used to describe impaired ability to recognize hemiplegia (generally on the left), the term is used more generically in common practice to refer to an unawareness of motor and cognitive deficits as well as a lack of awareness of illness (such as seen commonly among individuals with Alzheimer disease and schizophrenia).

3. **Course and prognosis.** Agnosia may be transient in the setting of mild focal cerebral insults (e.g., a small stroke), static in the setting of more severe focal cerebral insults (e.g., stroke, neoplasm, or traumatic contusion), or progressive (e.g., in neurodegenerative disorders).

B. **Neuropathogenesis.** As suggested in the preceding text, the development of agnosia is predicated on damage to or dysfunction of the posterior cortical white matter, or subcortical structures involved in sensory processing. Visual agnosia reflects impairment of unimodal (isotypic) visual association cortex or the white matter connecting primary visual and unimodal visual association cortex, in the ventral occipitotemporal-processing pathway. In particular, damage to the left ventral occipitotemporal visual processing pathway is associated with visual agnosia, and is often accompanied by a right visual field defect.[2] Prosopagnosia, however, is more commonly associated with bilateral lesions to the gray and/or white matter of the occipitotemporal gyri, and in particular, the inferior longitudinal fasciculus connecting the occipital and temporal cortices. Auditory agnosia reflects the effects of injury to unimodal auditory association cortex or the subcortical white matter connecting primary auditory cortex (*Heschl gyrus*) to unimodal auditory association cortex. Tactile agnosia reflects injury to unimodal sensory association cortex or the white matter connections between primary sensory cortex (*post-central gyrus*) and unimodal sensory association cortex.

C. **Diagnosis.** The identification of agnosia requires specific assessment of sensory function in the domain of impairment as well as the patient's ability to recognize stimuli presented in that domain. To make the diagnosis of agnosia, the clinician must first establish that primary sensory function is intact. Presentation of stimuli in the affected sensory domain (and relevant to the specific agnosia from which the patient is thought to suffer) is required. Visual, tactile, and nonverbal agnosias must also be distinguished from *anomia*; in the former, the patient is unable to identify the object in one sensory domain (e.g., visual), but is able to identify the object when presented in another domain (e.g., tactile, auditory); in the latter, the patient is able to recognize, copy, describe, and/or use the object correctly, but is unable to name it regardless of the manner in which it is presented. Impaired ability to name objects on the MMSE therefore entails clarification of that deficit as either agnosia or anomia. The diagnosis of pure-word deafness requires first identification of the inability to recognize language when presented verbally but preserved language recognition when presented in written form. Formal neuropsychological assessment may be useful for the characterization of the type and severity of agnosia. Identification of preserved recognition abilities through such testing may facilitate the development of compensatory strategies for agnosia.

D. **Treatment**
    1. **Optimize the physical health.** Maximizing treatment of underlying neurologic, psychiatric, or general medical conditions is a prerequisite to the prescription of treatments (nonpharmacologic and somatic) for agnosia.
    2. **Optimize the patient's environment and lifestyle.** Address environmental factors that exacerbate or maintain agnosia. Identifying and minimizing potential sources of overstimulation and/or distraction may permit patients with such problems to make the most effective use of their abilities. Organizing the environment and interactions so as to capitalize on preserved recognition

abilities may allow compensation for impairments. For example, providing tactile and/or auditory cues to individuals with visual agnosias may minimize the functional consequences of that impairment. Encouraging adequate rest and recovery after periods of intense or sustained mental effort also permits patients to maximize their functional abilities.

3. **Nonpharmacologic interventions.** There is limited evidence that nonpharmacologic interventions improve visual agnosia.[3,4] Although the evidence for the benefits of nonpharmacologic treatments of agnosia generally consists of small-scale, noncontrolled studies, the lack of evidence regarding the effectiveness of other therapies leads us to recommend cognitive rehabilitation interventions as the first-line treatments for agnosia. We recommend referral of individuals with agnosia to speech-language and occupational therapists with experience in the use of these interventions.

4. **Pharmacotherapy.** There are no FDA-approved pharmacotherapies for agnosias, and this type of cognitive impairments has not been the subject of pharmacologic treatment trials. Accordingly, we do not recommend any pharmacologic treatments for the agnosias.

References

1. Barton JJ. Disorders of face perception and recognition. *Neurol Clin.* 2003;21(2):521–548.
2. De Renzi E. Disorders of visual recognition. *Semin Neurol.* 2000;20(4):479–485.
3. Behrmann M, Marotta J, Gauthier I, et al. Behavioral change and its neural correlates in visual agnosia after expertise training. *J Cogn Neurosci.* 2005;17(4):554–568.
4. Burns MS. Clinical management of agnosia. *Top Stroke Rehabil.* 2004;11(1):1–9.

X. APRAXIA

A. **Clinical background**

1. **Occurrence and prevalence.** The development of apraxia (from Greek, *a-* "without" + *praxis-* "practice, action, doing") is a common consequence of stroke, severe TBI, and other acute neurologic conditions. Although the frequency of apraxia across all these conditions is not well established, estimates of poststroke apraxia range from 13% to 28%, and are more than twice as common following left-hemisphere than right-hemisphere stroke.[1–3] The development of poststroke apraxia is associated with greater stroke severity,[1,2] and may be more common among stroke survivors of advanced age.[2]

   Among the neurodegenerative and movement disorders, prominent ideomotor apraxia (defined in the subsequent text) is a hallmark feature of corticobasal degeneration, and is a relatively common feature of Alzheimer disease, dementia with Lewy bodies, Parkinson disease, frontotemporal dementia, and progressive supranuclear palsy.

Apraxia may also occur in a developmental form (i.e., *developmental apraxia*) in which it is present from birth and becomes evident as children fail to reach normal motor and/or speech milestones. This is a relatively rare disorder, not clearly associated with specific brain lesions, and its frequency is not well established.

2. **Phenomenology.** Apraxia refers to the inability to execute skilled purposeful movements on demand that cannot be attributed to basic sensory, language, or motor disturbances. Praxis requires the ability to integrate understanding of the requested task with the motor functions necessary for its execution. Apraxia may affect axial (buccofacial, truncal) movements, limb, and/or whole body movements.

Apraxia is most often classified into three types: *Limb-kinetic* (or *melokinetic*), *ideomotor*, and *ideational*. *Limb-kinetic apraxia* describes the inability to make finely graded, precise, individual finger movements on demand, leading to awkward and inaccurate finger movements. *Ideomotor apraxia* refers to the inability to perform gestural (pantomime) movements to verbal command despite preservation of the same movement in a naturalistic setting. This impairment may affect not only pantomime command but also spontaneous environmentally relevant movements. Ideomotor apraxia frequently involves both axial and limb movements. *Ideational apraxia* refers to the inability to carry out a complex sequence of movements despite preserved ability to correctly execute the individual components of that sequence. Ideational apraxia is most often seen in the setting of acute confusional states, dementias, and other disorders affecting frontal-subcortical function; these observations suggest that ideational apraxia overlaps conceptually and clinically with executive function and/or attention.[4]

Specific forms of apraxia include *oculomotor apraxia*, an impairment of saccadic initiation; *apraxia of eyelid opening*, an inability to initiate eyelid elevation in the absence of weakness of eyelid musculature; *buccofacial (orofacial) apraxia*, and inability to perform facial movements on command (e.g., winking, whistling, or blowing out a match) despite normal orofacial strength; *oral apraxia*, which overlaps conceptually and clinically with buccofacial apraxia, but is used to describe specifically an impairment of the ability to move the muscles of the mouth (i.e., lips, tongue) for non-speech purposes despite normal oral motor strength; *apraxia of speech*, a motor speech impairment in the absence of aphasia or dysarthria, the most severe form of which is *aphemia* (inability to articulate words despite normal language function); *swallowing (oropharyngeal) apraxia*, an inability to coordinate lingual, labial, and mandibular movements in the service of swallowing in the absence of muscular weakness in these areas; *limb apraxia*, which is generally used as a synonym for ideomotor apraxia affecting a limb (usually an arm); *apractic agraphia*, an impairment in writing letters and words despite normal sensorimotor function, visual feedback, and word and letter knowledge; *axial apraxia*, an impairment of axial rotation in the horizontal plane despite otherwise normal axial motor function; and *gait apraxia*, an inability to lift the feet from the floor despite preservation of alternating stepping action, often described as a "magnetic" gait. Two additional forms of apraxia are noteworthy: *Sympathetic apraxia*, an impairment of praxis on the nondominant body side among individuals with hemiparesis of the dominant body side; and *callosal apraxia*, an impairment of praxis on the nondominant body side despite normal praxis on the dominant body side resulting from injury to or infarction of the anterior portion of the corpus callosum.

Although impaired constructional ability and impaired ability to dress oneself are sometimes referred to as apraxias (i.e., *constructional apraxia* and *dressing apraxia*, respectively), these impairments are better regarded as manifestations of impaired visuospatial function (see subsequent text).

3. **Course and prognosis.** The course and prognosis of apraxia is highly variable: Apraxia may be transient and reversible manifestations of some conditions (e.g., mild stroke or TBI), a static problem in other contexts (e.g., developmental apraxia, severe stroke, or TBI), or progressive impairments in still others (e.g., neurodegenerative dementias). When apraxia develops outside the context of neurodegenerative and neurodevelopmental disorders, recovery, and functional outcome are influenced strongly by lesion type and location, age, education, and handedness, among other variables. In general, patients with apraxia due to cortical injuries tend to recover less fully than patients with apraxia following white matter or subcortical injuries.

Zwinkels et al.[3] observed significant correlations between apraxia and aphasia, impairments of visuospatial scanning, memory, attention, and executive function. Patients with apraxia perform significantly worse than the patients without apraxia on memory tasks, and require longer period of time to complete visuospatial scanning, attention, and language tasks. Accordingly, the presence of apraxia may adversely affect a broad range of other cognitive functions and contribute to functional disability.[5]

B. **Neuropathogenesis.** Given the variety of contexts where apraxia may develop, it is not surprising that multiple lesion locations (cortical, white matter, and subcortical; anterior and posterior) and types (e.g., vascular, traumatic, neoplastic, infections, neurodegenerative, etc.) may produce apraxia. However, praxis is generally regarded as a function of the dominant hemisphere, and the neuroanatomic substrates of praxis are located proximate to those serving the syntax and semantics of language. Limb-kinetic (melokinetic) apraxia is most commonly associated with lesions of the corticospinal tract contralateral to the affected hand; this observation has prompted suggestions that this form of apraxia may be more accurately understood as an elementary motor deficit rather than as a true apraxia. Leiguarda[6] suggests that the core deficit in ideomotor apraxia may be a deficit of movement representations encoded in the dominant hemisphere, possibly in premotor association areas; this might explain the common co-occurrence of ideomotor apraxia and nonfluent aphasia. By contrast, the core deficit in ideational apraxia is deficit in semantic knowledge for action, possibly encoded in a frontoparietal network subserving motor sequencing.

C. **Diagnosis.** The identification of limb-kinetic and ideomotor apraxia is predicated on assessment of motor function in the apraxic body area and also on comprehension of language, both of which must be intact to establish the presence of these apraxias. Testing for limb-kinetic apraxia involves commands requiring finely graded finger movements to command (e.g., "show me how you button a shirt; thread a needle; etc."). Testing for ideomotor apraxia involves commands requiring axial, limb, and whole body movements, because impairments may be present in only one of these areas. Pantomiming movement to command (e.g., "show me how you blow out a match; unscrew the lid of a jar; brush your hair; or take the stance of a boxer; etc.") is the most common manner of testing for ideomotor apraxia.

Ideational praxis requires intact motor function, language comprehension, as well as attention, working memory, and executive function. Accordingly, the identification of ideational apraxia requires concurrent assessment of these functions as well as performance of complex sequences on command. The 3-step command on the MMSE (i.e., "take this piece of paper in your hand, fold it in half, and place it on the table") is a test of ideational praxis. In clinical practice, it may be difficult to discriminate between ideational apraxia, memory or comprehension deficits, and the motor sequencing function commonly ascribed to executive function.

Several bedside assessments of praxis are available.[3,7] Although potentially useful, it is not clear that these assessments afford better sensitivity or specificity for apraxia than does a well-informed and thorough neurobehavioral assessment. When apraxia is identified at the bedside, formal assessment by a speech-language pathologist, occupational therapist, or neuropsychologist may be very useful for the identification of the type and severity of apraxia, and is required for the development of an adequate treatment plan for this problem.

D. **Treatment**
   1. **Optimize the physical health.** Maximizing treatment of underlying neurologic, psychiatric, or general medical conditions is a prerequisite to the prescription of treatments (nonpharmacologic and somatic) for apraxia.
   2. **Optimize the patient's environment and lifestyle.** Addressing environmental factors that exacerbate or maintain apraxia is essential. Identifying and minimizing potential sources of overstimulation and/or distraction may permit patients with such problems to make the most effective use of their abilities. Providing adequate time for completion of required tasks may allow individuals with mild apraxia to perform accurately and relatively independently. Modifying task demands by setting up items of a task (e.g., for hygiene, cooking, eating, transfers,

etc.) or modifying the need for such tasks (e.g., cutting hair short so as to obviate the need for its brushing; microwave use in lieu of stove-top cooking; etc.) may allow individuals with apraxia to maximize their functional independence. Keeping directions for tasks direct, simple, and concrete is essential for the success of such environmental and lifestyle adaptations. Encouraging adequate rest and recovery after periods of intense or sustained mental effort also permits patients to maximize their functional abilities.

3. **Nonpharmacologic interventions.** Three evidence-based reviews of cognitive rehabilitation suggest that compensatory strategy training is an effective treatment for apraxia following stroke and TBI.[8-10] Although the literature describing the effectiveness of compensatory strategy training for apraxia generally consists of small-scale, uncontrolled treatment trials, the lack of clearly effective pharmacologic treatments for apraxia lead us to conclude that compensatory strategy training should be regarded as the first-line treatment for this cognitive impairment. We recommend that patients with apraxia be referred for treatment to a speech-language pathologist, occupational therapist, or neuropsychologist experienced in the use of compensatory strategy training for apraxia.

4. **Pharmacotherapy.** There are no FDA-approved treatments for apraxia, and there is no established pharmacotherapy for apraxia when it occurs as an isolated cognitive impairment. Although several case reports suggest that dopaminergically active agents (i.e., amantadine, carbidopa/levodopa, and methylphenidate) may be useful for the treatment of apraxia, the literature is not sufficiently developed for us to recommend pharmacotherapy for apraxia.

References

1. Donkervoort M, Dekker J, van den Ende E, et al. Prevalence of apraxia among patients with a first left hemisphere stroke in rehabilitation centres and nursing homes. *Clin Rehabil.* 2000;14(2):130–136.
2. Pedersen PM, Jorgensen HS, Kammersgaard LP, et al. Manual and oral apraxia in acute stroke, frequency, and influence on functional outcome: The Copenhagen Stroke Study. *Am J Phys Med Rehabil.* 2001;80(9):685–692.
3. Zwinkels A, Geusgens C, van de Sande P, et al. Assessment of apraxia: Inter-rater reliability of a new apraxia test, association between apraxia and other cognitive deficits and prevalence of apraxia in a rehabilitation setting. *Clin Rehabil.* 2004;18(7):819–827.
4. Weintraub S. Neuropsychological assessment of mental state. In: Mesulam M-M, ed. *Principles of behavioral and cognitive neurology,* 2nd ed. Oxford: Oxford University Press; 2000:121–173.
5. Saeki S, Ogata H, Okubo T, et al. Return to work after stroke. A follow-up study. *Stroke.* 1995;26(3):399–401.
6. Leiguarda R. Limb apraxia: Cortical or subcortical. *Neuroimage.* 2001;14(1 Pt 2):S137–S141.

7. Almeida QJ, Black SE, Roy EA. Screening for apraxia: A short assessment for stroke patients. *Brain Cogn.* 2002;48(2–3):253–258.
8. Cicerone KD, Dahlberg C, Kalmar K, et al. Evidence-based cognitive rehabilitation: Recommendations for clinical practice. *Arch Phys Med Rehabil.* 2000;81(12):1596–1615.
9. Cicerone KD, Dahlberg C, Malec JF, et al. Evidence-based cognitive rehabilitation: Updated review of the literature from 1998 through 2002. *Arch Phys Med Rehabil.* 2005;86(8):1681–1692.
10. Cappa SF, Benke T, Clarke S, et al. EFNS guidelines on cognitive rehabilitation: Report of an EFNS Task Force. *Eur J Neurol.* 2005;12(9):665–680.

XI. VISUOSPATIAL DYSFUNCTION

A. **Clinical background**
   1. **Occurrence and prevalence.** Visuospatial function refers to a constellation of complex visual processing abilities, including spatial awareness and attention, awareness of self–other and/or self–object spatial relationships, visuospatial memory, and interpretation of and navigation within the extrapersonal space.

   Impairments of visuospatial function are common consequences of neurologic conditions affecting the nondominant (usually right) hemisphere. Visuospatial dysfunction is also a common feature of neurodegenerative disorders, and particularly those that involve posterior cortical structures (e.g., Alzheimer disease, dementia with Lewy bodies, and corticobasal degeneration, among others). Visuospatial dysfunction is also a prominent feature of the syndrome of posterior cortical atrophy. Despite the high frequency of visuospatial dysfunction across many dementia syndromes (frontotemporal dementia being a notable exception), impairment of this function is not included in the DSM-based diagnosis of dementia.

   2. **Phenomenology.** Visual attention permits awareness of the extrapersonal space as well as the ability to shift the focus of awareness from one extrapersonal event to another. The prototypical impairment of visual attention is *unilateral hemispace neglect.* This impairment refers to an inability to attend to sensory events in one hemispace (usually, but not always, the left hemispace) in the absence of elementary sensorimotor deficits that better account for this impairment. Although visual neglect may be the most obvious manifestation of impaired spatial attention, this impairment is often multimodal: It frequently involves hemi-inattention to auditory, somatosensory, and occasionally olfactory stimuli, and reduces motor exploration of the affected hemispace even on the unaffected side of the body.[1] In severe forms, unilateral neglect may result in complete inattention to the involved hemispace. Patients may shave, groom, and dress only the unaffected side; ignore food, reading material, and individuals in the affected hemispace; orient to the

unaffected hemispace in response to stimuli coming from the affected hemispace; and tonically rotate to the unaffected hemispace when sitting or supine. In more subtle forms, sometimes described as *unilateral hemi-inattention* rather than as neglect, impairments may not be identified easily by observation of spontaneous behavior but only by examination (see subsequent text).

Visuospatial memory impairment, also described as *topographic disorientation*, refers to an acquired inability to learn and/or retrieve information related to spatial relationships between places. For example, patients with impairment of topographic orientation may be unable to locate a building in a city, to describe either verbally or with a map the route from one location to another, or even to find their room at home.

Impairments of constructional ability are sometimes described as "constructional apraxia," but this is a misnomer. Performance on construction tasks (usually a figure copy of some sort) requires normal visual acuity, the ability to perceive the elements of the item to be copied, executive function to organize execution of the task, and the motor abilities to carry out the task. Assuming visual function and motor ability are normal, impaired constructional ability is better understood as a manifestation of spatial inattention (including unilateral neglect), executive dysfunction, or both.

Impairment of dressing ability is sometimes described as "dressing apraxia," but this too is a misnomer. Dressing requires the ability to align the axis of the body and/or limb with the garment to be donned. This requires normal visual acuity, the ability to perceive the elements of the item to be placed on the body, executive function to organize execution of the task, and the motor abilities to carry out the task. Assuming visual function and motor ability are normal, impaired dressing ability is better understood as a manifestation of spatial inattention (including unilateral neglect), executive dysfunction, or both.

3. **Course and prognosis.** The course and prognosis of visuospatial dysfunction is highly variable: Impairment may be transient and reversible manifestations of some conditions (e.g., mild stroke or TBI), a static (e.g., severe stroke or TBI), or progressive impairment (e.g., neurodegenerative dementias, posterior cortical atrophy). Functional outcome is influenced strongly by lesion type and location, age, education, and handedness, among other variables. In general, patients with cortically based visuospatial dysfunction tend to recover less fully than patients whose impairment is due to white matter or subcortical injury or dysfunction.

B. **Neuropathogenesis.** Visuospatial function is predicated on the integrity of a distributed neural network that includes elements of the reticular system, thalamus, superior colliculus, striatum, posterior parietal cortex, frontal eye fields, and parietal cortex. Visuospatial function displays a pattern of marked nondominant (right) hemispheric specialization, and the nondominant (right) parietal cortex appears to be an essential element of the network serving spatial attention and also constructional and dressing abilities. Nonetheless, hemi-inattention is occasionally, and usually transiently, seen following injury to the dominant (left) hemisphere. Impairment of any element of the network serving visuospatial function may produce deficits in this domain.

Visuospatial memory appears to have as a critical element a region of the parahippocampal gyrus known as the *parahippocampal place area* (PPA).[2] The PPA is selectively and automatically responsive to passively viewed scenes and weakly to single objects. The PPA encodes the geometry of the local environment, and thereby permits the development of memory for it (topographic orientation).

Deficits in the availability of acetylcholine and dopamine to the cortical and subcortical elements of the network serving visuospatial function may contribute to impairments in this domain of cognition.

C. **Diagnosis.** The diagnosis of visuospatial dysfunction entails a thorough examination of sensory (and especially vision and tactile) and motor function, attention, memory, language, recognition, praxis, and executive function. Impairment in each domain of neurobehavioral function may contribute to and/or confound the assessment of visuospatial function, and interpretation of performance on tests of visuospatial function must account for these factors.

Observation of the patient may be sufficient to identify unilateral hemispatial neglect. Bedside assessments of spatial attention often employ line bisection (e.g., patient is asked to mark the middle of several lines in different orientations), target cancellation tasks, searching tasks (e.g., finding by palpation a small object placed at various locations on a table), and reading tasks. Patients with severe unilateral hemispatial neglect will often bisect lines "off center" (biased toward the unaffected hemispace), and fail to cancel targets, search for objects, or read text in the affected hemispace. On constructional tasks (i.e., clock drawing, simple and complex figure copy), patients with severe unilateral hemineglect fail to assess material in the affected hemispace and therefore omit it from their drawings; alternatively, and particularly on clock drawing tasks, patients may draw the left hemispace (i.e., left half of the circle and numbers 7–11) up the midline of their drawings. Patients with mild unilateral hemispace neglect (unilateral hemi-inattention) show a similar pattern of impaired performance but of lesser severity. In these patients, assessment for extinction to bilateral simultaneous stimulation may be revealing: Patients may acknowledge the examiner's touch (stimulation) of either hand (or foot or face) independently, but fail to acknowledge (extinguish) stimulation of the contralesional hand to bilateral simultaneous stimulation.

Impaired visuospatial memory may be identified by asking the patients to locate a building in a city, to describe either verbally or with a map the route from one location to another or even to find their room at home or in the hospital.

Impairments of constructional ability may reflect unilateral hemispatial neglect, but may also occur in the absence of overt neglect. Bedside assessments of construction include drawing tasks as noted in the preceding text, as well as puzzle assembly and construction using blocks, sticks, or other objects. Poor performance on tasks of constructional ability in the absence of frank neglect and elementary sensorimotor deficits most often reflect impairments of either visuospatial function or executive function. Observing patients as they perform constructional tasks is essential for discriminating between visuospatial- and executive function-based constructional ability impairments. Impaired constructional ability based on executive dysfunction is evident in poor task planning and execution. By contrast, impaired constructional ability based on visuospatial dysfunction is evident in poor visual scanning of the item to be copied and often by impaired ability to appreciate that the object produces appears different than the item to be copied. It has also been suggested that the pattern of impairment differs between patients with right- and left-hemisphere lesions: Patients with right-hemisphere lesions employ a disorganized and "piecemeal" approach resulting in problems with the overall figure design, whereas patient with left-hemisphere lesions omit or misplace internal details in the copy of the figure.[3]

Identification of impaired dressing ability requires observation of the patient performing such tasks. However, a challenge to this ability can be devised by turning inside-out the sleeve of a coat or the leg of a pair of pants (outside of the patient's field of view), and then asking the patient to don the garment. Patients with impaired dressing ability based on visuospatial dysfunction are often unable to solve the problem presented by this maneuver.

D. Treatment

1. **Optimize the physical health.** Maximizing treatment of underlying neurologic, psychiatric, and general medical conditions is a prerequisite to the prescription of treatments (nonpharmacologic and somatic) for visuospatial dysfunction.

2. **Optimize the patient's environment and lifestyle.** Addressing environmental factors that exacerbate or maintain visuospatial dysfunction is essential. Identifying and minimizing potential sources of overstimulation and/or distraction may permit patients with such problems to make the most effective use of their abilities. Providing adequate time for completion of required tasks may allow individuals with visuospatial dysfunction to perform accurately and relatively independently. Modifying task demands by setting up items of a task (e.g., for hygiene, cooking, eating, transfers, etc.) in the unaffected hemispace, provides cues for attention to the affected hemispace, and reducing the risk of injury to the unattended hemispace, may allow individuals with visuospatial dysfunction to maximize their functional independence. Encouraging interaction with an individual with unilateral hemispace neglect to present to the

unaffected hemispace may facilitate social engagement. In the hospital, we place the patient's bed in the room such that the door is in their unaffected hemispace; this facilitates the patient's observation of their environment, and immediately places visitors into the patient's unaffected hemispace. Encouraging adequate rest and recovery after periods of intense or sustained mental effort also permits patients to maximize their functional abilities.

3. **Nonpharmacologic interventions.** Three evidence-based reviews of the world literature regarding cognitive rehabilitation conclude that the evidence is sufficient to merit recommending cognitive rehabilitation for visuospatial dysfunction.[4-6] We regard compensatory strategy training as the first-line intervention for visuospatial dysfunction. We recommend that patients with visuospatial dysfunction be referred for treatment to a speech-language pathologist, occupational therapist, or neuropsychologist experienced in the use of compensatory strategy training for this problem.

4. **Pharmacotherapy.** There are no FDA-approved treatments for visuospatial function, and there is no clearly established pharmacotherapy for visuospatial dysfunction when it occurs as an isolated cognitive impairment. Expert opinion based on reviews of clinical reports (mostly open-label) suggests that cholinesterase inhibitors, uncompetitive NMDA receptor antagonists, or catecholaminergically active agents may improve visuospatial dysfunction.[7] However, the literature is not sufficiently developed to recommend pharmacotherapy for isolated impairments of visuospatial function.

References

1. Mesulam M-M. Confusional state and spatial neglect. In: Mesulam M-M, ed. *Principles of behavioral and cognitive neurology*, 2nd ed. Oxford: Oxford University Press; 2000:174–256.
2. Epstein R, Kanwisher N. A cortical representation of the local visual environment. *Nature*. 1998;392:598–601.
3. Weintraub S. Neuropsychological assessment of mental state. In: Mesulam M-M, ed. *Principles of behavioral and cognitive neurology*, 2nd ed. Oxford: Oxford University Press; 2000:121–173.
4. Cicerone KD, Dahlberg C, Kalmar K, et al. Evidence-based cognitive rehabilitation: Recommendations for clinical practice. *Arch Phys Med Rehabil*. 2000;81(12):1596–1615.
5. Cicerone KD, Dahlberg C, Malec JF, et al. Evidence-based cognitive rehabilitation: Updated review of the literature from 1998 through 2002. *Arch Phys Med Rehabil*. 2005;86(8):1681–1692.
6. Cappa SF, Benke T, Clarke S, et al. EFNS guidelines on cognitive rehabilitation: Report of an EFNS Task Force. *Eur J Neurol*. 2005;12(9):665–680.
7. Sheppard DM, Bradshaw JL, Mattingley JB, et al. Effects of stimulant medication on the lateralisation of line bisection judgements of children with attention deficit hyperactivity disorder. *J Neurol Neurosug Psychiatry*. 1999;66(1):57–63.

XII. EXECUTIVE DYSFUNCTION

A. **Clinical background**

1. **Occurrence and prevalence.** Executive dysfunction is a common feature of many neurologic and neuropsychiatric disorders that affect the frontal cortex, subcortical structures, and the white matter connecting these areas. Among the neurodegenerative dementias, early and prominent impairment of executive function is a hallmark of frontotemporal dementia (FTD), in particular.[1] Executive dysfunction is increasingly appreciated as a manifestation of and predictor of disability in primary psychiatric disorders as well. Although the exact frequencies of executive dysfunction both within and across these conditions are not well established, they are common, contribute significantly to disability in multiple domains of everyday function, and increase caregiver burden.[2,3]

2. **Phenomenology.** Executive dysfunction may manifest as problems in one or more of the following functions: Categorization and abstraction; problem solving; self-direction; planning and organization of cognition and behavior; independence from external environmental contingencies; maintenance of and fluent shifting between information or behavior sets; and executive control of more "basic" cognitive functions such as attention, working memory, systematic memory searching and information retrieval, language (lexical fluency and functional communication), praxis, and visuospatial function. Judgment and insight are also generally considered executive functions, although the concept of "self-awareness" (that overlaps conceptually and clinically with insight) extends beyond this domain of cognitive function.

   Individuals with executive dysfunction may attend to salient features of a task or situation but not place those details into a larger and more useful context (i.e., they lose the "forest" for the "trees"), struggle to solve problems (i.e., to both recognize the nature of a problem and elaborate contextually relevant solutions), may manifest perseverative behaviors, fail to appreciate fully their present circumstances, and to anticipate consequences of their actions (i.e., demonstrate impaired judgment and insight).

   Impairments in executive function commonly co-occur with problems in attention and/or memory, and may be mislabeled by patients and caregivers as problems in these other domains. Executive dysfunction is also associated with impairments in other "frontally mediated" cognitive and behavioral functions, particular comportment and motivation. Comportment and motivational impairments are more commonly regarded as behavioral disturbances and not as disturbances of cognition *per se.* Although all these functions are sometimes grouped under the heading of "executive function," the treatment recommendations offered here will focus more specifically on the "cognitive" aspects of executive function and not on its behavioral elements.

3. **Course and prognosis.** Executive dysfunction may be a transient and reversible manifestations of some conditions (e.g., mild TBI, substance intoxication, and/or withdrawal states, chronic subdural hematoma, etc.), static problems in other conditions (e.g., severe traumatic or hypoxic-ischemic brain injuries, cerebrovascular disease, frontal neoplasm, etc.), or progressive impairments in still others (e.g., frontotemporal dementia, Parkinson and Huntington diseases, multiple sclerosis, or HIV/AIDS, etc.). Accordingly, the course and prognosis of such impairments varies with the underlying condition on which they are predicated.

B. **Neuropathogenesis.** Executive dysfunction may arise because of injury to or dysfunction of either the closed-loop or open-loop elements of the dorsolateral prefrontal-subcortical circuit.[4,5] The closed-loop elements of this circuit include Brodmann areas 9 and 10, anterior 11 and 12, and also 45–47 (on the dorsolateral surface of the frontal lobes); the dorsolateral head of the caudate nucleus; the lateral aspect of the globus pallidus interna and rostrolateral substantia nigra (elements of the "direct" circuit); the dorsal globus pallidus externa and lateral subthalamic nucleus (elements of the "indirect" circuit); the parvocellular portions of the ventral anterior and mediodorsal thalamus; and the white matter connections between these structures. The open-loop elements of this circuit include the other cortical areas that project to and from it (i.e., hippocampus, posterior cingulate cortex, posterior heteromodal association cortex, limbic, and paralimbic structures, etc.) and also the white matter connections between these other cortical areas and the dorsolateral prefrontal-subcortical circuit. These open-loop elements permit the dorsolateral prefrontal-subcortical circuit to integrate the processing of and interaction between more "basic" cognitive processes carried on elsewhere in the brain—in other words, to serve as the "executive in charge" of the brain areas serving other cognitive functions.

The white matter and subcortical elements of the dorsolateral prefrontal-subcortical circuit are anatomically segregated from but are in close proximity and reciprocally connected to those elements of the anterior cingulate- and the lateral orbitofrontal-subcortical circuits. These circuits serve motivation and comportment, respectively. Because of the anatomic proximity of the white matter and subcortical elements of these circuits, the types of injuries and diseases that compromise the function of one of the prefrontal-subcortical circuits often compromise the function of the other prefrontal-subcortical circuits.

The function of the prefrontal-subcortical circuits is dependent on a host of neurotransmitters including glutamate (serving as the primary excitatory neurotransmitter), acetylcholine, dopamine, norepinephrine, serotonin (serving various modulatory functions), and GABA (serving as the primary inhibitory neurotransmitter), among others. Executive dysfunction may arise as a direct effect of disruption of the neurochemical modulation of these circuits, whether due to toxic/metabolic perturbations, degeneration of the neuronal bodies in the various nuclei from which these neurotransmitter projections arise, or injury to and/or demyelination of those projections *en route* to their cortical and subcortical targets.

C. **Diagnosis.** Individuals with mild executive dysfunction and retained insight into such impairment may present independently for evaluation and treatment of that problem. In many conditions that produce executive dysfunction (i.e., severe TBI, many dementias), however, insight for that impairment may be limited or absent; in those contexts, others (e.g., relatives, friends, and employers, etc.) may present the patient for evaluation and treatment. In either case, the diagnosis first requires a careful description of the symptom of concern. As suggested in the preceding text, many individuals will use "memory problems," "forgetfulness," or "trouble concentrating" to describe impairments that are more accurately understood as difficulties with executive function. Thereafter, history should seek to identify the onset, course, and possible etiology of the "memory" impairment.

Physician evaluation of executive function is generally undertaken using one or more bedside assessment of cognition. The Frontal Assessment Battery[6] is particularly useful for such evaluations, and recently developed norms for this measure[7] may guide the interpretation of performance on this measure. The EXIT25,[8] for which normative data are available,[9] is also useful for the assessment of executive function at the bedside. It is important to note that the MMSE is not considered an adequate screening assessment of executive function, and its use for this purpose is discouraged.

In addition to bedside or office-based assessments, observation of performance in everyday life—directly and/or by a reliable informant—is essential for the identification of functionally significant deficits and also remaining strengths in executive function. The development of treatment strategies that generalize effectively beyond the clinical setting relies on such assessments.

When screening assessments and observation of daily function fail to adequately capture the types and severities of executive impairments reported by patients (or their caregiver), formal assessment is recommended. This assessment often includes not only formal neuropsychologic testing, but also occupational therapy and performance-based examinations. Following the other diagnostic principles (i.e., assessment of emotional or behavioral conditions; neurologic examination and neuroimaging; laboratory assessments; etc.) described in the preceding sections of this chapter is also recommended.

D. **Treatment**
1. **Optimize the physical health.** Maximizing treatment of underlying neurologic, psychiatric, or general medical conditions is a prerequisite to the prescription of treatments (nonpharmacologic and somatic) for impairments in executive function.
2. **Optimize the patient's environment and lifestyle.** Addressing environmental factors that exacerbate or maintain problems with executive function may be very useful. For example, identifying

and minimizing potential sources of overstimulation or distraction may permit patients with such problems to make the most effective use of their remaining executive abilities. Providing adequate time for completion of required tasks may allow individuals with impaired executive control of attention and processing speed impairments to perform more accurately and effectively on such tasks. Encouraging adequate rest and recovery after periods of intense or sustained mental effort may permit patients to maximize their functional abilities. Providing environmental cues, whether written or verbal, to facilitate retrieval of information may limit the functional consequences of memory impairments. Using direct, simple, and concrete communication with the patient, and encouraging the same of the patient, may also facilitate adaptation to functional with functional communication problems arising from executive dysfunction. Similarly, using simple and concrete verbal, written, or manual cues to assist with task performance may allow patients to function more independently despite executive dysfunction. Toward that end, written or electronic "day timers" (organizers) are often very helpful—so that these organizers are sometimes referred to by patients (and others) as their "peripheral brains."

3. **Nonpharmacologic interventions.** On the basis of expert review of the cognitive rehabilitation literature, the American Congress of Rehabilitation Medicine recommends compensatory strategy development for the treatment of executive dysfunction among individuals with TBIs, stroke, and other neurologic conditions.[10,11] Our experience suggests that these interventions may be useful in highly motivated patients with relatively mild impairments and preserved insight, particularly when compensatory strategies are tailored to generalize from the office to real-world contexts. We recommend compensatory strategy training for individuals with executive dysfunction due to neurologic disorders, and refer patients to speech therapists, occupational therapists, and neuropsychologists with expertise in the provision of such training.

    When patients present with more severe impairments, treatment may be directed instead at training caregivers to serve as the patient's "executive" for daily routines and to compensate entirely for the patient's impairments. This approach is particularly important when the patient's executive dysfunction requires direct supervision to remain safe at home or in other settings (e.g., to cope with unexpected emergencies that might threaten life or limb, or that leave him or her vulnerable to exploitation by unscrupulous individuals). We also recommend the provision of compensatory strategy training for caregivers of individuals with severe executive dysfunction by an experienced speech or occupational therapist or by a neuropsychologist.

    There is emerging evidence that cognitive rehabilitation interventions targeting executive dysfunction may improve the functional abilities of individuals with schizophrenia and other severe and persistent mental illnesses.[12] Although the literature is not developed sufficiently to recommend routine use of cognitive rehabilitation in this context, clinicians are encouraged to stay apprised of this rapidly developing area of nonpharmacologic intervention for the executive function impairments associated with mental illnesses.

4. **Pharmacotherapy.** There are no FDA-approved treatments for executive dysfunction. The neurochemistry of attention predicts that augmentation of cerebral catecholaminergic and cholinergic function, as well as augmentation or stabilization of glutamatergic function, may be useful targets for the treatment of executive dysfunction. The evidence regarding pharmacotherapy for executive dysfunction is composed of case reports, case series, small-scale open-label studies, and a few double-blind placebo-controlled trials.

Based on these reports, we recommend methylphenidate for the treatment of executive function when accompanied by impairments in arousal, attention, and/or processing speed. Treatment with methylphenidate generally begins with doses of 5 mg twice daily and is gradually increased in increments of 5 mg twice daily until either beneficial effect or medication intolerance is achieved. Most studies suggest that optimal doses of methylphenidate are in the range of 20 to 40 mg twice daily (i.e., 0.15–0.3 mg/kg/twice daily). This medication generally takes effect quickly (within 0.5–1 hour following administration), although this effect may wane after only a few hours. Therefore, the first issue in the administration of this agent is determining optimal dose and dosing frequency. Individuals requiring relatively high and frequent doses of methylphenidate may benefit from use of longer-acting preparations of this medication.

Mild increases in heart rate and/or blood pressure may occur during treatment with psychostimulants, although these tend to occur relatively infrequently in patients without other cardiac or vascular problems and are only rarely of sufficient magnitude to merit discontinuation of these agents. Serious adverse reactions to these medications are most often related to increases in cerebral dopamine, and to a lesser extent cerebral norepinephrine activity, and include paranoia, dysphoria, anxiety, agitation, and irritability. However, these adverse effects are in practice very uncommon at doses typically used to treat attention and speed of processing impairments. Although lowering seizure threshold is often cited as a risk associated with the use of these agents, this risk appears to be minimal, even among individuals with epilepsy. Clinicians are advised to familiarize themselves with prescribing information regarding side effects, drug interactions, and contraindications before using these agents for any purpose.

As noted earlier, careful pretreatment assessment of executive function and related impairments is essential. In the absence of objective assessment, reports of subjective improvement in cognition or daily function during treatment with these agents are frequently used as a measure of treatment response. However, subjective reports of improvement in the absence of improvement on objective measures of cogniton should prompt reevaluation of the etiology of those impairments. Because stimulants may improve mood, increase motivation, or lessen fatigue, discrepancy between subjective and objective measures of improvements may suggest that the primary problem lies in depression, apathy, fatigue, or some combination of these noncognitive problems.

When executive dysfunction is comorbid with impairments in memory (new learning and/or retrieval), we recommend cholinesterase inhibitors as our first-line pharmacologic intervention. Treatment with donepezil begins with 5 mg daily. If this dose is tolerated but does not produce improvements in attention after approximately 4 weeks of treatment, titration to 10 mg daily is generally undertaken. Slower dose titration may limit the development of treatment-emergent side effects that are gastrointestinal in nature. Rivastigmine and galantamine have shorter half-lives, and require twice daily dosing. Rivastigmine is generally started at 1.5 mg b.i.d. and increased in 1.5 mg b.i.d. increments every 4 weeks until maximal benefits are attained or treatment intolerance develops. Galantamine is generally started at 4 mg b.i.d. and increased in 4 mg b.i.d. increments until maximal benefits are attained or treatment intolerance develops. When the extended-release form of galantamine is used, treatment begins with 8 mg daily and is titrated in 8 mg increments until maximal benefits are attained or treatment intolerance develops.

All these agents produce, with variable frequency, headache, nausea, diarrhea, vomiting, fatigue, insomnia, muscle cramping, pain, and abnormal dreams. These side effects are frequently a consequence of overly rapid dose escalation, although they will occur in very few patients during treatment with standard dosing strategies. When intolerable side effects develop and/or persist during treatment with any of these agents, dose reduction is prudent. Such reductions may reduce adverse effects and permit patients to continue treatment. Clinicians are advised to familiarize themselves with prescribing information regarding other side effects, drug interactions, and contraindications before using these agents for any purpose. To date, there are no reports suggesting that the use of these agents in individuals with neurologic disorders is associated with a change (positive or negative) in seizure frequency. Nonetheless, remaining vigilant for the development of seizures and/or changes in seizure frequency is recommended.

Some patients will respond to stimulants alone, some to cholinesterase inhibitors alone, some to either or both classes of medication, and some to neither. In all cases, treatment of executive dysfunction remains a matter of empiric trial.

Atypical antipsychotic medications, and particularly olanzapine, quetiapine, and risperidone, appear to have a more favorable effect on executive function than do typical antipsychotics such as haloperidol,[13] an effect that merits consideration when treating patients with comorbid executive dysfunction and psychosis or agitation/aggression.

References

1. Neary D, Snowden JS, Gustafson L, et al. Frontotemporal lobar degeneration: A consensus on clinical diagnostic criteria. *Neurology*. 1998;51(6):1546–1554.
2. Fogel B. The significance of frontal system disorders for medical practice and health policy. *J Neuropsychiatry Clin Neurosci*. 1994;6:343–347.
3. Royall D, Cabello M, Polk M. Executive dyscontrol: An important factor affecting the level of care received by older retirees. *J Am Geriatr Soc*. 1998;46:1519–1524.
4. McDonald BC, Flashman LA, Saykin AJ. Executive dysfunction following traumatic brain injury: Neural substrates and treatment strategies. *Neurorehabilitation*. 2002;17:333–344.
5. Arciniegas DB, Beresford TP. Complex cognition. In: Arciniegas DB, Beresford TP, eds. *Neuropsychiatry: An introductory approach*. Cambridge: Cambridge University Press; 2001:52–74.
6. Dubois B, Slachevsky A, Litvan I, et al. The FAB: A frontal assessment battery at bedside. *Neurology*. 2000;55(11):1621–1626.
7. Appollonio I, Leone M, Isella V, et al. The Frontal Assessment Battery (FAB): Normative values in an Italian population sample. *Neurol Sci*. 2005;26(2):108–116.
8. Royall DR, Mahurin RK, Gray KF. Bedside assessment of executive cognitive impairment: The executive interview. *J Am Geriatr Soc*. 1992;40(12):1221–1226.
9. Royall DR, Palmer R, Chiodo LK, et al. Declining executive control in normal aging predicts change in functional status: The Freedom House Study. *J Am Geriatr Soc*. 2004;52(3):346–352.
10. Cicerone KD, Dahlberg C, Kalmar K, et al. Evidence-based cognitive rehabilitation: Recommendations for clinical practice. *Arch Phys Med Rehabil*. 2000;81(12):1596–1615.
11. Cicerone KD, Dahlberg C, Malec JF, et al. Evidence-based cognitive rehabilitation: Updated review of the literature from 1998 through 2002. *Arch Phys Med Rehabil*. 2005;86(8):1681–1692.
12. Kurtz MM. Neurocognitive rehabilitation for schizophrenia. *Curr Psychiatry Rep*. 2003;5(4):303–310.
13. Cuesta MJ, Peralta V, Zarzuela A. Effects of olanzapine and other antipsychotics on cognitive function in chronic schizophrenia: A longitudinal study. *Schizophr Res*. 2001;48(1): 17–28.

Chapter 4

GLOBAL COGNITIVE IMPAIRMENT: THE DEMENTIAS

Steven A. Rogers, Po H. Lu, Jeffrey L. Cummings

I. PRINCIPLES OF DEMENTIA AND NEUROPSYCHIATRIC SYMPTOMS

- A. **Definitions**
  1. Dementia syndromes are defined as acquired disorders of cognitive function, including impairment in memory and at least one other cognitive domain (aphasia, apraxia, agnosia, or executive functioning). These syndromes produce occupational or social disability, represent a significant decline from a previously higher level of functioning, and should not be present exclusively during the course of a delirium (Diagnostic and Statistical Manual of Mental Disorders, 4th edition; [DSM-IV]).
  2. Although neuropsychiatric symptoms are not part of the formal criteria for dementia, they are common in most dementing disorders and play a significant role in the diagnosis, course, severity, and treatment for many types of dementia. Over 90% of those with dementia experience behavioral and psychological symptoms at some point in the course of their illness, with most patients exhibiting a multiplicity of symptoms.
- B. **Principles of treatment for dementia.** In general, the treatment of dementia should follow the American Academy of Neurology's Practice Parameters for the Management of Dementia (2001), which integrates accurate assessment with pharmacologic and nonpharmacologic interventions.
  1. **Perform a comprehensive diagnostic evaluation**
     a. The purpose of diagnostic evaluation is to identify individuals with the dementia syndrome and distinguish the

specific subtype of dementia. Although dementia affects up to 50% of individuals above age 80, it remains undetected by 25% of physicians and 21% of family members.

b. A dementia evaluation is best performed in the outpatient setting, following the resolution of acute illnesses, delirium, and the treatment of depression. This evaluation starts with a full clinical interview that helps determine the course and symptoms of decline, complicating medical conditions, and presence of significant risk factors (i.e., family history of dementia, substance use, etc.). Considering the possibility of compromised insight, it is recommended that cognitive and functional deficits be substantiated by a caregiver.

c. Patients should be referred for more extensive neuropsychological assessment that examines general intellectual functioning, attention, language, visuospatial functioning, verbal and visual memory, executive functioning, and mood. Although neuropsychological testing takes a significant amount of time to administer, it can help determine the presence, degree, and pattern of a patient's cognitive deficits. The actual techniques used to assess these domains are somewhat discretionary, but educational and cultural factors should be considered.

d. A neurologic exam should assess gait disorders, focal abnormalities, and extrapyramidal signs. Likewise, routine laboratory tests, including blood cell count, glucose level, serum electrolyte level, blood urea nitrogen/creatinine levels, liver and thyroid function tests, syphilis serology, and vitamin B_{12} and folate levels, are necessary for differential diagnosis and ruling out reversible causes.

e. Both computed tomography (CT) scan and magnetic resonance imaging (MRI) are recommended for initial diagnostic evaluation to detect structural changes and to assess the level of atrophy in the brain. Although practical considerations of cost and accessibility influence which imaging procedure to use, a noncontrast CT scan is recommended to rule out reversible causes of dementia and the detection of cerebrovascular disease, whereas MRI may be more helpful in differential diagnosis of the types of degenerative dementia. Positron emission tomography (PET) or single proton emission computed tomography (SPECT) scans can identify metabolic and regional perfusion changes that are helpful in differential diagnosis, particularly between Alzheimer disease (AD) and frontotemporal dementia (i.e., hypometabolism or hypoperfusion of the temporal–parietal region and the posterior cingulate is supportive of the former although changes in the frontal and anterior temporal lobes are strongly suggestive of the latter).

2. **Implement a biopsychosocial treatment plan**
   a. The treatment of dementia is multimodal and guided by the stage of illness and specific symptoms manifested by the patient. Treatment begins with explicit education of family members and caregivers about the diagnosis, prognosis, and options for intervention, including sources of care and support.
   b. The particular type of intervention should involve a combination of pharmacologic interventions and psychosocial treatment for each target symptom. Cognitive and functional losses are typically addressed with cholinesterase inhibitors, vitamin E, and selegiline, whereas psychosis and other neuropsychiatric features are treated with antipsychotics, antidepressants, and other psychopharmacologic medications.
   c. Psychosocial interventions aim to improve quality of life and maximize function through psychotherapy, cognitive remediation, and stimulation therapies (i.e., music, changes in physical environment, pet therapy, etc.).
   d. The actual location of treatment is determined by the need to provide safe and effective interventions in the least restrictive setting. Individuals with dementia who are exhibiting psychotic, affective, or behavioral symptoms may need to be admitted to an inpatient facility. If there is an imbalance between the patient's clinical status and the caregivers' ability to supervise the patient and manage the burden of care, placement in a long-term care facility should be considered.
   e. Educational programs should be offered to family caregivers to improve caregiver satisfaction and delay the time to nursing home placement. The staff at long-term care facilities should be educated about dementia to minimize the unnecessary use of antipsychotic medications. This education should address basic principles of care, like keeping instructions simple, maintaining consistency and avoiding unnecessary change, and providing frequent reminders.
   f. There is no cure for dementia, but interventions that may significantly affect patient and caregiver quality of life are available. Specific treatment strategies for each type of dementia will be described in the subsequent text.

   References
   1. American Psychiatric Association. *Diagnostic and statistical manual of mental disorders*, 4th ed. Washington, DC: American Psychiatric Association; 1994.
   2. Doody RS, Stevens JC, Beck C, et al. Practice parameter: Management of dementia (an evidence-based review). *Neurology*. 2001;56:1154–1166.
   3. LoGiudice D. Dementia: An update to refresh your memory. *Intern Med J*. 2002;32:535–540.
   4. Vicioso BA. Dementia: When is it not Alzheimer disease. *Am J Med Sci*. 2002;324:84–95.

II. TYPES OF DEMENTIA

A. Alzheimer disease
1. **Clinical background and prevalence**
    a. Alzheimer disease is the most common form of dementia in the elderly, occurring in 6% of the population above age 65 and increasing by a factor of two with every 5 years of age after age 60.
    b. The onset generally occurs between ages 40 and 90, although most patients develop it after age 65. The average duration of the disease can vary from 5 to 20 years, and once acquired, it reduces life expectancy by half.
    c. Age is the primary risk factor for developing AD, although there is a slightly higher susceptibility for women, African Americans, and those with a history of head trauma and lower educational achievement. It is not certain why women may be at greater risk, although some researchers have posited a relationship between AD and hormonal imbalances. The increased risk in African Americans may be due to their vulnerability to vascular conditions. Individuals with head injury or lower education may have less cognitive reserve and a lower threshold for developing cognitive impairment.
    d. Genetically, AD is complex, heterogeneous, and follows an age-related dichotomy. Early onset familial AD, which typically presents before age 65, represents only a small fraction of all patients with AD (<5%) and is transmitted in an autosomal dominant fashion. Late-onset ("sporadic") AD (age 65 or older and represents most AD cases) follows the common disease/common variant hypothesis, which postulates that common disorders are governed by common deoxyribonucleic acid (DNA) variants that increase disease risk, but are insufficient to cause a specific disorder. Those with the apolipoprotein e4 (ApoE-4) are at a genetic risk for developing AD. The presence of even one copy of the ApoE-4 genotype may account for as much as 50% of the risk for developing AD, with increased risk as the number of allele copies increase. To date, only the e4 allele of the *apolipoprotein E* gene has been established as such a DNA variant, carrying a threefold risk for AD.
2. **Pathophysiology**
    a. The histopathologic hallmarks of AD include extracellular amyloid plaques, intracellular neurofibrillary tangles, and neuronal and synaptic loss.
    b. The putative process by which these features lead to dementia has been unified under the amyloid cascade hypothesis. The amyloid precursor protein (APP) is cleaved by β and γ secretase, leading to the production of β-amyloid peptides that are transported extracellularly and undergo an abnormal accrual and misfolding that leads to aggregation into

amyloid or neuritic plaques. In turn, this triggers a succession of events including abnormal *tau* protein phosphorylation and formation of neurofibrillary tangles, inflammation, oxidation, glutamatergic excitotoxicity, and loss of neurons, all of which further exacerbate the pathogenic process and lead to cell death. These latter processes have all been implicated in the pathophysiology of AD but are considered secondary consequences of the generation and deposition of Aβ.

   c. Neurochemical deficits in acetylcholine, norepinephrine, and serotonin, which are altered through the neurohistologic changes in the neurons and synapses, have been implicated most in the neuropsychiatric symptoms of AD. In particular, the apathy, agitation, and depression seen in AD may be partially attributed to the cholinergic–serotonergic imbalance and other alterations in the brain biochemistry.

3. **Diagnosis.** Once individuals present with symptoms of cognitive impairment, diagnosis of AD is based on the criteria established by the National Institute of Neurologic and Communicative Disorders and Stroke-Alzheimer Disease and Related Disorders Association.

   a. *Definite AD* is diagnosed when a prior clinical diagnosis of probable AD is confirmed by autopsy or biopsy.

   b. A diagnosis of *Probable AD* is made when there is no histopathologic confirmation available but individuals meet all clinical criteria for AD. Individuals must have gradually progressive deficits in memory and one other cognitive area, onset between ages 40 and 90, and the absence of delirium or other disorders that might account for the cognitive deficits.

   c. *Possible AD* is diagnosed when there is a gradually progressive cognitive deficit in one area without any other identifiable cause, or there is a complicating illness that could account for the dementia syndrome.

4. **Neuropsychiatric symptoms**

   a. More than 80% of patients with AD manifest neuropsychiatric symptoms, with apathy, depression, and agitation/aggression being the most common abnormalities.

   b. The apathy of AD is characterized by a lack of interest in formerly pleasant activities, reduced excitement for social activities, and a loss of social engagement and intimacy (see Chapter 1).

   c. Depression seems to develop early and persist throughout the course of AD. Some researchers suggest that depression is a prodromal risk factor that heralds the onset of AD, whereas others contend that depression is an early symptom that declines as insight becomes compromised (see Chapter 5).

   d. Symptoms of agitation/aggression are most prevalent during the middle and later stages.

e. Psychotic symptoms seem to operate in a quadratic relationship with disease stage, occurring primarily during the early and late stages of AD (see Chapter 7). Typical delusions include erroneous beliefs that others are stealing from them, delusions of infidelity, and beliefs consistent with Capgras syndrome.

5. **Treatment**

a. **Cholinesterase inhibitors**

(1) Cholinesterase inhibitors are the approved pharmacologic interventions for mild-to-moderate stages of AD and the first treatments approved by the U.S. Food and Drug Administration (FDA) for treatment of AD. Their mode of action is not to modify the progression of the disease, but rather to address the symptoms of AD by inhibiting the destruction of intrasynaptic acetylcholine, which increases the amount of acetylcholine available for neurotransmission.

(2) Currently, the four FDA-approved cholinesterase inhibitors are tacrine (Cognex), donepezil (Aricept), galantamine (Razadyne), and rivastigmine (Exelon). Owing to its hepatotoxic effects, tacrine is now rarely used. Even though the remaining three drugs differ in some pharmacologic aspects, double-blind, randomized controlled trials show how they have similar effects in improving global function and enhancing cognitive and behavioral functioning among individuals with AD.

(3) Donepezil is a pure acetylcholinesterase inhibitor. It has a half-life of 70 hours, and it is typically initiated at a dose of 5 mg daily and increased to 10 mg daily after 1 month. A review of 13 double-blind, randomized trials comparing donepezil to placebo, found a significant beneficial effect of donepezil on cognitive functioning, global status, and activities of daily living for patients with mild or moderate AD after 12, 24, and 52 weeks. Similarly, a review of seven double-blind, randomized controlled trials revealed significantly improved cognition, reduced loss of activities of daily living, improved quality of life, and delayed nursing home placement among those prescribed donepezil compared with placebo. Treatment with donepezil appears to reduce symptoms of agitation and behavioral disturbance among those with moderate-to-severe AD. The primary side effects include gastrointestinal problems, nausea, vomiting, and diarrhea.

(4) Galantamine has two modes of action, namely inhibiting acetylcholinesterase and modulating allosteric nicotinic receptors. Modulation of nicotinic receptors increases the release of acetylcholine and stimulates the release of other neurotransmitters responsible for

cognition. Two doses of 4 mg each are required daily due to its short half-life (5 hours), and this dosage is increased to 8 mg twice daily after 1 month. The extended release (Razadyne ER) formulation is administered once daily. On the basis of the review of six double-blind, randomized, controlled trials, patients with AD who received treatment with galantamine exhibited significantly better performances on cognition, global functioning, and behavioral measures compared with individuals receiving placebo. After 12 months of treatment with galantamine, most patients are 4.7 points better on the Alzheimer Disease Assessment Scale (ADAS-cog/11) than those who receive placebo, which suggests significant improvement in cognitive functioning. Potential side effects include nausea, diarrhea, and vomiting.

(5) Rivastigmine inhibits both acetylcholinesterase and butyrylcholinesterase. It is initiated at 1.5 mg twice daily and is eventually increased to 4.5 mg twice daily after 2 months. Compared with the other two cholinesterase inhibitors, rivastigmine tends to have more side effects. These include weight loss, nausea, and vomiting. However, it has beneficial effects on cognition, global functioning, activities of daily living, and the control and prevention of abnormal behaviors. When taken for a year, it significantly reduces cognitive decline compared with placebo. It appears to delay patients' overall global impairment, even after 5 years of treatment.

(6) All three cholinesterase inhibitors show similarly positive effects on cognition, global functioning, and activities of living, such that studies directly comparing these medications did not reveal significant differences in efficacy. The process of selection is one of considering the patient's optimal dosing schedule, the physician's familiarity with the agents, and the patient's preferences.

b. **Memantine**

(1) Memantine has more recently emerged as an effective pharmacologic intervention for the moderate-to-severe stages of AD.

(2) Memantine is posited to interfere with glutamatergic excitotoxicity. Glutamate is the primary excitatory neurotransmitter in the central nervous system (CNS) and subserves neurotransmission and plasticity. An extracellular increase in glutamate may excessively activate N-methyl-D-aspartate (NMDA) receptors, one subtype of glutamate receptors, and lead to intracellular accumulation of calcium that can initiate neuronal death cascades. Without blocking the physiologic activation of the NMDA receptor, memantine blocks the neural activity of prolonged glutamate release.

(3) Studies of memantine consistently reveal a beneficial effect on cognition, activities of daily living, and behavior for those with moderate-to-severe AD. Most common side affects are headache, dizziness, falls, somnolence, and confusion.

(4) Most individuals begin at 5 mg per day and increase the dose at weekly intervals until they reach the target dose of 10 mg twice daily.

c. **Antioxidants (vitamin E and selegiline)**

(1) Vitamin E and selegiline have recently emerged as potentially disease-modifying agents in the treatment of AD. In placebo-controlled, double-blind, multicenter trials, both the independent and combined effect of these agents delayed functional deterioration, nursing home placement, loss of activities of daily living, and progression to severe dementia in patients with moderate AD.

(2) Vitamin E is typically given at 2,000 units daily, and selegiline is administered at 5 to 10 mg per day. Their mechanism of action appears to protect lipids against oxidative stress and slow nerve cell damage, including damage associated with amyloid deposition.

(3) Selegiline may result in orthostatic hypotension as a side effect, but the low toxicity of both vitamin E and selegiline suggests that they may be useful agents in delaying the progression of disease among those in the moderate stages of AD.

All the cholinesterase inhibitors are of equal efficacy; choosing the medication depends greatly on the agent that the clinician is most familiar with. There are more side effects with rivastigmine; these can usually be managed by giving the agent with food and titrating slowly (increase by 1.5 mg b.i.d. every month). Patients are treated long term and discontinuation is considered when the physician and the family believe that the disease is so severe that a meaningful response is no longer likely. Any deterioration during the withdrawal period—functional, cognitive, behavioral—is evidence of continuing benefit, and the medication should be reinstated. Withdrawal is conducted by administering half the usual starting dose for 1 week and then stopping the agent.

d. **Psychosocial approaches**

(1) To the extent possible, these pharmacologic treatments should be paired with psychosocial interventions. Activity programs, changes in patients' physical environment, exposure to music and massage, and greater education for caregivers have all been associated with improvement in functional symptoms and mobilization of the patients' cognitive resources.

(2) Behavior therapy and reminiscence therapy may help patients with AD adjust to their illness, reduce problem

behaviors, and foster slight gains in mood and cognition. However, it is critical to match the level of therapeutic demand with patients' cognitive and functional capacities.

References

1. Bertram L, Tanzi RE. The genetic epidemiology of neurodegenerative disease. *J Clin Invest.* 2005;115: 1449–1457.
2. Birks J, Harvey R. Donepezil for dementia due to Alzheimer's disease. *Cochrane Database Syst Rev.* 2003;3:1–96.
3. Cummings JL. *The neuropsychiatry of Alzheimer's disease and related dementias.* Independence, KY: Taylor & Francis; 2003.
4. Cummings JL. Alzheimer's disease. *N Engl J Med.* 2004;351:56–67.
5. Desai AK, Grossberg GT. Diagnosis and treatment of Alzheimer's disease. *Neurology.* 2005;64:34–39.
6. Loy C, Schneider L. Galantamine for Alzheimer's disease (Review). *Cochrane Database Syst Rev.* 2004; 4:1–71.
7. McKhann G, Drachman D, Folstein M, et al. Clinical diagnosis of Alzheimer's disease: Report of the NNCDS-ADRDA work group under the auspices of Department of Health and Human Services Task Force on Alzheimer's Disease. *Neurology.* 1984;39:939–944.
8. Potyk D. Treatments for Alzheimer disease. *South Med J.* 2005;98(6):628–635.

B. Vascular dementia

1. **Clinical background and prevalence**

    a. Vascular dementia (VaD) is the second most common form of dementia. It occurs in 10% to 20% of patients with dementia and represents a constellation of cognitive and behavioral symptoms that are caused by cerebrovascular disease.

    b. The survival rates are generally worse compared with AD, and unlike the insidious onset and gradual progression of AD, VaD usually involves a relatively sudden onset and subsequent stepwise progression in cognitive decline.

    c. The primary risk factors for VaD are history of prior strokes, hypertension, diabetes, coronary artery disease and hyperlipidemia. Older African Americans may be at a slightly higher risk due to their high risk for stroke, and unlike AD, men are more likely to develop VaD than women.

2. **Pathophysiology**

    a. Cerebrovascular disease leads to either cortical or subcortical injury. Large vessel cerebrovascular disease and cardiac embolic events commonly contribute to multiple cortical infarcts and strategic-infarct dementias, whereas subcortical (small-vessel) disease, which usually results from hypertension and diabetes, produces periventricular white matter ischemia and lacunar strokes.

   b.   Hypertension and diabetes represent risk factors for athero-
        sclerosis of the small arterioles in the subcortical region and
        connections with the frontal lobe. MRI can differentiate the
        types of VaD and identify involved structures.

3. **Diagnosis**

   a.   Diagnosis of VaD depends on evidence of cerebrovascu-
        lar disease, signs of stroke on clinical observation and
        neuroimaging, and a compelling temporal relationship be-
        tween cognitive symptoms and the cerebrovascular event.
        This relationship is regarded as present if the dementia de-
        veloped within 3 months of a stroke, or if there was abrupt
        deterioration or fluctuation in the progression of cognitive
        function.

   b.   The cerebrovascular insult is often heterogeneous, such
        that three primary subtypes have been described: (a) Cor-
        tical (multi-infarct) dementia, (b) subcortical (small-vessel)
        dementia, and (c) strategic-infarct dementia.

   c.   The diagnosis of VaD is complicated by the high prevalence
        of vascular lesions in patients diagnosed with AD. This
        comorbidity has led to the construct of mixed dementia,
        where AD is complicated by the presence of cerebrovascular
        disease. When there is a mixed presentation of AD-type
        pathology and cerebrovascular symptoms, there may be
        cognitive decline before stroke, the course of decline may
        be insidious between strokes, and the phenotype includes
        the features of AD. This represents a distinct syndrome
        with unique clinical and neuropsychiatric features.

4. **Neuropsychiatric symptoms**

   a.   Depression is the hallmark neuropsychiatric symptom of
        VaD. This syndrome is partially due to the disruption
        of frontal-subcortical circuits that mediate disturbances in
        behavior and mood (see Chapter 5).

   b.   Apathy and aggression may also occur among those with
        VaD (see Chapter 1); psychosis and disinhibition are less
        common (see Chapter 7).

   c.   Deficits in cholinergic transmission, including abnormal-
        ities in nicotinic receptor binding, may contribute to the
        development of cognitive and neuropsychiatric impair-
        ment in VaD. This outcome is largely because cholinergic
        structures are vulnerable to ischemic damage.

5. **Treatment**

   a.   The primary area of management for VaD is the prevention
        of cerebrovascular injury. Antiplatelet medications, such as
        50 to 325 mg daily dose of aspirin, are the most widely
        used agents to prevent the recurrence of stroke. They also
        stabilize cognitive test performance and slow cognitive
        decline.

   b.   There is no FDA-approved treatment for the cognitive and
        behavioral features of VaD, hence prescribing cholinesterase
        inhibitors is off label, but there are data from controlled

trials supporting the use of these agents in other disorders with cholinergic deficits including VaD, in conjunction with management of cerebrovascular risk factors. Among patients with VaD, treatment with galantamine is associated with improved cognition, functional ability, and behavior. Similarly, those with VaD show slowed cognitive decline after taking rivastigmine. Trials using donepezil as a treatment for VaD reveal greater cognitive improvements after 5 months than those receiving placebo. The approach in starting and stopping cholinesterase inhibitors for VaD is the same as that for AD but these agents have cardiac effects and should be used with special caution in this population of patients.

c. Memantine also had a beneficial effect on cognition, behavior, and the reduction of agitation among individuals in trials with VaD.

d. A combination of vitamin E and C supplements may be associated with an 88% reduction in VaD frequency and the promotion of cognitive performance. Therefore, vitamins E and C may have a protective effect against the cerebrovascular injuries that lead to VaD, perhaps by inhibiting platelet aggregation and modulating immune responses.

e. Speech and language therapy can significantly benefit those with aphasia and dysarthria, just as physical therapy can provide gait retraining.

f. The methods of primary prevention against VaD include management of hypertension, stroke prevention, reduced stress, healthy diet (reduced low-density lipoprotein cholesterols), and a minimum of 8 hours of sleep. It also requires limiting stress, stopping smoking, and moderating one's consumption of alcohol or illicit substances.

References

1. Erkinjuntti T. Cognitive decline and treatment options for patients with vascular dementia. *Acta Neurologica Scandinavica*. 2002;106:15.

2. Erkinjuntti T, Kurz A, Small GW, et al. An open-label extension trial of galantamine in patients with probable vascular dementia and mixed dementia. *Clin Ther*. 2003;25:1765–1782.

3. Erkinjuntti T, Rockwood K. Vascular dementia. *Semin Clin Neuropsychiatry*. 2003;8(1):37–45.

4. Nyenhuis DL, Gorelick PB. Vascular dementia: A contemporary review of epidemiology, diagnosis, prevention, and treatment. *J Am Geriatr Soc*. 1998;46(11):1–22.

5. Roman GC. Defining dementia: Clinical criteria for the diagnosis of vascular dementia. *Acta Neurologica Scandinavica*. 2002;106:6.

6. Small GW, Erkinjuntti T, Kurz A, et al. Galantamine in the treatment of cognitive decline in patients with vascular dementia or Alzheimer's disease with cerebrovascular disease. *CNS Drugs*. 2003;17(12):905–914.

C. **Parkinsonian syndromes.** (see Chapter 9) The parkinsonian syndromes are a heterogeneous group of degenerative neurologic disorders that include symptoms of parkinsonism, often with additional or atypical clinical features (Mendez and Cummings, 2003; Mitra et al. 2003). The most common are Parkinson disease with dementia (PDD), dementia with Lewy bodies (DLB), progressive supranuclear palsy (PSP) and corticobasal degeneration (CBD).

D. **Parkinson disease with dementia**
1. **Clinical background and prevalence**
    a. Parkinson disease (PD) is a common and progressive degenerative movement disorder among older adults, afflicting 1.5% to 2.5% of those above age 70. It usually develops between 50 and 65 years of age and has an average duration of 8 years. The male-to-female ratio is 3:2, and it is less common in non-white populations.
    b. Dementia develops slowly and insidiously among 40% to 80% of individuals with PD. It is particularly common among those above age 65, with a 5% incidence of significant cognitive decline each year. This rate of decline contributes to reduced survival rates among those with PDD.
    c. The primary risk factors for PDD are advancing age, a history of cognitive decline, older age of onset of PD, lower educational attainment, depression, more severe extrapyramidal symptoms, and bilateral motor symptoms at the onset of PD. Greater frequency of dementia is observed in patients with akinetic rigidity than those with tremors.
2. **Pathophysiology**
    a. Idiopathic PD is characterized by degeneration of nigrostriatal dopaminergic neurons. This degeneration involves marked depigmentation, neuronal loss, and the aggregation of Lewy bodies in the substantia nigra, which result in dopaminergic deficiency.
    b. The presence of dementia in PD may occur following greater involvement of frontocortical areas and significant damage to the ascending dopaminergic, cholinergic, noradrenergic, and serotoninergic neuronal systems. Among those with PD, damage may be confined to nigroputaminal pathways, whereas the nigrocaudatal pathways are also implicated in PDD.
    c. Patients with PDD also have cortical changes that are similar to AD. Lewy bodies in the neurons of the cerebral cortex have the strongest correlation with the presence of dementia, but cortical neuronal loss, abnormal tau proteins in temporal and prefrontal cortices, and hypoperfusion in the posterior cortical regions are also present.
    d. There is an age-dependent dichotomy in the genetics of PDD. Most of those with early onset PDD show predominantly autosomal recessive modes of Mendelian

inheritance. The hereditability of late-onset PD is generally low, although there is an increased risk effect for the $\varepsilon 2$ apolipoprotein allele.

3. **Diagnosis**
   a. Idiopathic PD is diagnosed in the presence of a beneficial response to levodopa and at least two of the following symptoms: Resting tremor, bradykinesia, cogwheel rigidity, or postural reflex impairment.
   b. It is excluded in the presence of other known causes of parkinsonism.
   c. Most patients initially present with resting tremor and other cardinal symptoms of bradykinesia, rigidity, and postural instability. They may also exhibit shuffling gait and masked facies.

4. **Neuropsychiatric symptoms**
   a. PDD is frequently accompanied by depression, anxiety, and psychosis. Depression is common in 40% of those with PDD, particularly among those with greater cognitive impairment, early onset of PD, bradykinesia, and gait instability (see Chapter 9). It is distinct from idiopathic depression in that it is associated with increased dysphoria, pessimism, irritability, and sadness, but with minimal guilt and self-punitive ideation. Depression is also commonly accompanied by an anxiety disorder and may even be used to predict degree of disability in PD, although it is uncertain if it is a consequence of progressive physical impairment or the manifestation of neurochemical changes.
   b. Before the onset of the motor symptoms of PD, patients may present a distinct personality profile of obsessive and compulsive traits, including overcontrol, introversion, and inflexibility (see Chapter 11).
   c. Hallucinations also occur in 25% to 40% of patients with PD, although these are usually consequences of treatment by dopaminergic agents (see Chapter 7). They usually involve fully formed visual images that are silent, well-defined, and may involve movement. Although less frequent, hallucinations may be combined with delusions of paranoia or persecution.
   d. Sleep disorders are a common but frequently overlooked complication of PD. This disturbance includes reduced sleep quality, longer sleep latency, more nighttime awakenings, and daytime sleepiness. Between 20% and 40% of individuals with PD also have rapid eye movement (REM) sleep behavior disorder. This disorder may herald the onset of DLB.

5. **Treatment**
   a. The treatment of PD typically begins with dopaminergic therapy of parkinsonian motor symptoms. These symptoms are usually treated with levodopa and administered in

conjunction with a dopa-decarboxylase inhibitor to offset peripheral side effects. Dopamine agonists may also be used as monotherapy or adjunctives to levodopa.

b. Other agents can be administered to improve the cognitive symptoms of PD. There are no FDA-approved medications for the treatment of dementia in patients with PD, but we recommend the use of cholinesterase inhibitors on the basis of data of their efficacy from controlled trials and benign side effect profile. The antioxidant properties of selegiline may reduce the rate of cell loss in PD and delay the initiation of treatment with dopaminergic agents. Coenzyme Q also has promise as a neuroprotective agent.

c. Anticholinergic agents should be avoided because of the risk of increased confusion, delusions, and hallucinations.

d. For those who are intolerant or unresponsive to medication therapies, surgical intervention may be appropriate. Thalamotomy may reduce tremor activity, and pallidotomy or deep brain stimulation (DBS) of the internal globus pallidus may improve motor function and attention.

References

1. Aarsland D, Andersen K, Larsen JP, et al. Prevalence and characteristics of dementia in Parkinson's disease. *Arch Neurol.* 2003;60:387–392.
2. Dubois B, Pillon B. Cognitive deficits in Parkinson's disease. *J Neurol.* 1997;244:2–8.
3. Mendez MF, Cummings JL. *Dementia: A clinical approach,* 3rd ed. Philadelphia, PA: Butterworth-Heinemann; 2003.
4. Mitra K, Gangopadhaya PK, Das SK. Parkinsonism plus syndrome-A review. *Neurol India.* 2003;51:183–188.
5. Soukup VM, Adams RL. Parkinson's disease. In: Adams RL, Parsons OA, Culberston JL, et al. eds. *Neuropsychology for clinical practice: Etiology, assessment, and treatment of common neurologic disorders.* Washington, DC: American Psychological Association; 1996:243–270.
6. Stocchi F, Brusa L. Cognition and emotion in different stages and subtypes of Parkinson's disease. *J Neurol.* 2000;247:114–121.

E. **Dementia with Lewy bodies**
   1. **Clinical background and prevalence**
      a. DLB is a complex neuropsychiatric disorder composed of dementia, parkinsonism, and prominent neuropsychiatric symptoms. It accounts for 10% to 20% of dementias.
      b. The average age of disease onset is between 60 and 70, with a mean duration of 7.7 years.
      c. Men are at a slightly higher risk for developing DLB.
   2. **Pathophysiology**
      a. DLB is a synucleinopathy, characterized by abnormal functioning and aggregation of α-synuclein in the neurons. This aggregation leads to the formation of Lewy bodies

that become deposited in the brainstem nuclei, subcortical nuclei, and several neocortical areas.

b. Although the mechanism is unclear, the formation of Lewy bodies is associated with profound dysfunction of dopamingergic and acetylcholinergic systems. This dysfunction may partially account for the extrapyramidal motor symptoms inherent in DLB, and the imbalance between dopamine and acetylcholine may be related to the genesis of visual hallucination and cognitive fluctuation.

c. The identification of specific DLB genetic factors is uncertain and remains complicated by its unstable phenotypic classification.

3. **Diagnosis**

a. The central feature required for diagnosis of probable DLB is a progressive cognitive decline that interferes with social and occupational functioning, combined with the presence of two of three of the following core symptoms: (a) Fluctuating cognitive performance, (b) recurrent visual hallucinations, and (c) spontaneous motor features of parkinsonism. Presence of one core feature allows for a diagnosis of possible DLB.

b. Other supporting features include repeated falls, syncope, depression, delusions, REM sleep behavior disorder, and transient loss of consciousness.

c. To allow for differentiation from idiopathic PD, the clinical criteria for DLB also require the onset of dementia before the appearance of parkinsonism.

4. **Neuropsychiatric symptoms**

a. More than 75% of those with DLB report recurrent visual hallucinations (see Chapter 7), which correlates with Lewy bodies in the amygdala and parahippocampal gyrus. These hallucinations occur relatively early in the course of the disease and are usually detailed, well formed, and center on themes of animals and individuals intruding into the patient's home.

b. Delusions of misidentification often coexist with visual hallucinations.

c. Apathy and anxiety may occur early in the disease, but disinhibition and aggression are less common.

5. **Treatment**

a. Pharmacologic treatment usually entails treatment of the parkinsonian symptoms with dopaminergic agents and treatment of cognitive deficits with cholinesterase inhibitors.

b. Dopaminergic agents may provide partial relief from parkinsonism if administered in low doses, but they also carry a number of risks including the exacerbation of psychotic symptoms.

c. There are no FDA-approved medications for the treatment of cognitive symptoms in patients with DLB dysfunction.

Prescribing cholinesterase inhibitors for this type of dementia is off label, but acetylcholine dysfunction in DLB and data from clinical trials support the use of cholinesterase inhibitors for this population. When used at the dosages typical for AD, they reduce fluctuation in cognition, improve cognitive functioning, and reduce visual hallucinations, apathy, and anxiety. In fact, patients with DLB may have extreme adverse responses to antipsychotics and alternatives such as cholinesterase inhibitors should be tried first in these patients to quell behavioral abnormalities. There are no differences in how these drugs are used; refer to the preceding section on AD for specific treatment recommendations.

d.   Education is also critical to help patients and families understand the characteristic symptoms of DLB. The reduction of environmental risk factors, like loose carpets and poor lighting, as well as active participation in physiotherapy and exercise programs can minimize patients' risk for falls. The treatment of potentially treatable sensory impairments, like poor hearing or vision, may also reduce hallucinations and falls.

References

1.   Barber R, Panikkar A, McKeith IG. Dementia with lewy bodies: Diagnosis and management. *Int J Geriatr Psychiatry*. 2001;16:12–18.
2.   Del Ser T, McKeith I, Anand R, et al. Dementia with lewy bodies: Findings from an international multicentre study. *Int J Geriatr Psychiatry*. 2000;15:1034–1045.
3.   McKeith I, Del Ser T, Spano P, et al. Efficacy of rivastigmine in dementia with lewy bodies: A randomised, double-blind, placebo-controlled international study. *Lancet Neurol*. 2000;356:2031.
4.   McKeith I, Mintzer J, Aarsland D, et al. Dementia with lewy bodies. *Lancet Neurol*. 2004;3:19–28.
5.   Mosimann UP, McKeith IG. Dementia with lewy bodies–diagnosis and treatment. *Swiss Med Wkly*. 2003; 133:131–142.

F.   **Progressive supranuclear palsy**

1.   **Clinical background and prevalence**

a.   The incidence rate for progressive supranuclear palsy (PSP) is generally low, affecting approximately 6 out of 100,000 individuals and twice as many men than women, with an average onset age of 63.

b.   More than half of afflicted patients are initially misdiagnosed, usually as having idiopathic PD.

2.   **Pathophysiology**

a.   The cognitive and neuropsychiatric symptoms are consistent with the dysfunction of the frontal-subcortical circuitry underlying the neuropathology of PSP.

b.   MRI and PET studies have consistently revealed frontotemporal and midbrain atrophy, hypometabolism of frontal lobes and subcortical structures, and high concentrations of neurofibrillary tangles in the basal ganglia.

   c. Unlike DLB, PSP is regarded as a tauopathy rather than an α-synucleinopathy because the neurofibrillary tangles are composed of abnormally phosphorylated tau proteins. Disruption of the medial and orbitofrontal subcortical circuits may contribute to the high prevalence of apathy and disinhibition seen in PSP.

3. **Diagnosis**

   a. Among the distinguishing features for probable PSP are vertical supranuclear palsy and prominent postural stability, including a fall within the first year of onset, at the age of 40 or after.

   b. Other supportive features include bradykinesia, axial rigidity, limitation of vertical saccades, and pseudobulbar palsy.

4. **Neuropsychiatric symptoms**

   a. More than 90% of patients with PSP experience apathy and approximately 30% display disinhibition (see Chapters 1 and 11).

   b. Depression and anxiety may be present but are less common (see Chapters 5 and 6).

5. **Treatment**

   a. For both PSP and CBD, treatments target symptoms and are minimally effective, probably because of the widespread involvement of dopaminergic and nondopaminergic neurotransmitter systems, as well as the compromise of multiple subcortical and cortical systems in these diseases.

   b. There is no effective treatment for PSP or CBD; cholinesterase inhibitors are not efficacious. Clinicians can offer palliative therapeutic approaches to improve quality of life or survival, like treating the dysphagia and addressing parkinsonian symptoms with dopaminergic agents. In general, dopaminergic agents such as levodopa or amitriptyline have only mild and brief effects on severe motor dysfunction, but the lack of observed benefit helps to rule out idiopathic PD.

   c. There are promising emerging therapeutic approaches, including strategies that limit free radical production and oxidative stress, as well as biologic therapies that may slow the advance of PSP and CBD by preventing the aggregation of tau.

References

1. Lauterbach EC. The neuropsychiatry of Parkinson's disease and related disorders. *Psychiatr Clin North Am.* 2004;27:801–825.

2. Litvan I. Diagnosis and management of progressive supranuclear palsy. *Semin Neurol.* 2001;21:41–48.

3. Litvan I, Mega MS, Cummings JL, et al. Neuropsychiatric aspects of progressive supranuclear palsy. *Neurology.* 1996;47:1184–1189.

4. Litvan I, Phipps M, Pharr VL, et al. Randomized placebo-controlled trial of donepezil in patients with progressive supranuclear palsy. *Neurology.* 2001;57(3): 467–473.
5. Aarsland D, Litvan I, Larsen JP. Neuropsychiatric symptoms of patients with progressive supranuclear palsy and Parkinson's disease. *J Neuropsychiatry Clin Neurosci.* 2001;13:42–49.
6. Pahwa R. Parkinson's disease and Parkinsonian syndromes: Progressive supranuclear palsy. *Med Clin North Am.* 1999;83:369–379.

G. Corticobasal degeneration
  1. **Clinical background and prevalence**
      a. CBD is a tauopathy and it is characterized by steadily progressive motor and cognitive disturbances.
      b. Individuals with CBD experience insidious and progressive unilateral akinesia and rigidity, as well as asymmetry in motor or sensory deficits, such as dystonia, myoclonus, alien limb syndrome, or asymmetric loss of voluntary limb control.
      c. Most patients initially present with limb clumsiness, akinesia, rigidity, and apraxia, although they may be accompanied by cortical sensory loss and an action and postural tremor.
      d. CBD is slightly more predominant in women and occurs in five to seven cases per 100,000, with a mean age of onset of 63.
  2. **Pathophysiology**
      a. Symptoms of CBD may be related to the cortical degeneration in superior frontoparietal regions.
      b. There is prefrontal and parietal atrophy, severe cortical neuronal loss, and abnormal tau protein inclusions in the substantia nigra and basal ganglia. These abnormalities are often circumscribed and are most severe contralateral to the clinically afflicted side.
  3. **Neuropsychiatric symptoms**
      a. Individuals afflicted with CBD exhibit elevated levels of apathy but also have significant depression and irritability.
      b. Anxiety, disinhibition, and psychosis are less common among those with CBD, although symptoms of obsessive-compulsive behavior occasionally emerge in the form of indecisiveness, repetitive acts, or preoccupation with perfectionism.
  4. **Treatment**
      a. See "Treatment" section for PSP.
      b. Occupational therapy can help patients maintain some degree of functional independence by providing customized devices, like utensils with long handles. Speech therapy may also offer practical exercises to optimize speech function.

References

1. Litvan I, Cummings JL, Mega M. Neuropsychiatric features of corticobasal degeneration. *J Neurosurg Psychiatry.* 1998;56:717–721.
2. Mitra K, Gangopadhaya PK, Das SK. Parkinsonism plus syndrome—A review. *Neurol India.* 2003;51:183–188.
3. Stover NP, Watts RL. Corticobasal degeneration. *Semin Neurol.* 2001;21:49–58.

H.   Frontotemporal lobar degeneration

    1.   **Clinical background and prevalence**

        a.   Frontotemporal lobar degeneration (FTLD) is a constellation of syndromes that includes frontotemporal dementia (FTD), semantic dementia (SD), and primary non-fluent aphasia (PNA) and is marked by a profound alteration of language, cognition, and character and social conduct.

        b.   The onset is usually insidious and occurs earlier than AD, typically between the ages of 45 and 65. Once the disease has developed, it assumes a gradual and progressive course.

    2.   **Pathophysiology**

        a.   Collectively, the three subtypes of FTLD share the common feature of a disproportionate atrophy and hypometabolism of the frontal and temporal structures.

        b.   The heterogeneity among these subtypes suggests potential differences in histopathology; however, research has narrowed the neuropathologic changes responsible for FTLD to neuronal loss, microvacuolation, and gliosis associated in many cases with abnormal tau-positive inclusions. In FTD, this pathology may lead to bilateral atrophy of the frontal and anterior temporal lobes.

        c.   In PNA, the corresponding atrophy is asymmetric, chiefly involving the left frontotemporal lobes, whereas the atrophy in SD is typically bilateral involving anterior temporal regions.

        d.   Tau mutations represent the first and most obvious candidates for understanding the genetics of FTLD. There is a significant risk effect associated with the APOE-2 allele and the 3-repeat and 4-repeat tau of the *MAPT* gene.

    3.   **Diagnosis**

        a.   FTD is marked by a profound change in character and disordered social conduct. Its core diagnostic features include an insidious onset and gradual progression, an early decline in interpersonal decorum, disinhibition in interpersonal conduct, and both emotional blunting and a loss of insight.

        b.   PNA refers to a disorder of expressive language that is manifested in nonfluent spontaneous speech, together with some combination of agrammatism, phonemic paraphasias, or anomia. Other cognitive and social skills are intact early in the disease process, although there may be additional speech and language difficulties, like stuttering, impaired repetition, or alexia.

   c. Patients with SD have fluent and syntactically correct spontaneous speech, but their speech is empty and anomic. They have difficulty comprehending the meaning of words and experience prosopagnosia and/or associative agnosia.

4. **Neuropsychiatric symptoms**

   a. Despite the importance of the cognitive features, it is the neuropsychiatric and behavioral symptoms of FTLD that frequently lead patients to evaluation. In fact, behavior and personality changes frequently precede cognitive changes in the FTLD syndrome.

   b. Compared with patients having AD, those with FTD evidence greater disinhibition and apathy. It is not uncommon for these patients to express disinhibition by making lewd remarks, laughing in inappropriate situations, or engaging in inappropriate behaviors.

   c. Emotionally, they are often blunted and stifled in their capacity for demonstrating joy, sadness, or empathy. Those with FTD also report less depression than those with SD.

5. **Treatment**

   a. Currently there is no established pharmacologic treatment for dementia in patients with FTLD. There is no specific abnormality of the presynaptic cholinergic system, so cholinesterase inhibitors are not indicated.

   b. We recommend the use of selective serotonin reuptake inhibitors (SSRIs) (i.e., zoloft) and specific behavioral interventions to treat the neuropsychiatric and behavioral symptoms. Strategies include cognitive remediation for social misconduct and stereotypy, dietary restrictions to offset the risk of weight gain from hyperorality, and reality orientation and adherence to standard routines to compensate for lack of insight and to guard against the dangers of disinhibition.

   c. Considering the level of distress that patients and caregivers experience from these neuropsychiatric symptoms, it is increasingly important to incorporate neuropsychiatric treatment into the overall treatment plan for patients with FTLD.

References

1. Hodges JR. Frontotemporal dementia (pick's disease): Clinical features and assessment. *Neurology.* 2001;56(11): 1–8.

2. Mourik JC, Rosso SM, Niermeijer MF, et al. Frontotemporal dementia: Behavioral symptoms and caregiver distress. *Dement Geriatri Cogn Disord.* 2004;18: 299–306.

3. Neary D, Snowden JS, Gustafson L, et al. Frontotemporal lobar degeneration: A consensus on clinical diagnostic criteria. *Neurology.* 1998;51(6):1–20.

4. Ratnavalli E, Brayne C, Dawson K, et al. The prevalence of frontotemporal dementia. *Neurology.* 2002;58(11): 1–12.
5. Rosen HJ, Gorno-Tempini ML, Goldman WP, et al. Patterns of brain atrophy in frontotemporal dementia and semantic dementia. *Neurology.* 2002;58(2):1–20.
6. Srikanth S, Nagaraja AV, Ratnavalli E. Neuropsychiatric symptoms in dementia-frequency, relationship to dementia severity and comparison in Alzheimer disease vascular dementia and frontotemporal dementia. *J Neurol Sci.* 2005;236:43–48.

I. **Prion diseases**
   1. **Clinical background and diagnosis**
      a. Although the incidence of prion diseases is relatively rare, they have recently been in the forefront of public attention in light of the new form transmitted from cows with bovine spongiform encephalopathy ("mad cow disease").
      b. Prion diseases represent a group of rare fatal spongiform encephalopathies that can result from mutations, polymorphisms, or transmission of the *prion protein* gene (*PrP*) or corresponding protein.
      c. Currently, four human illnesses are recognized as prion disorders, the most important of which is Creutzfeldt-Jakob disease (CJD). Kuru, Gerstmann-Straussler-Scheinker disease, and fatal familial insomnia constitute the other forms of prion disease.
      d. Probable CJD is diagnosed by a history of rapidly progressive dementia, typical periodic complexes on electroencephalgrams (EEGs), and at least two of the following: Myoclonus, visual or cerebellar signs, pyramidal/extrapyramidal signs, or akinetic mutism.
      e. Unfortunately, the vague and nonspecific nature of symptoms often leads to misdiagnosis and the absence of a complete evaluation until individuals are in the moderate to advanced stages.
   2. **Neuropsychiatric symptoms.** Apathy, depression, and emotional lability are common during the prodromal and early phases.
   3. **Treatment.** Currently, there are no proven treatments for any of the prion diseases, although psychotropic agents may reduce behavioral disturbances, which are heterogeneous and include anxiety, depression, delusion, emotional lability, agitation, and apathy.
   References
   1. Mendez MF, Cummings JL. *Dementia: A clinical approach,* 3rd ed. Philadelphia, PA: Butterworth-Heinemann; 2003.

III. DEMENTIA FROM INFECTIOUS AGENTS

A. **Human immunodeficiency virus–associated dementia**
   1. **Clinical background and prevalence**
      a. Human immunodeficiency virus–associated dementia (HAD) is the most common viral dementia and represents

a chronic, neurodegenerative syndrome that occurs in the later stages of human immunodeficiency virus (HIV) infection when immunodeficiency has developed.

b. It affects 15% to 20% of patients with acquired immunodeficiency syndrome (AIDS) and carries a prognosis of 2 to 12 months, with an average 6-month survival rate without treatment.

c. Other infectious causes of dementia include neurosyphilis, Lyme disease, and Whipple disease.

2. **Pathophysiology**

a. The profile of HAD has been likened to subcortical dementia because a significant part of the disease process involves the infection of subcortical brain structures, like the basal ganglia, substantia nigra, and deep white matter.

b. HAD results from high HIV viral loads that enter the CNS and infect monocytes and macrophages, which are subsequently activated to release toxins that cause meningitis and eventual dendritic and synaptic damage and neuronal death.

3. **Diagnosis**

a. To meet criteria for HAD, individuals must be HIV-1 seropositive and display an acquired abnormality in motor functioning or a decline in motivation/emotional control, as well as deficits in at least two cognitive domains.

b. Neuroimaging and neuropsychologic testing are often the first step in determining the cognitive and behavioral alterations that reflect HAD. The presence of HAD on neuroimaging is supported by atrophy with diffuse loss of gray matter volume, selective loss in caudate regions, and periventricular white matter lesions.

4. **Neuropsychiatric symptoms**

Some patients have neuropsychiatric features like agitation, mania, obsessive-compulsive behavior, and persecutory delusions and auditory hallucinations. As the disease advances, increased apathy emerges.

5. **Treatment**

a. Patients should receive highly active antiretroviral therapy (HAART), a combination treatment that pairs azidothymidine (AZT) with reverse transcriptase inhibitors and protease inhibitors. HAART may lengthen survival time to 44 months.

b. Cholinergic agents have also been used in traumatic brain injury and postviral syndromes though these are typically clinical observations and are not supported by any clinical trial studies. If used, procedures for prescribing are the same as that employed for treatment of patients with AD (see preceding text).

References

1. Adams MA, Ferraro FR. Acquired immunodeficiency syndrome dementia complex. *J Clin Psychol*. 1997;53(7): 767–778.
2. Baldewicz TT, Leserman J, Silva SG, et al. Changes in neuropsychological functioning with progression of HIV-1 infection: Results of an 8-year longitudinal investigation. *AIDS Behav*. 2004;8(3):345–355.
3. Rausch DM, Stover ES. Neuroscience research in AIDS. *Neuro-Psychopharmacol Biol Psychiatry*. 2001;25:231–257.
4. Reger M, Welsh R, Razani J, et al. A meta-analysis of the neuropsychological sequelae of HIV infection. *J Int Neuropsychol Soc*. 2002;8:410–424.

B. **Non-human immunodeficiency virus causes of dementia from infectious agents: Viral encephalitis**
   1. Viral encephalitis is an inflammation of the brain parenchyma. In the acute phase, it produces illness with fever and alterations of consciousness, with 55% of patients having mild-to-severe cognitive deficits after the acute stage and 15% eventually developing dementia.
   2. Herpes simplex encephalitis is the most common sporadic viral encephalitis, with common features of seizures, fever, aphasia, and mental abnormalities. Currently, the mortality rate from herpes simplex encephalitis is up to 75%.
      a. Because the medial temporal and orbitofrontal regions are severely damaged in herpes simplex encephalitis, there is anterograde memory dysfunction, personality change, motor deficits, aphasia, amnestic syndrome, and epilepsy. Some patients develop the Kluver-Bucy syndrome, panic and anxiety disorders, manic behavior, and affective disorders.
      b. Acyclovir has emerged as a significant treatment for the infection that can decrease impairment and mortality rates to 19%, with greatest prognosis if initiated within 4 days of the onset of symptoms.
   3. Other causes of viral encephalitis include subacute sclerosising panencephalitis, progressive rubella panencephalitis, progressive multifocal leukoencephalopathy, and fungal causes of meningitis.
   4. As in HIV, cholinergic agents have been used in postviral syndromes and found to be efficacious in clinical observations but there is no clinical trial data. Same procedures as that used for treatment of patients with AD should be employed (see preceding text).

References

1. Hokkanen L, Launes J. Cogntiive outcome in acute sporadic encephalitis. *Neuropsychol Rev*. 2000;10:151–167.
2. Mendez MF, Cummings JL Dementia from conventional infectious agents. In: *Dementia: A clinical approach*. Philadelphia, PA: Butterworth-Heinemann; 2003.

IV. TOXIC AND METABOLIC CAUSES OF DEMENTIA

A. Toxic dementias
  1. Alcohol-related dementia
    a. Dementia can arise from a variety of chemical agents and environmental toxins, including alcohol.
    b. Although light-to-moderate levels of alcohol consumption have been associated with reduced risk for dementia, heavy alcohol intake can result in alcohol-related dementia (ARD). It is more apparent in the elderly than young adults, and it appears earlier in women even with less consumption.
    c. ARD is diagnosed when (a) a clinical diagnosis of dementia has been made at least 60 days after the last exposure to alcohol, (b) the individual has consumed over 35 drinks per week for >5 years, and (c) the period of significant alcohol use is within 3 years of the initial onset of dementia. Supportive features include ataxia or peripheral sensory polyneuropathy, cognitive improvement beyond 60 days of abstinence, and alcohol-related hepatic, pancreatic, gastrointestinal, or cardiovascular disease. It is important to gather an extensive clinical history of alcohol use, incorporating family, friends, and past medical records to ensure accuracy.
    d. ARD is a mildly and minimally progressive disorder that creates executive and memory deficits associated with both cortical and subcortical neuropathology. It is characterized by poor working memory, decreased verbal fluency, poor visuospatial functioning, reduced verbal memory, and impaired abstraction. However, abstinence can result in a partial reversal of neuropsychological deficits, creating a potentially reversible form of dementia.
  2. Wernicke-Korsakoff syndrome
    a. In Wernicke-Korsakoff syndrome, poor nutritional intake associated with alcohol dependence results in severe thiamine deficiency. This frequently engenders the classic clinical triad of ophthalmoplegia, ataxia, and mental confusion (Wernicke encephalophathy), followed by prolonged amnestic disorder (Korsakoff syndrome).
    b. The Korsakoff element is characterized by confabulation, executive deficits, an inability to learn new material, and poor recall for information learned up to several years before onset.
    c. The natural treatment for Wernicke-Korsakoff syndrome is thiamine administration. If thiamine is administered within hours of the acute onset of Wernicke encephalopathy and subsequently maintained, these abnormalities may gradually resolve over the next several days.
    d. There are no FDA-approved medications for treatment of ARD, but considering that thiamine deficiency may be correlated with reduced cortical acetylcholine,

acetylcholinesterase inhibitors may have partial benefit in cognitive functioning in patients with ARD. Refer to the section on treatment of AD for prescribing procedures.

References
1. Oslin D, Atkinson RM, Smith DM, et al. Alcohol related dementia: Proposed clinical criteria. *Int J Geriatr Psychiatry.* 1998;13:203–212.
2. Schmidt KS, Gallo JL, Ferri C, et al. The neuropsychological profile of alcohol-related dementia suggests cortical and subcortical pathology. *Dement Geriatr Cogn Disord.* 2005;20:286–291.

B. **Acquired metabolic dementias**
1. Chronic hypoxia results in insufficient oxygen to the brain and the development of an ischemic dementia that manifests a frontal-subcortical profile.
2. Sleep apnea represents one hypoxemic cause of cognitive deficits due to recurrent nocturnal oxygen desaturation and hypercapnia. It occurs in above 30% of older populations, with greater prevalence in men. It typically results in daytime somnolence, attention deficits, and memory impairment. Depression and anxiety are also common. Treatment involves continuous positive airway pressure and tricyclic compounds that suppress REM sleep when desaturation and apneas occur.
3. Diabetes mellitus and glucose metabolism can increase risk for dementia due to metabolic and vascular changes related to chronic hyperglycemia and deficits in insulin action. Correction of hypoglycemia will halt progression, but not reverse existing deficits.
4. Deficiencies in vitamins may disrupt normal cellular metabolism and give rise to symptoms of dementia. B_{12} deficiency frequently results from autoimmune chronic atrophic gastritis, malnutrition, or malabsorption. It can cause demyelinating myelopathy, psychomotor slowing, cognitive confusion, memory defects, and psychiatric symptoms, including neurologic depression and occasional psychosis.
5. Diagnosis of B_{12} deficiency is determined by serum B_{12} levels below 200 pg per mL. Treatment consists of administering 1000 μg of vitamin B_{12} daily for 10 days, weekly for a month, and monthly thereafter. Although neurologic improvement will usually occur within a few days of therapy, the dementia syndrome remains irreversible and permanent deficits usually remain.
6. Other metabolic causes of dementia include sodium abnormalities, hypo- and hyperthyroidism, Cushing disease, and other conditions.

References
1. Bliwise DL. Is sleep apnea a cause of reversible dementia in old age? *J Am Geriatr Soc.* 1996;11:1407–1408.
2. Rita M, Paola T, Rodolfo A, et al. Vitamin B12 and folate depletion in cognition: A review. *Neurol India.* 2004;52: 310–318.

C. Normal pressure hydrocephalus
  1. **Clinical background and diagnosis**
     a. Normal pressure hydrocephalus (NPH) is distinguished by the clinical triad of gait disturbance, urinary incontinence, and cognitive impairment that presents as a dementia syndrome.
     b. It accounts for not <5% of dementia cases and typically occurs during the sixth and seventh decades of life.
     c. Gait instability is usually the earliest and most prominent symptom, characterized by slow gait, short and shuffling steps, and wide-based stance. This is followed by urinary urgency and incontinence.
  2. **Pathophysiology**
     a. The basic physiologic disturbance in NPH is an abnormal balance between cerebrospinal fluid (CSF) production and CSF absorption.
     b. Scarring or fibrosis may obscure absorptive interfaces and interfere with CSF flow, creating a pressure gradient that leads to decreased CSF production. This new pressure distends the ventricles, compresses the periventricular parenchyma, and deforms white matter tracks that instigate gait abnormalities, incomplete bladder control, and difficulties with processing speed.
     c. For two thirds of patients, there is a discoverable etiology for NPH, with subarachnoid hemorrhages, cranial traumas, and meningitis being the most frequent causes.
  3. **Neuropsychiatric symptoms**
     a. Most patients with NPH present as emotionally indifferent or disengaged, although a subset of them may display emotional lability, hostility, and paranoid psychoses.
     b. They are frequently apathetic and appear depressed and bradyphrenic, but they lack depressive thought content.
  4. **Treatment**
     a. NPH represents one of the few potentially reversible causes of dementia, making it imperative to engage in diagnosis and referral at the slightest suspicion of the disorder.
     b. Diagnostic testing is critical in differentiating from other profiles of dementia and other movement disorders. NPH is implicated when routine spinal taps and lumbar punctures reveal normal levels of CSF protein and glucose, a white blood cell count of five or fewer cells per mcL, and an opening pressure of <200 mm H_2O. Placement of an intracranial pressure monitor can determine episodic waves of high pressure that are characteristic of NPH. Cranial neuroimaging studies (CT scan and MRI) frequently lend to a diagnosis when they reveal enlarged ventricles without commensurate cortical atrophy.
     c. The most common therapy for NPH is ventriculoperitoneal shunting, where CSF is drained from one lateral ventricle to the sterile peritoneal cavity. After shunt surgery,

approximately 60% of patients with NPH show improvement in activities of daily living, urinary control, and ambulation, with 50% showing improvement in the first month.

d. However, considering the potential side effects of shunting (i.e., subdural hematomas, infections, epilepsy), it is strongly recommended to those with a short history of mental deterioration, a known secondary cause for hydrocephalus, substantial improvement after CSF taps, and strong indications of NPH on diagnostic testing.

References
1. Hebb AO, Cusimano MD. Idiopathic normal pressure hydrocephalus: A systematic review of diagnosis and outcome. *Neurosurgery.* 2001;49:1166–1186.
2. Vanneste JAL. Diagnosis and management of normal-pressure hyrdocephalus. *J Neurol.* 2000;247:5–14.
3. Verrees M, Selman W. Management of normal pressure hydrocephalus. *Am Fam Phys.* 2004;70:1071–1078, 1085–1086.

D. **Treatment for the neuropsychiatric symptoms of dementia**
1. The neuropsychiatric and behavioral features of dementia are the most troubling to patients and family members. These behavioral features may include negative symptoms like apathy/indifference, as well as positive symptoms like depression, anxiety, agitation, psychosis, and disinhibition. Behavioral symptoms are highly prevalent among patients in clinics, research centers or nursing homes, and occur in 90% of those individuals with dementia living in the community.[1] These symptoms not only accelerate cognitive deterioration and functional impairment, but they are also associated with increased burden and psychological morbidity of caregivers, earlier institutionalization and residential placement, and increased medical care and costs.

2. It is critically important to explore the neuropsychiatric symptoms associated with different types of dementia, as well as their pathophysiology and corresponding treatment.

a. **Psychotropic agents**
   (1) Atypical antipsychotics or mood-stabilizing anticonvulsants are frequently given to patients with agitation or psychosis. The former is the treatment of choice due to the adverse side effects of conventional neuroleptic agents and limited efficacy of mood-stabilizing anticonvulsants (see Chapter 7).
   (2) In clinical trials, administration of olanzapine and risperidone significantly reduced symptoms of psychosis and agitation in patients with AD, VaD, and PDD (Mendez & Cummings, 2003).[2]
   (3) Atypical antipsychotics do not confer a significant benefit to the neuropsychiatric symptoms and hallucinations among those with DLB. Approximately

one half of patients with DLB who are treated with neuroleptics develop severe side effects.

(4) Despite their potential efficacy in managing neuropsychiatric symptoms, the benefits of atypical antipsychotics need to be carefully weighed against their potential adverse effects. The FDA reported a nearly twofold increase in rate of death among elderly patients with dementia who were treated for their neuropsychiatric symptoms with atypical antipsychotic medication. On the basis of a review of 17 placebo-controlled studies of olanzapine, aripiprazole, risperidone, and quetiapine, the agency reported a 4.5% mortality rate among elderly patients with dementia who were treated with these medications compared with a 2.6% mortality rate among patients treated with a placebo.[3]

(5) Apathy may respond to psychostimulants or related agents, such as methylphenidate, dextroamphetamine, or modafanil (see Chapter 1).

(6) To treat the depression that accompanies VaD, PDD, and other dementias, most clinicians elect to use SSRIs, which are preferred above tricyclic antidepressants due to the latter's anticholinergic side effects (see Chapter 5).

(7) SSRIs are also the treatment of choice for the disinhibition and repetition syndromes that characterize FTLD (see Chapter 11).

(8) Clinicians have used trazadone and other SSRIs for treatment of agitation, which has met with mixed success.

b. **Cholinesterase inhibitors**

(1) Considerable evidence is emerging to suggest that treatment with cholinesterase inhibitors may reduce neuropsychiatric symptoms. Central to these findings is the idea that many neuropsychiatric symptoms are linked to brain regions that have substantial cholinergic dysfunction.[4]

(2) A study found that 294 patients with moderate-to-severe AD exhibited improvement in depression, agitation, and apathy after 24 weeks of receiving donepezil.[5] Among those receiving standard treatments of galantamine for mild-to-moderate AD, there are pronounced reductions in psychosis, apathy, agitation, and depression. Similar findings have been reported with rivastigmine.

(3) Patients with DLB are generally less apathetic, less agitated, and experience fewer hallucinations and delusions after taking rivistigmine. Those taking rivastigmine are twice as likely as those on placebo to

show more than 30% improvement in hallucinations and psychosis.

(4) Rivastigmine is associated with improvement in cognition, hallucinations, and sleep disturbance among those with PDD.

(5) These findings suggest that cholinesterase inhibitors may have not only cognitive and functional effects, but also psychotropic effects.

References

1. Ikeda M, Fukuhara R, Shigenobu K, et al. Dementia associated mental and behavioural disturbances in elderly people in the community: Findings from the first Nakayama study. *J Neurol Neurosurg Psychiatry.* 2004;75:146–148.
2. Mulsant BH, Gharabawi GM, Bossie CA, et al. Correlates of anticholinergic activity in patients with dementia and psychosis treated with risperidone or olanzapine. *J Clin Psychiatry.* 2004;65(12):1708–1714.
3. Kuehu BM. FDA warns antipsychotic drugs may be risky for elderly. *JAMA.* 2005;293(20):2462.
4. Cummings JL, Back C. The cholinergic hypothesis of neuropsychiatric symptoms in Alzheimer's disease. *Am J Geriatr Psychiatry.* 1998;6(2):64–78.
5. Gauthier S, Feldman H, Hecker J, et al. Efficacy of donepezil on behavioral symptoms in patients with moderate to severe Alzheimer's disease. *Int Psychogeriatr.* 2002;14(4):389–404.

c. **Nonpharmacologic interventions**
(1) When developing a biopsychosocial treatment plan for the neuropsychiatric symptoms of dementia, it is important to incorporate nonpharmacologic interventions. These types of treatments may have particular utility with the neuropsychiatric and behavioral features of dementia.
(2) Some common neuropsychiatric symptoms of dementia may be responses to needs that have not been met, poor learning, or greater responsiveness to one's environment. To the extent this is true, the best treatment of these neuropsychiatric symptoms may be to match a patient's target symptom with a corresponding intervention, which may occasionally involve addressing the patient at a psychological level, rather than intervening exclusively at a biologic level.
(a) Simple changes in a patient's physical environment, like removing distracting stimuli, creating natural environments using audiotapes of nature, or personalizing one's environment and offering multimodal sensory stimulation, can significantly reduce agitation and aggression.[1]

(b) Many patients experience reduced agitation and improved depression by participating in activity programs like a walking program, reminiscence groups, interactions with pets, or simulated social interactions with other adults.[2]

(c) Music, massage, and light therapies all alleviate some of the neuropsychiatric symptoms of agitation, depression, and aggression.

(d) Although the capacity for learning is limited in patients with dementia, cognitive and behavioral interventions can help reduce disinhibition, restructure thoughts that may be contributing to depression, and reduce agitation by increasing personal structure.

(e) It is essential to provide education and treatment services to caregivers, including developing psychoeducational programs, discussing community resources, and encouraging personal therapy.

References

1. Cohen-Mansfield J. Nonpharmacologic interventions for inappropriate behaviors in dementia. *Am J Geriatr Psychiatry.* 2001;9(4): 361–381.

2. Opie J, Rosewarne R, O'Connor DW. The efficacy of psychosocial approaches to behaviour disorders in dementia: A systematic literature review. *Aust N Z J Psychiatry.* 1999;33:789–799.

V. CONCLUSION

When formulating and implementing these interventions, it is important to keep in mind that the actual content or format of the intervention are not crucial. It is the customization of one's interventions according to the interests, history, and needs of the individual patient that creates effective treatment. In essence, these interventions attempt to respect the emotions that may accompany neuropsychiatric symptoms, insure that patients and caregivers are truly heard and understood, and intervene in a personal and compassionate way.

Chapter 5

DISTURBANCES OF MOOD, AFFECT, AND EMOTION

C. Edward Coffey

I. BACKGROUND

A. **Definitions**

1. *Mood* refers to the feeling state that one is experiencing at a particular moment in time, and its qualities can be either positive (e.g., happiness, or relief) or negative (e.g., sadness, anger, disgust; apprehension, fear, terror, etc.).

2. The term "mood" is not synonymous with the term *affect*, which refers to the behavioral domain in which the mood is expressed. Affect can be conceptualized quantitatively by the range (flat or narrow to broad), intensity (shallow to deep), and stability of mood (rigid to labile), and qualitatively by the appropriateness (congruence with situation or thought content) and relatedness of the mood. Mood is the content of affect. Mood is to affect as weather is to climate.

3. *Emotion* may be defined as the moods, affects, and related physiologic states that are associated with specific thoughts, ideas, or stimuli (particularly reinforcing stimuli).

4. Emotions have many functions including interpersonal (e.g., communication, or social bonding), cognitive (e.g., by affecting a perception or cognitive evaluation, by facilitating storage or recall of a memory, etc.), and motivation and preparation for action (including elicitation of autonomic and endocrine responses), all of which have survival value.

B. **Classification of mood syndromes and disorders.** Disturbances of mood include *depression, mania/hypomania,* and *anxiety*. These terms can be used to describe a normal mood, a clinical syndrome, or a group of specific disorders (Table 5.1).

TABLE 5.1   Classification of Mood and
Mood Episode Syndromes

Depression
- Normal sadness
- Adjustment disorder
- Bereavement
- Major depressive episode
    Secondary
    Primary

Elated Mood and Mania/Hypomania
- Normal happiness
- Manic episode
    Secondary
    Primary
- Mixed episode
    Secondary
    Primary
- Hypomanic episode
    Secondary
    Primary

1.   **Depressed mood and the major depressive syndrome**
     a.   As a *normal (nonpathologic) ubiquitous mood state*, feelings of
          depression are synonymous with feeling sad, blue, down,
          or unhappy. Such feelings are common following a loss or
          disappointment, and typically last only hours to days. More
          severe depressive symptoms may occur in the setting of
          significant stress. The term *adjustment disorder* is used when
          a recent (within 3 months) stressor produces symptoms that
          do not meet criteria for a mood disorder (see subsequent
          text). The loss of a loved one may result in even more severe
          depressive symptoms (this mood state is called *bereavement*),
          but in such settings would not be diagnosed as a major
          depressive disorder unless the symptoms are especially
          severe or prolonged. Bereavement that lasts longer than
          12 months is called a *pathologic grief reaction*, and may be
          seen when the survivor was excessively dependent upon
          the deceased, or is unable to grieve adequately or to obtain
          emotional and other (e.g., financial) support.
     b.   The clinical syndrome of a *major depressive episode* is defined
          by either *abnormal* sadness or loss of interest or pleasure,
          occurring for most of the time for at least 2 weeks, to-
          gether with four or more of the following symptoms:
          Weight loss or decrease in appetite, insomnia or hyper-
          somnia, psychomotor agitation or retardation, fatigue or
          loss of energy, feelings of worthlessness or inappropriate
          guilt, impaired concentration and thinking, and recurrent

thoughts of death or suicide. All these symptoms must cause clinically significant distress or functional impairment.

2. **Elated mood and the manic/hypomanic syndromes**

   a. Elated mood states (elation, exaltation, euphoria, and ecstasy) are normal when life is going well, or when major goals are achieved, as well as in states of love, sexual pleasure, and religious fervor and transcendence.

   b. The clinical syndrome of a *manic episode* is defined by *abnormally* elated (or irritable) mood lasting for at least 1 week, together with three or more of the following symptoms: Inflated self-esteem or grandiosity, decreased need for sleep, talkativeness, flight of ideas or racing thoughts, distractibility, increased psychomotor activity, and excessive involvement in pleasurable activities. All these symptoms must cause clinically significant distress or functional impairment.

   c. Mania may present in a milder form (known as a *hypomanic episode*) or together with a major depressive episode (known as a *mixed episode*).

3. **Mood disorders (Table 5.2)**

   a. Disorders of mood are conceptualized by their presumed etiology. *Secondary mood disorders* are those that are presumed to be a direct physiologic effect of either a substance (e.g., medication, toxin, or drug of abuse) or a general medical (including neurologic) condition. All other disorders are referred to as *primary mood disorders*.

   b. Primary disorders of mood are classified as either *depressive disorders* or *bipolar disorders* (DSM-IV).

      (1) The essential feature of *depressive disorders* is one or more episodes of major depression *without* a history of either manic or hypomanic episodes. There are three

TABLE 5.2   Classification of Mood Disorders

Secondary Mood Disorders
- Substance-induced mood disorder
- Mood disorder due to a general medical (including neurologic) condition

Depressive Disorders
- Major depressive disorder
- Dysthymic disorder
- Depressive disorder NOS

Bipolar Disorders
- Bipolar I disorder
- Bipolar II disorder
- Cyclothymic disorder
- Bipolar disorder NOS

NOS, not otherwise specified.

depressive disorders—major depressive disorder (characterized by one or more episodes of major depression), dysthymic disorder (characterized by at least a 2-year history of depressed mood that does not meet diagnostic criteria for major depression), and depressive disorder not otherwise specified (NOS) (Table 5.2).

(2) The essential feature of *bipolar disorders* is the presence of one or more manic or hypomanic episodes, usually (but not always) with a history of major depressive episodes. There are three bipolar disorders–bipolar disorder with manic (type I) or hypomanic (type II) episodes (usually with major depression), cyclothymic disorder (characterized by at least a 2-year history of numerous hypomanic episodes and depressed mood that does not meet diagnostic criteria for major depression), and bipolar disorder NOS (Table 5.2).

4. **Affective lability and dissociation of mood and affect**

   a. Although not classified as a syndrome in the Diagnostic and Statistical Manual of Mental Disorders, 4th edition (DSM-IV), *affective lability* ("emotional incontinence") is common in a manic episode and in several neuropsychiatric disorders, particularly in patients with mental retardation (see Chapter 16) or frontal lobe dysfunction (see Chapters 3 and 12). Patients with affective labililty are typically irritable and may shift rapidly from positive (happiness, or euphoria) to negative (sadness, or anger) mood states. These emotional outbursts are usually short lived, and the affect is congruent with the mood (e.g., the patient both appears and feels angry).

   b. A lack of congruence between affect and mood is known as *pathologic affect* (or pseudobulbar affect), a condition which characterizes some neuropsychiatric disorders. These patient's may laugh or cry excessively in a situation that is not consistent with such an emotional reaction, and when questioned will deny they feel the emotional intensity they are displaying. Dissociation of mood and affect is most commonly seen in patients with bilateral lesions of the upper brainstem and diencephalon. The pathophysiology of this condition is not known but may involve a disturbance in brainstem motor nuclei involved in emotional expression, and in regulatory neurons that project to the cortex.

5. **Anxiety.** These mood states and related disorders are common in neuropsychiatric disorders and are discussed in Chapter 6.

6. **Apathy and emotional blunting.** These mood states and related disorders are common in neuropsychiatric disorders and are discussed in Chapter 1.

C. **Epidemiology**

   1. Depressive symptoms and syndromes are reported to be two to three times more common in patients with certain neurologic disorders than in control or reference populations (Table 5.3).

**TABLE 5.3   Prevalence of Depression
in Patients with Neurologic Disease**

Poststroke	~5–40%
Alzheimer disease	~20–50%
Parkinson disease	~10–50%
Huntington disease	~40%
Traumatic brain injury	~33%
Multiple sclerosis	~25%
Epilepsy	~55%

The precise prevalence rates are difficult to establish given wide methodologic variation in the published reports, but in general, depressive *symptoms* are more common than depressive *syndromes* in patients with neurologic illness.

2. *Euphoria and mania/hypomania* have been described in patients with a variety of neurologic disorders but again, the precise prevalence rates are difficult to establish given methodologic variation in the published reports, many of which are case reports or small case series. The highest rates of euphoria and mania/hypomania have been reported for patients with Huntington disease (~9%), traumatic brain injury (TBI) (~9%), multiple sclerosis (0 to 67%), and epilepsy (~5%). Mania occurring for the first time in an elderly individual should raise suspicion of an associated medical or neurologic disorder.

D. **Prognosis.** Very little literature exists on the course and prognosis of mood disorders associated with a neurologic illness. These limited data are consistent, however, in suggesting that *depression* following a neurologic illness may persist for months and even years after onset, and its presence may increase both the morbidity and mortality of the illness (see subsequent text on discussion of specific illness). Even less is known about the course and prognosis of *mania/hypomania* associated with a neurologic illness.

II. NEUROBIOLOGY AND PATHOPHYSIOLOGY OF MOOD

A. **Normal emotion.** The neurobiology of normal emotional behavior is not fully understood. One model posits that emotional experiences are mediated by interplay between subcortical regions (e.g., hypothalamus, or amygdala) and higher brain centers. In response to emotionally relevant stimuli, *subcortical systems* (particularly the hypothalamus) coordinate autonomic, endocrine, and skeletomotor responses (arousal) that alter the internal milieu and prepare the organism to respond appropriately (fight or flight). *Cortical (prefrontal cortex, cingulate, or parahippocampal) systems* respond by filtering the stimuli and assessing their significance to the organism. Although this assessment is presumably based on learning and memory, it may also be affected by the relative contributions to the assessment of the left (positive emotional valence) and right (negative emotional valence) cerebral hemispheres. Once the assessment is made, these cortical systems communicate with the subcortical systems to enhance or suppress the somatic responses (the right hemisphere appears to drive cortical arousal by activating the reticular activating system). This bidirectional processing between cortical and subcortical systems, may be mediated in part by the *limbic system* (particularly the *amygdala*), which is also critically involved in mediating both inborn and learned emotional responses. It is this "cross talk" between neocortical and subcortical systems together with the somatic feedback from the periphery, which appear to mediate the *experience* of a particular emotion.

The communication between these cortical and subcortical systems is accomplished primarily by chemical neurotransmitters, the activity of which may impact the emotional state because of mediation of arousal (norepinephrine), motivation and reward (dopamine), and mood and impulsivity (serotonin).

B. Depressive disorders

1. **Major depression.** The pathophysiology of major depression is not fully understood. Depression may be the result of genetically determined (primary mood disorders have a strong genetic predisposition) defects in neurotransmitter function (particularly serotonin and norepinephrine) that may occur *de novo* or in response to psychosocial stress (the *stress-diathesis model*). We do not understand the mechanisms that cause these presumed neurotransmitter disturbances. Depression is associated with a myriad of neurobiologic disturbances (sleep, neuroendocrine, neurotransmitter; immunologic, and cerebral structure, blood flow, and metabolism, particularly of frontal-subcortical regions), most of which are consistent with an exaggerated stress response. We do not know whether these changes reflect causal associations or epiphenomena.

2. **Depression in patients with a neurologic illness.** The pathophysiology of depression in patients with neurologic illness is not known, but is likely to be heterogeneous. Depression may reflect some combination of an emotional reaction to deficits from the neurologic illness (e.g., an adjustment disorder with depressed mood), a recurrence of a preexisting mood disorder, a result of other neurologic or general medical problems, or a direct effect of the neurologic illness on brain systems that mediate emotion.

   Studies in patients with brain disease suggest a relation between depression and lesions of particular brain regions including the left frontal-subcortical regions (cerebrovascular disease, or TBI), the basal ganglia (Parkinson disease, or Huntington disease), and the anterior limbic system (complex partial epilepsy, or multiple sclerosis) (discussed in the subsequent text).

C. Mania/hypomania

1. **Manic episode.** The pathophysiology of mania/hypomania and bipolar disorder are not known. Most of what is known is similar to that described for major depression.

2. **Mania/hypomania in patients with a neurologic illness.** Mania/ hypomania is seen much less frequently in association with brain disease than is depression. Studies in patients with brain disease suggest a relation between mania and lesions of the right cortical (orbitofrontal or basotemporal cortex) or right subcortical (thalamus, head of the caudate) regions (discussed in the subsequent text).

III. MANAGEMENT

A. **Principles of management.** In general, the management of mood disorders in patients with neurologic illness (regardless of whether the depression is considered to be "secondary" to the neurologic illness) should follow the Principles of Management recommended by the American Psychiatric Association (APA) (2000, 2002) for patients with primary mood disorders.
   1. **Perform a diagnostic evaluation**
      a. The diagnosis of a mood disorder in patients with neurologic illness is challenging. Some controversy exists about the most appropriate method for diagnosing mood syndromes in patients with neurologic or general medical conditions, because some of the signs or symptoms (e.g., weight loss, and insomnia) may result from the general medical or neurologic illness. Still, most data support the validity of an *"inclusive" approach* (i.e., counting depressive symptoms regardless of whether they may be related to the general medical illness). An additional diagnostic challenge relates to the assessment of symptoms that require verbal expression (e.g., sadness, hopelessness, etc.) in patients who cannot speak (e.g., due to an aphasia). In such cases, it may be necessary to give greater weight to clearly manifest *signs* of the mood disorder (e.g., crying, irritability, weight gain, sleep disturbance, etc.).
      b. The *mood disorder should be defined* as being a depressive disorder, a bipolar disorder, an adjustment disturbance, or a mood disorder secondary to a neurologic illness. The judgment that the mood disorder is *secondary* to the neurologic illness requires confirmation of a neurologic illness, evidence that the mood disorder is a "direct physiologic consequence" of that illness, and evidence that the mood disorder is not better accounted for by another mental disorder (see differential diagnosis in the preceding text). Determining whether the mood symptoms are "a direct physiologic consequence" of the neurologic illness may be very challenging indeed, as there are no clear rules for establishing such an association. A potential relation is suggested by a temporal association between the neurologic illness's onset, exacerbation, or remission and that of the mood disorder (e.g., the depression begins shortly after the stroke); atypical features of the mood disorder; or a well

established relation between the mood disorder and the neurologic illness.

c. *Laboratory tests* are indicated only to confirm the presence of a general medical disorder or substance use disorder (as suggested by the history or examination), or to characterize its status.

d. Evaluate and address *comorbidity*, particularly anxiety disorders, substance use disorders, and personality disorders.

e. Evaluate the *safety* of the patient and others. It is essential to assess the patient's risk of suicide or homicide.

2. **Implement a biopsychosocial treatment plan**

a. Determine and continually evaluate the *treatment setting* (inpatient vs. outpatient) based on the patient's clinical status, available support systems, and ability to care adequately for self and cooperate with treatment.

b. We do not know whether mood disorders in patients with a neurologic illness require treatment different from that for primary mood disorders. As such, treatment of these mood disorders generally employs established treatments for primary mood disorders, although the data supporting such use are limited (see subsequent text). We recommend a *biopsychosocial model*, that is the combined use of appropriate biologic (somatic) treatments (including acute phase and continuation/maintenance phase treatment), psychological treatments, and social interventions.

c. Evaluate and address *functional impairments* (e.g., in interpersonal relationships, work and living conditions, and other health-related needs).

d. Provide *education and support to the patient and family*.

e. Enhance *treatment adherence* (e.g., by simplifying the treatment regimen, minimizing the cost of treatment, education about side effects, etc.).

f. Address early signs of *relapse*.

g. *Coordinate the care* with other clinicians. Patients with a neurologic disorder will typically be receiving care from multiple clinicians, including an internist, a neurologist or neurosurgeon, a rehabilitation medicine specialist, a physical therapist, or speech therapist. Coordination of care among these many providers is essential to ensure that the care is safe and effective.

B. **Management of depression in patients with neurologic illness**

1. **Post-stroke depression**

a. **Clinical background**

(1) The 1-year *prevalence* of depression in patients with stroke varies from approximately 5% to 40%, with half of them manifesting a full major depressive episode and the other half exhibiting less severe symptoms ("minor depression").

(2) The *occurrence* of post-stroke depression (PSD) appears to be related to a personal or family history of mood

disorder, premorbid cortical atrophy, stroke location (left frontal-subcortical), and degree of functional impairment.

(3) The *phenomenology* of PSD is similar to that of a primary major depressive episode.

(4) During the *course and prognosis*, depression appears to typically last approximately 9 to 10 months, but symptoms may persist for longer periods especially in patients with cortical lesions and marked functional impairment. PSD is associated with greater impairment in activities of daily living, greater cognitive impairment, and greater (three to five times) long-term mortality. Of interest, depressive symptoms are also a prospective risk factor for stroke. Effective treatment of depression appears to reduce mortality or improve the outcome after stroke.

b. **Pathogenesis of post-stroke depression.** The *pathophysiology* of depression in patients with stroke is not known, but is likely to be heterogeneous.

c. **Diagnosis**

(1) The diagnosis is clinical and is based on the presence of criteria for a mood disorder. The diagnosis is often difficult, however, given the overlap of depressive symptoms with symptoms of stroke, or in patients with aphasia, denial/neglect, or severe dementia. Information from caregivers may greatly assist diagnosis.

(2) Post stroke apathy syndromes have to be ruled out (see Chapter 1).

(3) Hypothyroidism has to be ruled out.

d. **Treatment**

(1) *Optimize the physical health* of the patient and ensure that all underlying general medical and neurologic disorders have been optimally treated, including the provision of pain management.

(2) *Optimize the patient's environment and lifestyle,* including the promotion of exercise and a regular sleep–wake cycle. Caregivers should be instructed in *behavioral management* of the patient's behavioral problems, including prevention and modification of adverse behaviors. Caregivers should also be monitored closely for development of depression in themselves.

(3) Consider brief, structured psychotherapy (e.g., cognitive-behavioral therapy or interpersonal therapy) in patients with mild to moderately severe depression and who are able to participate in the treatment. Although its effectiveness has not been formally studied in patients with PSD, it is very safe and its efficacy is well established for acute phase treatment in primary mood disorders.

TABLE 5.4   Selected Antidepressant Treatments

Medication	Starting Dose	Dosing Range
Selective Serotonin Reuptake Inhibitors		
• Citalopram (Celexa)	10–20 mg/d	Up to 100 mg/d
• Sertraline (Zoloft)	12.5–25 mg/d	Up to 200 mg/d
Tricyclic Antidepressants		
• Nortriptyline (Pamelor; Aventyl)	10 mg at bedtime	50–75 mg (therapeutic serum level = 50–150 ng/mL)
Others		
• Buproprion (Wellbutrin)	75–150 mg buproprion/d	Up to 400 mg/d
• Venlafaxine (Effexor)	25 mg two to three times daily	Up to 375 mg/d
Brain Stimulation Procedures		
Electroconvulsive therapy	NA	
Vagus nerve stimulation	NA	
Transcranial magnetic stimulation	Experimental	
Deep brain stimulation	Experimental	

NA, not applicable.

(4) Implement somatic therapy if depression is severe or persists despite the steps listed in the preceding text. There are no U.S. Food and Drug Administration (FDA)-approved somatic treatments for PSD. Therapeutic options are the same as for major depressive disorder, that is antidepressant (Table 5.4) or mood-stabilizing medication, or electroconvulsive therapy (ECT).

(5) Treat initially with *citalopram* based on its safety and tolerability, as well as its efficacy as demonstrated in two small randomized controlled trials of patients with PSD. *Sertraline* is a reasonable alternative. It should be noted that serotonin reuptake inhibitors (SRIs) should be used with caution in patients with subarachnoid hemorrhage, where they are associated with vasospasm.

Nortriptyline is a reasonable second-line agent (efficacy demonstrated in two small randomized controlled trials of PSD), provided there are no contraindications (e.g., heart block, cardiac arrhythmia, narrow angle glaucoma) or concerns regarding sedation or orthostatic hypotension.

(6) Consider ECT in patients with PSD who are severely ill (e.g., melancholic, psychotic, suicidal) and in need of rapid clinical improvement, or who are unresponsive

to or intolerant of psychotropic medications. A small uncontrolled (primarily retrospective) clinical literature supports the safety, tolerability, and efficacy of ECT in such patients, although randomized controlled data are lacking. Several modifications in ECT technique may be required, however, based on the patient's medical/neurologic status and concerns about cognitive side effects.

(7) Give patients with psychotic symptoms an *antipsychotic medication* in addition to the antidepressant medication, although there are no controlled data on such use in patients with PSD. Atypical antipsychotic medications are generally preferred given their safety, but should be used sparingly given their small risk in the elderly of stroke and death (see Chapters 4 and 7).

(8) Continue successful acute treatment (medication or ECT) for at least 6 to 9 months. Of note, antidepressant treatment of PSD is associated with a lower mortality over the ensuing 9 years.

References

1. American Psychiatric Association: Practice guideline for the treatment of patients with major depressive disorder (revision). *Am J Psychiatry.* 2000;157: 1–45.
2. American Psychiatric Association: Practice guideline for the treatment of patients with bipolar disorder (revision). *Am J Psychiatry.* 2002;159(Suppl 4):1–50.
3. Coffey CE, Kellner CH. Electroconvulsive therapy. In: Coffey CE, Cummings JL, eds. *Textbook of geriatric neuropsychiatry*, 2nd ed. Washington, DC: American Psychiatric Press; 2000:829–859.
4. Robinson RG. The neuropsychiatry of mood disorder. In: Schiffer RB, Rao SM, Fogel BS, eds. *Neuropsychiatry*, 2nd ed. Philadelphia, PA: Lippincott Williams & Wilkins; 2003:724–749.
5. Whyte EM, Mulsant BH. Post stroke depression: epidemiology, pathophysiology, and biologic treatment. *Biol Psychiatry.* 2002;52:253–264.

2. **Depression in patients with Alzheimer disease**
   a. **Clinical background**
      (1) Depression is seen in approximately 20% to 50% of patients with Alzheimer disease (AD), with about half manifesting a full major depressive episode and the other half exhibiting minor depression.
      (2) No consistent *risk factors* have been identified. There is controversy over whether depression is more common early or late in the illness or in those patients with a family history of mood disorder, and whether it is related to the ApoE 4 or serotonin transporter genes.
      (3) The *phenomenology* of major depression in patients with AD appears to be characterized by more cognitive

disturbance, more psychotic symptoms, less sleep disturbance, and less feelings of worthlessness or excessive guilt, relative to patients without dementia.

(4) The *natural history* of depression in AD is not fully known. Depression may be the initial symptom of dementia, and may even be a risk factor for later development of AD in the elderly and in those with mild cognitive impairment. Depressive symptoms in patients with AD may persist for months, and are associated with greater physical and cognitive impairment (and hence earlier placement in higher levels of care), increased mortality or suicide, and greater caregivers burden. Effective treatment of depression may therefore reduce mortality or improve the functional status of patients with dementia, although there are no definitive data on this issue.

b. **Pathogenesis**

(1) The *pathophysiology* of depression in patients with AD is not known, but is likely to be heterogeneous.

(2) *Abnormal neurotransmission* may be involved, in that postmortem studies of patients with AD have found a relation between depression and loss of noradrenergic neurons in the locus ceruleus, and with loss of dorsal raphe serotonergic nuclei.

(3) Depression in patients with AD does not appear to be related to the severity of the dementia nor the patient's insight into having AD.

c. **Diagnosis**

(1) The diagnosis is clinical and is based on the presence of criteria for a mood disorder. The diagnosis is often difficult, however, given the overlap of depressive symptoms with symptoms of dementia, or in patients with aphasia, denial/neglect, or severe dementia. Information from caregivers may greatly assist diagnosis.

(2) Apathy syndromes have to be ruled out (Chapter 1).

(3) Hypothyroidism has to be ruled out (check thyroid-stimulating hormone [TSH] and thyroxine [T4]).

d. **Treatment**

(1) *Optimize the physical health* of the patient and ensure that all underlying general medical disorders have been optimally treated, including pain management.

(2) Optimize the patient's *environment and lifestyle*, including the promotion of exercise and a regular sleep–wake cycle. Caregivers should be instructed in *behavioral management* of the patient's behavioral problems, including prevention and modification of adverse behaviors. Controlled studies have shown that caregivers can be successfully trained to reduce patient depression.

(3) Monitor caregivers closely for development of depression in themselves.

(4) Use *psychotherapy* which is supported by controlled data, including individual (particularly cognitive-behavioral therapy) and group (including formal support groups) psychotherapy.

(5) Optimize the use of *cholinesterase inhibitors* (see Chapter 4). Controlled data suggest that these agents may improve neuropsychiatric symptoms (including depression) and functional status, as well as cognition.

(6) Implement somatic therapy if depression is severe or persists after these initial steps. There are no FDA-approved somatic treatments for depression in patients with dementia. Therapeutic options are the same as for major depressive disorder, that is antidepressant or mood-stabilizing medication, or ECT.

(7) Treat initially with *sertraline* or *citalopram*, based on their safety and tolerability, as well as their efficacy as demonstrated in a small number of randomized controlled trials.

   Venlafaxine is a reasonable second-line agent (given the well-described pathologic deficit in norepinephrine-producing neurons in patients with AD), but its efficacy in patients with dementia has not been demonstrated. Medications with anticholinergic side effects (e.g., tricyclic antidepressants) should be used cautiously, as their anticholinergic properties may worsen the memory impairment, in addition to other adverse effects.

(8) Consider ECT in depressed patients with AD who are severely ill (e.g., melancholic, psychotic, or suicidal) and in need of rapid clinical improvement, or who are unresponsive to or intolerant of psychotropic medications. A small uncontrolled (primarily retrospective) clinical literature supports the safety, tolerability, and efficacy of ECT in such patients, but controlled randomized data are lacking. Several modifications in ECT technique may be required, however, based on the patient's medical/neurologic status and concerns about cognitive side effects. ECT does not appear to worsen the underlying dementing process.

(9) Give patients with psychotic symptoms an *antipsychotic medication* in addition to the antidepressant medication, although there are no controlled data on this issue. Atypical antipsychotic medications are generally preferred given their safety, but should be used sparingly given their small risk in the elderly of stroke and death.

(10) Continue successful acute therapy for at least 6 to 9 months.

References
1. Coffey CE, Kellner CH. Electroconvulsive therapy. In: Coffey CE, Cummings JL, eds. *Textbook of*

geriatric neuropsychiatry, 2nd ed. Washington, DC: American Psychiatric Press; 2000:829–859.

2. Holmes C, Wilkinson D, Dean C, et al. The efficacy of donepezil in the treatment of neuropsychiatric symptoms in Alzheimer disease. *Neurology*. 2004; 63:214–219.

3. Lee HB, Lyketsos CG. Depression in Alzheimer disease: Heterogeneity and related issues. *Biol Psychiatry*. 2003;54:353–362.

4. Lyketsos CG, Olin J. Depression in Alzheimer disease: Overview and treatment. *Biol Psychiatry*. 2002;52:243–252.

5. Teri L, Gibbons LE, McCurry SM, et al. Exercise plus behavioral management in patients with Alzheimer disease. *JAMA*. 2003;290:2015–2022.

6. Zubenko GS, Zubenko WN, McPherson S, et al. A collaborative study of the emergence and clinical features of the major depressive syndrome of Alzheimer disease. *Am J Psychiatry*. 2003;160: 857–866.

3. **Depression in patients with Parkinson disease**
   a. **Clinical background**
      (1) Depression is the most common neuropsychiatric disturbance in Parkinson disease (PD), with a *prevalence* of approximately 10% to 50%. Roughly half of affected patients will meet criteria for major depression, with the remainder meeting criteria for dysthymia.

      (2) *Risk factors* for depression in patients with PD include psychosis and degree of cognitive impairment, but there are conflicting data on whether it is related to physical impairment. The incidence of hypothyroidism is increased in patients with PD (perhaps due to inhibited release of TRH by levodopa stimulation of the pituitary) and may contribute to both the depressive and cognitive symptoms. Testosterone deficiency, present in up to 25% of men over age 60, may also contribute to depression and other nonmotor symptoms in patients with PD.

      (3) The *phenomenology* of depression in patients with PD is similar to that in patients with primary major depression, except that the former may be less likely to experience guilt, self-blame, and a sense of failure. Psychotic symptoms may be seen in 20% or more of patients, with hallucinations more common than delusions. The potential etiologies of these symptoms are complex (see Chapter 9).

      (4) During the *course and prognosis*, depression may appear to precede the onset of the movement disorder by several years. Depression (both major and minor) in patients with PD is associated with more personal suffering, faster progression of physical symptoms,

greater disability, and greater decline in both cognitive skills and ability for self-care. The risk of suicide in depressed patients with PD has not been defined (patients with PD do not have an increased occurrence of suicide relative to the general population). Effective treatment of depression may improve the functional status of patients with PD, although there are no definitive data on this issue.

b. **Pathogenesis**

(1) The pathophysiology of depression in patients with PD is not known, but is likely to be heterogeneous. Certainly, the *stress* of the illness and related disability is a contributing factor.

(2) Brain imaging and *neurochemical* studies suggest that patients with PD and depression may have degeneration in dopamine and serotonin systems believed to be important in mood. Recent data suggest that the risk of depression is increased in patients with PD who have elevated plasma homocysteine levels or the low-activity allele of the serotonin transporter gene-linked polymorphic region 5HT-TLPR.

(3) *Hypothyroidism* may be a contributing factor.

c. **Diagnosis**

(1) The diagnosis is clinical and is based upon the presence of criteria for a mood disorder. The diagnosis is often difficult, however, given the overlap of depressive symptoms with symptoms of parkinsonism, or in patients with denial/neglect or severe dementia. Information from caregivers may greatly assist diagnosis.

(2) Apathy syndromes have to be ruled out (Chapter 1).

(3) Hypothyroidism has to be ruled out (check TSH and T4).

(4) *Deep brain stimulation* of the subthalamic nucleus for PD is associated with acute, transient mood changes, as well as more persistent and severe depression (including suicide) in some patients. Patients with a personal or family history of suicide may be at high risk for this complication.

d. **Treatment**

(1) *Optimize the physical health of the patient* and ensure that all underlying general medical disorders (particularly hypothyroidism, testosterone deficiency) have been optimally treated, including pain management.

(2) *Optimize the patient's environment and lifestyle,* including the promotion of exercise and a regular sleep–wake cycle. Caregivers should be instructed in *behavioral management* of the patient's behavioral problems, including prevention and modification of adverse behaviors.

Caregivers should also be monitored closely for development of depression themselves.

(3) *Optimize treatment of the movement disorder* (see Chapters 9 and 10). Dopamine replacement therapy is only a weak antidepressant, however, and it may cause other neuropsychiatric symptoms, most notably psychosis, delirium, and agitation.

(4) Consider brief, structured *psychotherapy* (e.g., cognitive-behavioral therapy or interpersonal therapy) in patients with mild to moderately severe depression and who are able to participate in the treatment. Although its effectiveness has not been formally studied in patients with PD, it is very safe and its efficacy is well established for acute phase treatment in primary mood disorders.

(5) Consider somatic therapy if depression is severe or persists after these initial interventions. There are no FDA-approved somatic treatments for depression in PD. Therapeutic options are the same as for major depressive disorder, namely, antidepressant or mood-stabilizing medication, or ECT.

(6) Treat initially with *citalopram* or *sertraline* based on their tolerability and the results of prospective open label trials. Worsening of motor symptoms has been reported in a few patients on SRIs, however, and SRIs should be used with caution in patients receiving deprenyl (a selective inhibitor of MAO-B) given a potential risk of adverse reactions similar to serotonin syndrome or hypertensive crisis. Sexual side effects are common with SRIs and may worsen sexual dysfunction that is experienced by many patients with PD. If there is inadequate response to first-line treatment, then switching to *buproprion* is recommended, given its dopaminergic properties and its relatively lower incidence of sexual side effects. *Venlafaxine* is a reasonable alternative. Both *amoxapine and lithium* should be avoided because they can worsen parkinsonism.

(7) Consider *ECT* in depressed patients with PD who are severely ill (e.g., melancholic, psychotic, suicidal) and in need of rapid clinical improvement, or who are unresponsive to or intolerant of antidepressant medications. A small uncontrolled (primarily retrospective) clinical literature supports the safety, tolerability, and efficacy of ECT in such patients, but randomized controlled data are lacking. Several modifications in ECT technique may be required, however, based on the patient's medical/neurologic status and concerns about cognitive side effects. Of note, controlled studies

indicate that ECT may also improve the motor symptoms of parkinsonism, irrespective of its effect upon mood.

(8) Base the treatment of concomitant psychotic symptoms in patients with parkinsonism, which is complex, upon a thorough assessment of the potential causative factors (e.g., medication-induced vs. depression with psychotic features vs. dementia with Lewy bodies, etc.) (see Chapters 7 and 9). Atypical antipsychotic medications are generally preferred given their safety, but should be used sparingly given their small risk in the elderly of stroke and death.

(9) Continue successful acute therapy (psychotropic medication or ECT) for at least 6 to 9 months, although there are no controlled data on this issue.

References
1. Coffey CE, Kellner CH. Electroconvulsive therapy. In: Coffey CE, Cummings JL, eds. *Textbook of geriatric neuropsychiatry*, 2nd ed. Washington, DC: American Psychiatric Press; 2000:829–859.
2. McDonald W, Richard IH, DeLong MR. Prevalence, etiology, and treatment of depression in Parkinson disease. *Biol Psychiatry*. 2003;54:363–375.
3. Okum MS, Watts RL. Depression associated with Parkinson disease. *Neurology*. 2002;58(Suppl 1):S63–S70.
4. Troster AI, Fields JA, Koller WC. Pardinson disease and parkinsonism. In: Coffey CE, Cummings JL, eds. *Textbook of geriatric neuropsychiatry*, 2nd ed. Washington, DC: American Psychiatric Press; 2000:559–600.

4. **Depression in patients with Huntington disease**
   a. **Clinical background**
   (1) The *prevalence* of mood disorders in Huntington disease (HD) is approximately 40%, with 30% developing major depression and 10% bipolar disorder (usually type II).
   (2) The *phenomenology* of depression in HD is similar to that of primary major depression. Conflicting findings have been reported regarding the relation of depression to the cognitive and motor symptoms of HD. In addition, depression may precede the motor manifestations of HD by several years, and may occur in patients with minimal motor symptoms who are unaware they are affected.
   (3) The impact of depression on outcomes in HD has not been well studied, but the occurrence of *suicide* is increased in patients with HD relative to the general population. Effective treatment of depression may improve the functional status of patients with HD

and reduce the risk of suicide, although there are no definitive data on these issues.

b. **Pathogenesis**

(1) The *pathophysiology* of depression in patients with HD is not known, but is likely to be heterogeneous.

(2) The early onset of depression in many patients suggests that it may be related to *degeneration of the caudate nucleus and related circuits*, because they are also affected early in the disease. Mood symptoms apparently do not correlate with CAG repeat length.

(3) The *stress* of a fatal disease no doubt is a contributing factor, but other patients may develop depression before they are aware of the diagnosis or before they experience motor symptoms.

c. **Diagnosis**

(1) The diagnosis is clinical and is based on the presence of criteria for a mood disorder. The diagnosis is often difficult, however, in patients with dementia or denial/neglect. Information from caregivers may greatly assist diagnosis.

(2) Apathy syndromes have to be ruled out (see Chapter 1).

d. **Treatment**

(1) *Optimize the physical health of the patient* and ensure that all underlying general medical disorders have been optimally treated, including pain management.

(2) *Optimize the patient's environment and lifestyle,* including the promotion of exercise and a regular sleep–wake cycle. Caregivers should be instructed in *behavioral management* of the patient's behavioral problems, including prevention and modification of adverse behaviors. Caregivers should also be monitored closely for development of depression in themselves.

(3) *Optimize treatment of the movement disorder* (see Chapter 10).

(4) Consider brief, structured *psychotherapy* (e.g., cognitive-behavioral therapy or interpersonal therapy) in patients with mild to moderately severe depression and who are able to participate in the treatment. Although its effectiveness has not been formally studied in patients with HD, it is very safe and its efficacy is well established for acute phase treatment in primary mood disorders.

(5) Consider somatic therapy if depression is severe or persists after these initial interventions. There are no FDA-approved somatic treatments for depression in HD. Therapeutic options are the same as for major depressive disorder, that is antidepressant or mood-stabilizing medication, or ECT.

(6) Treat initially with *citalopram* or *sertraline* based on their tolerability and efficacy as demonstrated in case

reports. Sexual side effects are common with SRIs and may worsen sexual dysfunction that is experienced by many patients with HD. Nortriptyline is recommended if the SRIs are ineffective.

For patients with HD and bipolar depression, we recommend lamotrigine or valproic acid.

Lithium is generally avoided because patients with HD are at risk for dehydration and may therefore develop lithium toxicity.

(7) Consider ECT in depressed patients with HD who are severely ill (e.g., melancholic, psychotic, or suicidal) and in need of rapid clinical improvement, or who are unresponsive to or intolerant of psychotropic medications. A small-uncontrolled (primarily retrospective) clinical literature supports the safety, tolerability, and efficacy of ECT in such patients, but randomized controlled data are lacking. Several modifications in ECT technique may be required, however, based on the patient's medical/neurologic status and concerns about cognitive side effects.

(8) Continue successful acute therapy for at least 6 to 9 months, although there are no controlled data on this issue.

(9) Treat concomitant psychotic symptoms in patients with HD with antipsychotic medications (see Chapters 7 and 10). Atypical antipsychotic medications are generally preferred given their safety, but should be used sparingly given their small risk in the elderly of stroke and death.

References

1. Coffey CE, Kellner CH. Electroconvulsive therapy. In: Coffey CE, Cummings JL, eds. *Textbook of geriatric neuropsychiatry*, 2nd ed. Washington, DC: American Psychiatric Press; 2000:829–859.

2. Paulsen JS, Ready RE, Hamilton JM, et al. Neuropsychiatric aspects of Huntington disease. *J Neurol Neurosurg Psychiatry*. 2001;71:310–314.

3. Ranen NG. Psychiatric management of Huntington disease. *Psychiatr Ann*. 2002:32:105–110.

5. **Depression in patients with traumatic brain injury**

   a. **Clinical background**

      (1) The 1-year *prevalence* of depression in patients with TBI is at least 33%, and the lifetime prevalence has been estimated at approximately 18%.

      (2) Potential *risk factors* for depression in patients with TBI include a personal history of psychiatric disorder (mood and anxiety disorders), impaired social functioning, and lesions of the left basal ganglia and left dorsolateral cortex. There are conflicting data on the relation of depression to the severity of the TBI, or

to functional (including cognitive) impairment following TBI.

(3) The *phenomenology* of depression in patients with TBI is similar to that in patients with primary major depression, except that the former may have higher rates of comorbid anxiety (~75%) and aggressive behavior (~55%).

(4) The *longitudinal course* of depression following TBI is variable, with some patients experiencing only transient syndromes lasting a few weeks perhaps (a result of neurochemical changes provoked by the TBIs) and others experiencing a more persistent disorder lasting several months (perhaps more related to physical or cognitive impairment?). Major depression in patients with TBI is associated with cognitive impairment, as well as with significantly poorer social functioning at 6- and 12-month follow up. Treatment of depression may improve these outcomes, but there are no data on this issue.

b. **Pathogenesis**

(1) The *pathophysiology* of depression in patients with TBI is not known, but is likely to be heterogeneous.

(2) *Stress* related to the injury and its physical, cognitive, and emotional sequelae may be a contributing factor, particularly in those with a personal history of mood disorder or who develop depression several months after the injury.

(3) Some have speculated that depression (particularly acute depression occurring after the brain injury) may also relate to the neuropathologic changes of TBI, including deactivation of lateral and dorsal prefrontal cortical regions, and increased activation of ventral lateral and paralimbic systems including the amygdala.

c. **Diagnosis**

(1) The *diagnosis* of major depression in patients with TBI is clinical.

(2) There may be considerable overlap of symptoms with those of the *postconcussive syndrome, apathy syndrome* (see Chapter 1), and *personality syndromes* (see Chapter 12).

(3) Comorbid *substance use/abuse* is common.

d. **Treatment**

(1) *Optimize the physical health of the patient* and ensure that all underlying general medical and neurologic disorders have been optimally treated, including the provision of pain management.

(2) *Optimize the patient's environment and lifestyle,* including the promotion of exercise and a regular sleep–wake cycle. Caregivers should be instructed in *behavioral*

management of the patient's behavioral problems, including prevention and modification of the adverse behaviors. Caregivers should also be monitored closely for development of depression in themselves.

(3) Consider brief, structured *psychotherapy* (e.g., cognitive-behavioral therapy or interpersonal therapy) in patients with mild to moderately severe depression and who are able to participate in the treatment. Although its effectiveness has not been formally studied in patients with TBI, it is very safe and its efficacy is well established for acute phase treatment in primary mood disorders.

(4) Consider somatic therapy if depression is severe or persists after these initial interventions. There are no FDA-approved somatic treatments for depression in patients with TBI. Therapeutic options are the same as for major depressive disorder, namely, antidepressant medication or ECT.

(5) Treat initially with *sertraline*, based on its tolerability and the results of a single placebo-controlled, single-blind, nonrandomized trial. *Citalopram* is a reasonable alternative. In patients who fail to respond, *desipramine* is an alternative (supported by a small randomized, single-blind, placebo-controlled trial), although its use may be associated with seizures (tricyclic antidepressants [TCAs] lower seizure threshold).

Case reports and small clinical series also support the use of *psychostimulants*, including dextroamphetamine (8 to 60 mg daily), methylphenidate (10 to 60 mg daily), and pemoline (56 to 75 mg daily). These medications are given twice daily, with the last dose at least 6 hours before bedtime to prevent insomnia. Treatment is begun at lower doses, with gradual escalation. Patients should be monitored closely for evidence of abuse or toxicity, including anxiety, dysphoria, headaches, insomnia, irritability, anorexia, dyskinesias, cardiovascular symptoms, and frank psychotic symptoms.

(6) Consider ECT in depressed patients with TBI who are severely ill (e.g., melancholic, psychotic, or suicidal) and in need of rapid clinical improvement, or who are unresponsive to or intolerant of antidepressant medications. A small uncontrolled (primarily retrospective) clinical literature supports the safety, tolerability, and efficacy of ECT in such patients, but randomized controlled data are lacking. Several modifications in ECT technique may be required, however, based on the patient's medical/neurologic status and concerns about cognitive side effects.

(7) Give patients with psychotic symptoms an *antipsychotic medication* in addition to the antidepressant medication, although there are no controlled data on this issue. Atypical antipsychotic medications are generally preferred given their safety, should be used sparingly given their small risk in the elderly of stroke and death.

(8) Continue successful acute therapy for at least 6 to 9 months, although there are no controlled data on this issue.

References

1. Coffey CE, Kellner CH. Electroconvulsive therapy. In: Coffey CE, Cummings JL, eds. *Textbook of geriatric neuropsychiatry*, 2nd ed. Washington, DC: American Psychiatric Press; 2000:829–859.
2. Fields RB, Cisewski D, Coffey CE. Traumatic brain injury. In: Coffey CE, Cummings JL, eds. *Textbook of geriatric neuropsychiatry*, 2nd ed. Washington, DC: American Psychiatric Press; 2000:621–653.
3. Silver JM, McAllister TW, Yudofsky SC. *Textbook of traumatic brain injury*. Washington, DC: American Psychiatric Press; 2005.

6. **Depression in patients with multiple sclerosis**
   a. **Clinical background**
   (1) Depression is approximately twice as common in patients with multiple sclerosis (MS) relative to patients with other chronic illnesses (particularly for women), with an estimated 1-year *prevalence* of at least 25% and a lifetime prevalence of up to 50%.
   (2) Potential *risk factors* for depression in patients with MS include younger age, lesion volume on magnetic resonance imaging (MRI) (particularly in the left frontal region and left arcuate fasciculus), cortical (especially left anterior temporal) atrophy, and various psychosocial factors (stress, coping ability, social support, uncertainty about the future, etc.) related to disease severity and disability.
   (3) The *phenomenology* of depression in patients with MS appears similar to that of patients with primary major depression, although this issue has not been well studied.
   (4) The *longitudinal course* of depression in patients with MS has not been thoroughly studied. Major depression has a negative impact on quality of life and treatment adherence in patients with MS, and is a risk factor for suicide. The risk of suicide is high in patients with MS (up to seven times that of the general population), and is associated with major depression, alcohol abuse, and social isolation. Therefore, effective treatment of the depression may improve the functional status and well-being of patients with MS.

b. **Pathogenesis**
(1) The *neurobiology* of depression in patients with MS is not known, but is likely to be heterogeneous.
(2) *Stress* is a contributing factor, as MS is a disease of the young, which is unpredictable, can cause devastating disability, and which is without cure currently.
(3) Brain imaging studies implicate atrophy, lesion burden, and involvement of frontal-subcortical and anterior temporal systems.
(4) Depression may also be related to *treatment* of MS, particularly with interferon or steroids.

c. **Diagnosis**
(1) The *diagnosis* of depression in patients with MS is clinical.
(2) All patients should be thoroughly and continuously assessed for risk of *suicide*.
(3) Depression secondary to *medications* should be considered in the differential diagnosis, particularly in patients receiving interferon or corticosteroids. In patients with depression, glatiramer may be a preferred drug for treatment of relapse.
(4) Affective lability (see subsequent text), fatigue syndrome, or apathy syndrome has to be ruled out.

d. **Treatment**
(1) *Optimize the physical health of the patient* and ensure that all underlying general medical disorders have been optimally treated, including the provision of pain management.
(2) *Optimize the patient's environment and lifestyle*, including the promotion of exercise and a regular sleep–wake cycle. Caregivers should be instructed in *behavioral management* of the patient's behavioral problems, including prevention and modification of the adverse behaviors. Caregivers should also be monitored closely for development of depression in themselves.
(3) Consider *psychotherapeutic interventions* (supported by controlled trials), including disease education (particularly for caregivers), as well as individual (particularly cognitive-behavioral therapy, that is supported by an open study), group (including formal support groups), and family therapy.
(4) Consider somatic therapy if depression is severe or persists after these initial interventions. There are no FDA-approved somatic treatments for depression in patients with MS. Therapeutic options are the same as for major depressive disorder, that is antidepressant medication or ECT.
(5) Treat initially with *sertraline*, based on its tolerability and the results of open studies. *Citalopram* is

a reasonable alternative. In patients who fail to respond, *desipramine* may be considered (supported by a small randomized, placebo-controlled study).

(6) Consider ECT in depressed patients with MS who are severely ill and in need of rapid clinical improvement, or who are unresponsive to or intolerant of antidepressant medications. A small uncontrolled (primarily retrospective) clinical literature supports the safety, tolerability, and efficacy of ECT in such patients, but randomized controlled data are lacking. Several modifications in ECT technique may be required, however, based on the patient's medical/neurologic status and concerns about cognitive side effects.

(7) Give patients with psychotic symptoms an *antipsychotic medication* in addition to the antidepressant medication, although there are no controlled data on this issue. Atypical antipsychotic medications are generally preferred given their safety, but should be used sparingly given their small risk in the elderly of stroke and death.

(8) Continue successful acute therapy for at least 6 to 9 months, although there are no controlled data on this issue.

References
1. Mohr DC. Treatment of depression in multiple sclerosis: Review and meta-analysis. *Clin Psychol Sci Prac.* 1999;6:1–9.
2. Mohr DC, Classen C, Barrera M. The relationship between social support, depression and treatment for depression in people with multiple sclerosis. *Psychol Med.* 2004;34:533–541.

7. **Depression in patients with epilepsy**
   a. **Clinical background**
   (1) Psychiatric disorders are common in patients with epilepsy, and of these disorders depression is perhaps the most common. Depressive *symptoms* may occur peri-ictally (before, during, or after the ictus), but typically these mood symptoms are brief and do not require treatment per se, as they will resolve with improvement in seizure control. Depressive *disorders* occur interictally, and include major depression, dysthymia, or rarely bipolar disorder.

   (2) The precise *prevalence* of interictal major depression is unknown, but may occur in 30% to 50% of patients with epilepsy. Of interest, the risk of epilepsy may also be increased in patients with depression.

   (3) No consistent *risk factors* have been identified for interictal major depression. Conflicting findings have been reported regarding the relation of depression to male gender, sinistrality, family history of mood disorder, psychosocial stressors, seizure frequency/severity, or presence of a neurologic disorder causing the epilepsy.

    (4) The *phenomenology* of interictal major depression appears to differ from that of primary major depression, with fewer "neurotic" traits (e.g., anxiety, guilt, rumination, somatization, hopelessness, or low self-esteem) and more psychotic symptoms. Atypical pain symptoms may also be present.

    (5) The *longitudinal course* of major depression in patients with epilepsy has not been sufficiently studied. At least some patients tend to suffer from dysthymia between episodes of major depression. Depression in patients with epilepsy is associated with greater utilization of health resources and a poorer quality of life. Effective treatment of depression may improve the functional status and well-being of patients with epilepsy, although this issue has not been well studied.

b. **Pathogenesis of interictal major depression**

    (1) The pathogenesis of interictal major depression is not known. Several factors may be involved.

    (2) The importance of *temporal lobe involvement* is suggested by the higher frequency of major depression in patients with temporal lobe seizures and complex partial seizures, compared with patients with other forms of epilepsy. Laterality (left greater than right) of epileptic focus as a possible pathogenetic factor is controversial.

    (3) Abnormal *neurotransmission* may be involved in the comorbidity of epilepsy and major depression. In animal models, seizures are associated with low levels of norepinephrine and high levels of serotonin.

    (4) Depression may be related to *treatment* of the epilepsy, including polypharmacy with anticonvulsant medication, the use of certain anticonvulsant medications (particularly barbiturates, phenytoin, primidone, vigabatrin, and all y-aminobutyric acid [GABA] agonists), and folate deficiency resulting from most anticonvulsant medications (especially those that induce liver enzymes). Withdrawal of antiepileptic medications may also be associated with depression, as well as anxiety and psychosis. Depression may also occur after (typically 3 to 6 months) temporal lobe surgery for epilepsy, particularly in patients with a history of mood disorder, and especially if seizures persist. No consistent relation has been found between post-surgery depression and side of surgery.

    (5) Depression in patients with epilepsy is certainly related to numerous *psychosocial factors*, including the burden of chronic disease, the stigma of epilepsy, the loss of autonomy (e.g., driving, occupational limitations, etc.), and impaired interpersonal relations (e.g., anticonvulsant induced loss of libido).

  c. **Diagnosis**

    (1) The diagnosis is clinical and is based on the presence of criteria for a mood disorder.

    (2) Peri-ictal depressive symptoms have to be ruled out, as these do not typically require treatment (see preceding text).

    (3) Depressive symptoms secondary to antiepileptic medications have to be ruled out (see preceding text).

  d. **Treatment**

    (1) *Optimize the physical health of the patient* and ensure that all underlying general medical disorders have been optimally treated, including the provision of appropriate pain management. In particular, the *treatment of epilepsy* should be optimized. Antiepileptic polypharmacy should be minimized, and the use of antiepileptics with relatively low dysphorogenic properties should be considered (see preceding text).

    (2) *Optimize* the patient's *environment and lifestyle*, including the promotion of exercise and a regular sleep–wake cycle. Caregivers should be instructed in *behavioral management* of the patient's behavioral problems, including prevention and modification of the adverse behaviors. Caregivers should also be monitored closely for development of depression in themselves.

    (3) Consider *psychotherapeutic interventions*, including disease education, as well as individual (particularly cognitive-behavioral therapy), group (including formal support groups), and family therapy, although the efficacy of such interventions has not been formally studied.

    (4) Consider somatic therapy if depression persists after these initial interventions. There are no FDA-approved somatic treatments for depression in patients with epilepsy. Therapeutic options are the same as for major depressive disorder, that is antidepressant or mood-stabilizing medications, or ECT.

    (5) Choose antidepressant medication guided by its side effect profile (particularly its effect on seizure threshold) and risk of interactions with concomitant medications, because it is assumed (although not proved) that all antidepressants are equally efficacious in treating depression in patients with epilepsy. We recommend *sertraline*, based on its apparent minimal impact upon seizure threshold and its low risk of pharmacokinetic interactions, as well as the results of several open clinical trials demonstrating efficacy for major depression in patients with epilepsy. *Citalopram* is an acceptable alternative. *Venlafaxine* is a reasonable second-line choice if sertraline or citalopram are ineffective. There is only

one published randomized controlled trial of antidepressant medication in epilepsy, and it found that 12 weeks of nomifensine (that is no longer available) was superior to amitriptyline.

(6) Avoid certain antidepressants (buproprion, maprotiline, and amoxapine) as they are *proconvulsant* in particularly vulnerable patients. Tricyclic antidepressants may also lower seizure threshold, but their use does not appear to worsen seizure control unless plasma levels are high, the dose is escalated rapidly, there are concomitant drugs with proconvulsant properties, or the patient has either cerebral pathology, an abnormal electroencephalography (EEG), and personal and family history of epilepsy. Less is known about the effects of newer antidepressants on seizure threshold.

(7) Consider *pharmacokinetic interactions* of antidepressant and antiepileptic drugs. Those anticonvulsants that induce liver enzymes (particularly phenobarbital, primidone, phenytoin, and carbamazepine) can lower plasma levels of paroxetine and the tricyclic antidepressants. Conversely, certain antidepressants (fluoxetine, fluvoxamine, and paroxetine) inhibit the cytochrome P-450 enzyme system and can induce toxic levels of phenytoin and carbamazepine. Sertraline and citalopram have far fewer pharmacokinetic interactions with antiepileptic drugs.

(8) Consider ECT in patients with epilepsy and major depression who are severely ill (e.g., melancholic, psychotic, or suicidal) and in need of rapid clinical improvement, or who are unresponsive to or intolerant of psychotropic medications. A small uncontrolled (primarily retrospective) clinical literature supports the safety, tolerability, and efficacy of ECT in such patients, but randomized controlled data are lacking. Several modifications in ECT technique may be required, however, based on the patient's medical/neurologic status and concerns about cognitive side effects. Of note, the anticonvulsant properties of ECT may help improve seizure control.

(9) Manage *bipolar depression* in patients with epilepsy with lamotrigine or ECT. Lithium is a second choice, because of its proconvulsant properties and its propensity for inducing delirium especially when used in combination with carbamazepine. *Mania* in patients with epilepsy may be managed with a mood-stabilizing antiepileptic medication (e.g., valproic acid) and an antipsychotic medication, or with ECT.

(10) Base the treatment of concomitant *psychotic symptoms* in patients with epilepsy and major depression upon a thorough assessment of the potential causative factors

(e.g., medication-induced vs. depression with psychotic features vs. other), as discussed in Chapter 8. Atypical antipsychotic medications are generally preferred given their safety, but should be used sparingly given their small risk in the elderly of stroke and death.

(11) Continue successful acute therapy for major depression in patients with epilepsy for at least 6 to 9 months, although there are no controlled data on this issue.

(12) In July 2005, the FDA approved vagus nerve stimulation (VNS) therapy as an add-on long-term treatment for adults with treatment-resistant chronic or recurrent depression. Whereas VNS may be considered as a treatment option for depression in patients with epilepsy, its role in patients with other neurologic illnesses remains to be defined.

References

1. Coffey CE, Kellner CH. Electroconvulsive therapy. In: Coffey CE, Cummings JL, eds. *Textbook of geriatric neuropsychiatry*, 2nd ed. Washington, DC: American Psychiatric Press; 2000:829–859.
2. Kanner AM. Depressive in epilepsy. *Biol Psychiatry*. 2003;54:388–398.
3. Krystal AD, Coffey CE. Neuropsychiatric considerations in the use of electroconvulsive therapy. *J Neuropsychiatry Clin Neurosci*. 1997;9:283–292.
4. Mendez MF. Epilepsy. In: Coffey CE, Cummings JL, eds. *Textbook of geriatric neuropsychiatry*. Washington, DC: American Psychiatric Press; 2000:655–667.
5. Prueter C, Norra C. Mood disorders and their treatment in patients with epilepsy. *J Neuropsychiatry Clin Neurosci*. 2005;17:20–28.

C. **Management of mania/hypomania in patients with neurologic disease**

1. Mania/hypomania has been described in patients with a variety of neurologic disorders, most commonly epilepsy (some studies suggest a relation to nondominant temporal lobe epilepsy), stroke (associated with a family history of mood disorder, premorbid mild subcortical atrophy, and stroke location [right basotemporal cortex]), TBI, multiple sclerosis, Huntington disease, and tumor. The occurrence of mania/hypomania in patients with neurologic illness in not precisely known, but appears to be rarer than depression.

2. There are no FDA-approved treatments, nor any randomized controlled treatment trials of mania in patients with neurologic disease.

   a. Follow the APA guidelines for bipolar disorder (APA 2002), which call for treatment of mania with a mood stabilizer (valproate or lithium) and an antipsychotic medication. Lithium is generally avoided in patients with epilepsy due to its potential proconvulsant properties, and antipsychotic medications should likewise be used cautiously because they also lower seizure threshold.

  b. Concomitant psychosocial and psychotherapeutic interventions are also reasonable considerations, although these have not been studied.

  c. ECT should be considered in manic patients with epilepsy who are severely ill and in need of rapid clinical improvement, or who are unresponsive to or intolerant of pharmacotherapy. Several modifications in ECT technique may be required, however, based on the patient's medical/ neurologic status. Of note, the anticonvulsant properties of ECT may help improve seizure control.

  d. Effective acute treatment should be continued for 6 to 9 months, although the antipsychotic medication should be discontinued unless required for control of persistent psychosis or prophylaxis against recurrence.

D. **Management of affective lability ("emotional incontinence") and pathologic affect.** There are no FDA-approved somatic treatments for affective lability or pathologic affect associated with neurologic disorders, and only a few studies have examined this issue prospectively. Both nortriptyline and citalopram have been found to be effective in small randomized controlled trials of pathologic affect following stroke. Amitriptyline was found effective for pathologic affect in a randomized controlled trial of 12 patients with MS. A recent 17-center, double-blind, randomized, controlled clinical trial found that AVP-39 (a combination of quinidine 30 mg and dextromethorphan 30 mg orally) was effective in relieving pathologic affect and improving quality of life in patients with amyotrophic lateral sclerosis (ALS) (ALS). A similar study is under way in patients with pathologic affect and MS. Case reports support the use of tricyclic antidepressants, SRIs, levodopa, and mood stabilizers for pathologic affect in various neurologic disorders.

References

1. American Psychiatric Association. Practice guideline for the treatment of patients with bipolar disorder (revision). *Am J Psychiatry.* 2002;159(Suppl 4):1–50.

2. Brooks BR, Thisted RA, Appel SH, et al. Treatment of pseudobulbar affect in ALS with dextromethorphan/quinidine. *Neurology.* 2004;63:1364–1370.

3. Schiffer RB, Herndon RM, Rudick RA. Treatment of pathological laughing and weeping with amitriptyline. *NEJM.* 1985;312: 1480–1482.

Chapter 6

ANXIETY

Robert G. Robinson, Jess G. Fiedorowicz

I. BACKGROUND

A. Definitions

1. *Anxiety* refers to a vague, often unpleasant, emotion associated with a sense of apprehension, arousal, or tension. Karl Jaspers described the experience of abnormal anxiety as "free-floating and unattached" and associated with a "feeling of restlessness." Anxiety symptoms may be consciously experienced as psychological symptoms (anticipation, apprehension, arousal, dread, fear, worry, irritability, insomnia, inattention) or as physical (somatic) symptoms (nausea/dyspepsia, dry mouth, racing heart, palpitations, shortness of breath, sweating, tremor, muscular tension).

2. Anxiety is universally experienced and normal anxiety is thought to be adaptive as illustrated by the Yerkes–Dodson law demonstrating an "inverted U" relationship between arousal and performance. Anxiety may also be a manifestation of a neuropsychiatric disorder.

3. Anxiety is commonly divided into state and trait anxiety. State anxiety refers to anxiety in the setting of a specific stressor, whereas trait anxiety refers to an enduring pattern of high anxiety at baseline or a tendency to respond with exaggerated anxiety in mildly stressful situations. Clinically, the boundary between state and trait anxiety is often blurred.

4. Phenomenologically, the construct of anxiety assumes a breadth of symptoms including situational anxiety, general anxiety, panic attacks, phobic states, obsessions, and compulsions. *General anxiety* is distinguished from situational anxiety by the perceived lack of a sufficient stressor. *Panic attacks* are discrete episodes of limited duration with prominent psychological and physical anxiety symptoms in conjunction with a sense of impending doom. *Phobias* consist of involuntary fears out of proportion to the object of fear leading to avoidance of that object. *Obsessions* represent recurring, intrusive thoughts, or images. Obsessions may be linked to compulsions, which are

TABLE 6.1   Classification of Anxiety Disorders of Particular Relevance to Neuropsychiatry

Generalized anxiety disorder	Persistent anxiety and worry out of proportion to circumstances
Obsessive-compulsive disorder	Obsessions and compulsions of clinically sufficient severity and duration
Panic disorder	Recurrent, spontaneous panic attacks accompanied by fear of repeated attacks

repeated actions driven by a desire to relieve an anxiety preceding the action and compelling the completion of the action.

B. **Classification and epidemiology of anxiety syndromes.** This chapter will focus on state anxiety syndromes associated with neurologic conditions. The anxiety syndromes with the strongest association are detailed in Table 6.1.

C. **Normal anxiety contrasted with generalized anxiety disorder**
   1. Anxiety is ubiquitous in human mental life and plays a role in maintaining arousal and response to environmental stress. Individuals differ dimensionally on baseline levels of anxiety as well as in their ability to mount an anxious response to a stressor. The ability to be aroused by threatening aspects in the environment condones clear survival advantages.
   2. Individuals who have excessive anxiety at baseline or display exaggerated responses to relatively unthreatening or only moderately arousing events may be categorized as suffering from a *generalized anxiety disorder* (GAD). Criteria for GAD include persistent, excessive, and uncontrollable worries over a period of at least 6 months and encompassing multiple aspects of one's life, not limited to a single activity or event and not confined to a specific aspect of another psychiatric disorder such as, worrying about having a serious illness in hypochondriasis. This anxiety is clinically significant and associated with symptoms such as edginess, fatigue, impaired concentration, irritability, restlessness or sleep disturbance, and particularly, initial insomnia. Physical symptoms associated with generalized anxiety may include muscular tension, a sense of a racing pulse, sweating, headaches, and nausea.
   3. The diagnosis of anxiety disorder due to a general medical condition with generalized anxiety is applied by convention when a clinically significant syndrome of excessive general anxiety is deemed to be the result of a medical condition. The presence of a temporal relationship with the condition, atypical features, and an evidence base of an association between the specific condition and generalized anxiety support the diagnosis.
   4. The lifetime prevalence of GAD in the general population is approximately 2% to 5%. The point prevalence is approximately 1% to 2%.

D. Obsessive-compulsive disorder

1. Significant obsessions and compulsions are not commonly experienced in the general population. In addition to occurring in those with obsessive-compulsive disorder (OCD), they may arise in the context of affective syndromes, psychotic disorders, and in those with trait obsessionality such as in obsessive-compulsive personality disorder, in which case these symptoms are less likely to be perceived as intrusive or unreasonable.

2. OCD is characterized by either obsessions or compulsions that are recognized as excessive or unreasonable. The symptoms are associated with significant clinical impairment through psychological distress, consumption of time, or impairment in function. Common obsessions include fear of contamination, fear of harming oneself or others, overwhelming concern with neatness or order, fear of making a mistake, fear of losing something, fear of embarrassing oneself, and persistent thinking about a specific image, number, sound, or word. Common compulsions include washing, checking, counting, repeating words or actions, arranging items in a specific order, and collecting or hoarding items no longer needed. Compulsive symptoms are often recognized as voluntary acts arising from oneself although they are typically not perceived as willful. Individuals often feel a desire to resist compulsions, albeit a seemingly futile desire at times.

3. The diagnosis of anxiety disorder due to a general medical condition with obsessive-compulsive symptoms is applied by convention when a preponderance of clinically significant obsessions and compulsions are deemed to be the result of a medical condition. The diagnosis is supported by the presence of a temporal relationship with the condition, atypical features, and an evidence base of an association between the specific condition and a syndrome of obsessions and compulsions.

4. The lifetime prevalence of OCD in the general population is approximately 2% to 2.5%. Peak incidence occurs around 20 years of age with more than half developing the illness before 25 years of age.

E. Panic disorder

1. Panic attacks may occur in the setting of a depressive syndrome, schizophrenia, phobias, GAD, OCD, or with separation anxiety. Panic attacks elicited by a specific situation are typically differentiated from spontaneous panic attacks.

2. Panic disorder is defined by convention as the presence of spontaneous, recurrent panic attacks followed by a fear of repeated attacks for at least 1 month. The panic attack is classically sudden in onset and typically reaches maximum intensity within 10 minutes. The duration of a panic attack can vary from minutes to hours although panic attacks typically last 10 to 20 minutes. Given the intensity of the event, the reported duration may overestimate the actual duration. In addition to intense fear or anxiety, patients may experience a rapid even pounding heart rate, sweating, shaking, tremor, shortness of breath,

hyperventilation, a choking sensation, chest discomfort, nausea, dyspepsia, lightheadedness, unsteadiness, derealization, depersonalization, sense of losing control, sense of going crazy, sense of impending doom or death, paresthesia, or chills. Panic disorder may be accompanied by agoraphobia, a fear of situations where escape may be difficult should a panic attack occur.

3. The diagnosis of anxiety disorder due to a general medical condition with panic attacks is applied by convention when panic attacks predominate and are deemed to be the result of a medical condition. The diagnosis is supported by the presence of a temporal relationship between panic attacks and the medical condition, atypical features, and an evidence base of an association between the specific condition and panic attacks.

4. The lifetime prevalence of panic disorder in the general population is approximately 1% to 2%. Rates have been found to be as high as 1% to 6% in primary care clinics and 17% to 25% in those presenting to an emergency department with chest pain. Rates are also thought to be elevated in neurology clinics, particularly among those referred for evaluation of dizziness and vestibular function.

F. **Post-traumatic stress disorder**

1. By current criteria, post-traumatic stress disorder (PTSD) follows the experiencing or witnessing of a traumatic event where threatened death, serious injury, or the physical integrity of self or others evoked fear, helplessness, or horror.

2. PTSD then involves persistently experiencing that traumatic event, avoiding stimuli associated with the traumatic event, and symptoms of hyperarousal such as hypervigilance or an exaggerated startle response. The symptoms must result in significant distress or impairment and must last for more than 1 month (otherwise operationalized as acute stress disorder). PTSD is considered chronic if symptoms persist for more than 3 months.

References

1. American Psychiatric Association. *Diagnostic and statistical manual of mental disorders*, 4th ed. Text Revision. Washington, DC: American Psychiatric Association; 2000.
2. Sadock BJ, Sadock VA. *Kaplan & Sadock's comprehensive textbook of psychiatry*, 7th ed. Philadelphia, PA: Lippincott Williams & Wilkins; 2000.
3. Sims A. *Symptoms in the mind: An introduction to descriptive psychopathology*, 3rd ed. London: WB Saunders; 2003.

II. NEUROBIOLOGY AND PATHOPHYSIOLOGY OF ANXIETY

A. **Normal anxiety**

1. The neurobiology of normal anxiety remains to be fully elucidated. There are two systems of anxiety that probably overlap: A "defense system" directed to making an immediate response to a threat and a "behavioral inhibition" system, which suppresses

potentially dangerous behaviors. Sensory input is relayed by the dorsal thalamus to the modality-appropriate cortical areas. Upon reaching secondary association cortex for a particular modality, information is relayed to emotion and memory centers in the amygdala, hippocampus, entorhinal cortex, orbitofrontal cortex, and anterior cingulate. Further, neural circuits orchestrating anxiety are organized at various levels throughout the brain. Brainstem regions appear to mediate somatic anxiety symptoms. Midbrain regions such as the periaqueductal gray and locus coeruleus are prominently involved in simple reflexive responses. Intermediate regions such as the amygdala and septohippocampal systems manage practiced responses. Cortical regions such as the paralimbic cortex appear to address more cognitively demanding situations.

2. The clinical efficacy of pharmaceuticals targeting γ-aminobutyric acid (GABA), serotonin (5-HT), and norepinephrine (NE) systems has promulgated interest in the role of these neurotransmitter systems in anxiety. Generally speaking, increased GABA release attenuates anxiety and increased NE release augments anxiety. The role of 5-HT is less straightforward and likely involves an adaptive or modulating role.

B. **Generalized anxiety**
1. GAD is thought to result from a dysfunction or change in the set point of the aforementioned anxiety systems.
2. Acute increases in 5-HT levels which are presumed to be treatment induced have been associated with increased anxiety; however, chronic increases are believed to be associated with diminished anxiety.

C. **Obsessions and compulsions**
1. Cortico-subcortical-thalamic-cortical circuits, particularly the orbitofrontal circuit appears to be dysfunctional in OCD. It has been demonstrated that patients with OCD have significantly more gray and less white matter than those without OCD. The onset of OCD may be immediately preceded by streptococcal infection in children (Pediatric Autoimmune Neuropsychiatric Disorders Associated with Streptococcal infections, [PANDAS]), encephalitis, head injury, or damage to the striatum.
2. OCD has been linked to disruption in serotonergic pathways involving the basal ganglia and orbitofrontal cortex.

D. **Panic attacks**
1. The locus coeruleus, a noradrenergic nucleus, has been identified in playing a prominent role in the etiology of panic. Positron emission tomography (PET) evidence has further identified involvement of the hippocampal and parahippocampal regions.
2. A dysregulation of noradrenergic systems, particularly the locus coeruleus, has been implicated in the pathogenesis of panic attacks. A shift in the "set point" of the benzodiazepine receptor has been proposed as a contributing factor in panic disorder.

Sodium lactate, hypercapnia, and cholecystokinin may provoke panic.

References

1. Sandford JJ, Argyropoulos SV, Nutt DJ. The psychobiology of anxiolytic drugs. Part 1: Basic neurobiology. *Pharmacol Ther*. 2000;88(3):197–212.
2. Argyropoulos SV, Sandford JJ, Nutt DJ. The psychobiology of anxiolytic drugs. Part 2: Pharmacological treatments of anxiety. *Pharmacol Ther*. 2000;88(3):213–227.

III. MANAGEMENT

A. **Principles of management.** The evidence base for the specific treatment of anxiety in patients with neurologic illness is limited. In the absence of compelling data from a study specific to a particular neurologic condition, it is generally advisable to follow the treatment guidelines for patients with primary anxiety disorders when appropriate. The American Psychiatric Association has published practice guidelines in panic disorder (1998) and for acute stress disorder and PTSD (2004). Cochrane reviews exist for "Antidepressants for generalized anxiety disorder (2003)" and "Pharmacologic management for agitation and aggression in people with acquired brain injury (2003)."

B. **Performing a comprehensive diagnostic evaluation**
   1. The importance of a *comprehensive examination* (psychiatric, medical, and neurologic) of patients with neuropsychiatric disorders cannot be overemphasized. This examination should include a history, mental status examination, and physical examination. Although an interdisciplinary approach is advantageous, the primary responsibility for the complete examination should not be delegated. Information from outside informants such as family members or primary care providers is essential, particularly to ascertain the patient's premorbid function, premorbid personality, and the temporal relationship between the onset of anxiety symptoms and the neurologic illness. Given the often insidious onset of anxiety symptoms and frequent impairments in the patient's historical abilities secondary to neuropsychiatric illness, it may be difficult to delineate the relationship between anxiety symptoms and the illness. A prudent approach is to clearly separate observations from interpretations. One must avoid assuming "who wouldn't be anxious with condition X" and postpone such explanation until formulating the case. Although often tempting, it is inadvisable to reflexively disregard a patient's psychological suffering as a normal reaction. Such an approach need not underestimate the tragedy of the neurologic illness, but may rather call attention to the comorbid anxiety. A rigorous and thorough elucidation of phenomenology is vital for an accurate assessment while further fostering the development of an empathic therapeutic relationship.
   2. Medical and psychiatric *comorbidity* should be thoroughly assessed, including alcohol and other substance abuse, personality

vulnerabilities, and frank personality disorders. Mood disorders are a common cause of anxiety and occur with increased frequency in those with anxiety disorders. Anxiety may occur as a consequence of asthma, central nervous system (CNS) infection, dehydration, fever, hyperventilation, metabolic abnormalities, mitral valve prolapse, myocardial infarction, neurosyphilis, pheochromocytoma, respiratory illness, thyroid disease, and other endocrine conditions. Alcohol, amphetamines, anabolic steroids, caffeine, cocaine, ecstasy, γ-hydroxybutyrate, inhalants, and phencyclidine (PCP) commonly produce clinically significant anxiety symptoms with intoxication and habitual use. Withdrawal from alcohol, barbiturates, benzodiazepines, cocaine, sedative/hypnotics and opiates may be associated with significant anxiety and agitation. Medications may be associated with anxiety and a thorough review of current and recent medications should be performed. Anxiety may also occur as an adverse reaction to medications including but not limited to acyclovir, antiretrovirals (esp. efavirenz), bronchodilators, corticosteroids, interferons, interleukin-2, isoniazid, lidocaine, pentamidine, procaine, sympathomimetics, and stimulants.

3. *Laboratory tests* may be required to follow up on any concerns elucidated during the comprehensive evaluation. The laboratory workup is, of course, guided by clinical suspicion as well as the estimated prevalence rate of the condition screened and will therefore appropriately vary from one patient or one setting to another. Because of the relatively high prevalence of thyroid abnormalities and a strong association with anxiety, a thyroid-stimulating hormone (TSH) test should be obtained as a screening test in patients with GAD or panic disorder if thyroid abnormalities have not been ruled out because of the onset of anxiety symptoms. Additionally, any patient who is neuropsychiatric, with a constellation of symptoms suggestive of thyroid disease including a change in the frequency of bowel movements, hair changes, skin changes, soft or brittle nails, sweating, temperature intolerance, tremor, or weight change should be screened for thyroid abnormalities with a minimum TSH. A complete medical panel may reveal hypercalcemia associated with hyperparathyroidism, liver abnormalities suggestive of alcoholism (i.e., elevated aspartate aminotransferase [AST]/alanine aminotransferase [ALT] ratio), or reflections of other endocrine disorders. Other tests should include a complete blood count, erythrocyte sedimentation rate (ESR), vitamin B_{12} level, folate level, and a rapid plasma reagin (RPR). The rate of medical comorbidities with neuropsychiatric illness is high enough to warrant such screening if not already performed.

4. No definitive practice guidelines exist for the use of *neuroimaging* in the evaluation of patients with anxiety in the setting of a neuropsychiatric condition. Structural neuroimaging (i.e., computed tomography [CT] scan or magnetic resonance

imaging [MRI]) should be obtained when the onset of anxiety symptoms begins after age 50, as follow-up of any abnormalities from the neurologic exam suggestive of intracranial pathology, or in the setting of a temporal association between symptoms and head trauma.

5. Performing a *risk assessment*, which includes a suicide risk assessment as well as assessment of general dangerousness to self or others is important.

C. **Formulating the case**

1. A comprehensive *formulation* should summarize the salient aspects of the history and physical examination. It may be helpful to organize one's diagnostic thinking into a biopsychosocial or an etiopathic model. Aspects of the patient's presentation can be organized into those that are likely the result of brain disease, the provocation of psychological vulnerabilities, the product of maladaptive behaviors, or demoralization from a tragic illness or other life events.

2. The *neuropsychiatric diagnosis* is a product of the formulation. It may be difficult to judge whether the anxiety disorder is primary or occurs secondary to the neurologic illness. The diagnosis of anxiety disorder secondary to a general medical condition is supported by the presence of a temporal relationship between the anxiety syndrome and the neurologic condition, atypical features, and an evidence base of an association between the specific neurologic condition and an anxiety disorder. Neurologic conditions associated with specific anxiety syndromes are detailed in Table 6.2.

D. **Implementing a treatment plan**

1. The determination of *treatment setting* (outpatient, partial hospitalization, or inpatient) is based on multiple factors, including but not limited to severity of illness, level of function, strength of family and social supports, and treatment compliance. The

TABLE 6.2   Neurologic Conditions Associated with Specified Anxiety Syndromes

Generalized anxiety disorder	Dementia, epilepsy, Huntington disease, multiple sclerosis?, Parkinson disease, restless legs syndrome, stroke, traumatic brain injury
Obsessive-compulsive disorder	Huntington disease?, Parkinson disease?, stroke (involving basal ganglia), traumatic brain injury, Tourette syndrome, Sydenham's chorea
Panic disorder (with or without agoraphobia)	Migraine headache, epilepsy, Lyme disease?, Parkinson disease, restless legs syndrome, traumatic brain injury
Post-traumatic stress disorder	Traumatic brain injury

?, association not fully established.

decision regarding treatment setting is a fluid one and must be reassessed on a regular basis. In the outpatient setting, the frequency of outpatient visits should be titrated to patient need.

2. Given the subjective nature of anxiety symptoms, having a *benchmark* to monitor progress and treatment effectiveness is necessary. This may include a scale such as the Yale-Brown Obsessive Compulsive Scale (Y-BOCS), a target symptom or symptoms, a functional assessment, or an outside informant's impression. Titration of psychiatric medications for anxiety disorders can be a prolonged process and it can be difficult for patients or providers to recall how current symptoms and function compare to prior months or previous treatment. The assessment of treatment effects is further complicated in neurodegenerative disorders where treatment effects must be inferred from a projected course of worsening illness.

3. The patient's personality and cognitive *strengths and vulnerabilities* should be assessed. Counseling and education may help patients capitalize on strengths and attend to vulnerabilities. Function-oriented guidance, delineation of prognosis and expectations, and exploration of means of coping with illness and handicap serves to combat demoralization for the patient and family.

4. Address avoidance behaviors, substance use (including caffeine), and other maladaptive *behaviors* proactively. Substance abuse or dependence is optimally managed in a structured substance abuse program.

5. Implementing a biopsychosocial treatment plan.
   a. Patients should be instructed to eliminate or at least limit caffeine and alcohol use.
   b. Psychotherapeutic approaches include cognitive-behavioral, supportive, and psychodynamic.
   c. Medications commonly prescribed for anxiety include selective serotonin reuptake inhibitors (SSRIs), venlafaxine, tricyclic antidepressants (TCAs), and benzodiazepines.

6. Treatment outcomes and compliance should be routinely monitored. Any worsening in illness or decline in adherence should be dealt with proactively.

References
1. McHugh PR, Slavney PR. *The perspectives of psychiatry*, 2nd ed. Baltimore and London: The Johns Hopkins University Press; 1998.

IV. GENERALIZED ANXIETY IN PATIENTS WITH NEUROLOGIC ILLNESS

A. Generalized anxiety disorder general treatment pearls
   1. Psychotherapeutic approaches to GAD include cognitive-behavioral, supportive, and psychodynamic. Cognitive-behavioral approaches have been well studied and should be employed when expertise is available. Specific behavioral approaches include relaxation techniques and biofeedback.

TABLE 6.3   Selected Psychiatric Medications for Treatment of Generalized Anxiety Disorder

Medication	Starting Dose	Usual Dosing Range
Tricyclic Antidepressants		
Nortriptyline (Pamelor, Aventyl HCl)	25 mg/d	Typically 50–150 mg qhs (dosed to 50–150 ng/mL)
Selective Serotonin Reuptake Inhibitors		
Citalopram (Celexa)	10–20 mg/d	20–60 mg/d
Escitalopram[a] (Lexapro)	10 mg/d	10–20 mg/d
Paroxetine[a] (Paxil)	10 mg/d	40 mg/d
Sertraline (Zoloft)	25–50 mg/d	100–200 mg/d
Other Antidepressants		
Mirtazapine (Remeron, Remeron SolTab)	15 mg/d	15–45 mg qhs
Venlafaxine[a] (Effexor XR)	75 mg/d	150–300 mg qd
Antipsychotics		
Olanzapine (Zyprexa)	2.5–5 mg/d	2.5–10 mg/d
Other		
Diphenhydramine (Benadryl)	25 mg	25–50 mg q4 hours as needed
Pindolol (Visken)	5–10 mg/d	10–60 mg/d
Propranolol (Inderal)	60–80 mg/d	80–520 mg/d

[a]U.S. Food and Drug Administration indication for generalized anxiety disorder.

    2.   Patients should be instructed to eliminate or at least limit caffeine and alcohol use.

    3.   Medications commonly prescribed for primary GAD include SSRIs, venlafaxine, TCAs, buspirone, and benzodiazepines. Starting and target doses are detailed in Table 6.3. Long-term treatment is required for many patients. To limit adverse reactions, including a possible initial worsening in anxiety, antidepressants must often be initiated at low doses and titrated slowly.

B. **Poststroke anxiety**

    1.   **Clinical background**

        a.   Approximately one fourth of patients, after acute stroke, meet criteria for GAD. Nearly another one fourth of patients will go on to develop clinically significant generalized anxiety. Approximately half of all poststroke patients with anxiety will have a clinically significant depressive syndrome (major or minor).

        b.   The *occurrence* of poststroke anxiety is not associated with acute social, cognitive, or physical impairment, but it is associated with later impairment in activities of daily living and a more limited social support network. Early onset poststroke anxiety, as defined by occurring within the first 3 months, is associated with a history of psychiatric disorder. Late-onset poststroke anxiety, arising more than 3 months after stroke, has not been associated with a previous psychiatric history. The use of stimulants to treat poststroke apathy may precipitate or contribute to anxiety.

c.   The *phenomenology* of poststroke anxiety is similar to that of a primary anxiety disorder. The phenomenology of early-onset and late-onset poststroke anxiety are also similar.

d.   Poststroke anxiety may last several months to years. When comorbid with depression, poststroke anxiety is associated with a longer duration of depression and greater functional and social impairment.

2.   **Pathogenesis of poststroke anxiety.** The *pathophysiology* of poststroke anxiety remains unclear. The combination of depression and anxiety has been associated with left frontal cortical lesions. Poststroke anxiety without depression has been associated with right hemisphere lesions.

3.   **Diagnosis.** As in primary anxiety disorders, the diagnosis is clinical and based on the presence of consensus criteria. The diagnosis may be impeded by the presence of a comorbid depression, aphasia, anosognosia, or dementia. Observations of family and other caretakers may assist in making the diagnosis.

4.   **Treatment**

a.   The clinician should optimize treatment and rehabilitate the patient, provide adequate pain management, and treat any underlying medical conditions.

b.   *Environmental modifications* should be implemented, including a daily routine with structured activities and good sleep hygiene. *Behavioral management* techniques should be employed by staff and taught to the family for any agitation secondary to anxiety.

c.   Although *psychotherapy* has not been explicitly studied in poststroke anxiety, cognitive behavior therapy (CBT) should be considered given its efficacy in patients with primary anxiety disorders.

d.   *Somatic therapy* should be implemented if anxiety is severe or persists despite the steps listed in the preceding text. There are no U.S. Food and Drug Administration (FDA)-approved somatic treatments for poststroke anxiety. Therapeutic options are the same as for primary anxiety disorders.

e.   *Nortriptyline* titrated slowly from 25 to 75 mg per day should be administered based on data from the treatment of poststroke depression comorbid with GAD. Tolerance and subsequent titration of nortriptyline may be limited by sedation, orthostatic hypotension, and anticholinergic side effects such as dry mouth, constipation, urinary retention, and blurry vision. In patients where nortriptyline is either not desired or contraindicated such as during acute recovery after myocardial infarction, *escitalopram* 10 mg per day or *venlafaxine* up to 300 mg per day are reasonable alternatives based on safety profile and efficacy in primary anxiety disorders.

f. *Benzodiazepines* are commonly prescribed in the treatment of primary generalized anxiety. However, benzodiazepines have not been studied in patients with stroke and carry significant risk of side effects and adverse events such as falls. In addition, tolerance is developed to benzodiazepines, which may result in rebound anxiety and withdrawal symptoms when prescribed for more than 4 weeks. Given these safety concerns and the high comorbidity of depression with poststroke anxiety, a course of treatment with an antidepressant is preferable.

g. Only one in four patients with early onset generalized anxiety recover by 1 year following the stroke. Most of the remaining experience a chronic course defined as at least 2 years' duration. Therefore, long-term treatment is required for many patients with poststroke anxiety similar to a primary GAD. We recommend continuing effective acute therapy for at least 1 year in responders. Partial responders or those whose symptoms return during subsequent taper may require chronic antidepressant treatment.

References

1. Astrom M. Generalized anxiety disorder in stroke patients: A 3 year longitudinal study. *Stroke.* 1996;27:270–275.
2. Castillo CS, Schultz SK, Robinson RG. Clinical correlates of early-onset and late-onset poststroke generalized anxiety. *Am J Psychiatry.* 1995;152(8):1174–1179.
3. Kimura M, Tateno A, Robinson RG. Treatment of poststroke generalized anxiety disorder comorbid with poststroke depression: Merged analysis of nortriptyline trials. *Am J Geriatr Psychiatry.* 2003;11(3):320–327.

C. **Generalized anxiety in patients with dementia, including Alzheimer disease**

1. **Clinical background**

a. Neuropsychiatric symptoms including agitation, anxiety, apathy, delusions, depression, hallucinations, and insomnia are commonly seen with dementia, including in the early stages of dementia and those with mild cognitive impairment. The population-based *cumulative prevalence* of general anxiety symptoms in dementia has been estimated at 25% with a 10% cumulative prevalence in those with mild cognitive impairment. Smaller studies have demonstrated anxiety symptoms in as many as 70% of those with dementia. Although the presence of anxiety symptoms is remarkably common in dementia, studies using the threshold of meeting diagnostic criteria for GAD have found a point prevalence of 5% to 6%. These rates may underestimate prevalence with anxiety symptoms, because such symptoms may be masked by the widespread use of psychotropic drugs in this population. Although some studies have shown a greater frequency of anxiety symptoms in vascular dementia over Alzheimer disease (AD), this finding has not been borne out in population-based studies.

b. The *occurrence* of anxiety in AD has been associated with depression, dementia severity, and age at onset. The presence of anxiety is also associated with impairments in activities of daily living (independent of age), increased nighttime awakenings, and overt aggression. Anxiety may adversely affect patient and caregiver quality of life. Anxiety in dementia has not been associated with age, gender, or ethnicity.

c. Given cognitive limitations in this population, comparing the *phenomenology* to that of primary anxiety disorders is difficult. Aggressive and agitated behaviors may occur more commonly and may be precipitated by a challenging situation, an unfamiliar environment, social isolation, or lack of routine.

d. Given the chronic nature of generalized anxiety and the progressive course of dementia, long-term treatment is typically warranted.

2. **Pathogenesis of anxiety in dementia.** The *pathophysiology* of anxiety in dementia remains unclear and understudied. Depression has been associated with damage to noradrenergic or serotonergic nuclei. Aggression has been associated with damage to serotonergic nuclei with relative preservation of dopaminergic regions. Anxiety often occurs with depression and may result in agitation or aggression. Anxiety may be a symptom of the underlying dementia or a psychological response to cognitive and functional deterioration.

3. **Diagnosis.** As in primary anxiety disorders, the diagnosis is clinical. The diagnosis may be impeded by cognitive limitations or obscured by comorbid depression. Observations of family and other caretakers may assist in making the diagnosis.

4. **Treatment**

a. The clinician should optimize treatment and rehabilitation of the dementia, provide adequate pain management, and treat any underlying medical conditions. *Cholinesterase inhibitors* may be continued, as they demonstrate a modest benefit in general neuropsychiatric outcomes (although their effects on anxiety symptoms per se have not been studied).

b. *Behavior management* training for addressing anxiety-related agitation may empower families and staff although improving outcomes. Distraction may be useful.

c. *Environmental and psychosocial interventions* may limit the anxiety associated with challenging situations, unfamiliar environments, isolation, or limited structure.

d. Ensuring an adequate *support network* for the patient and family is important. Given the stress associated with caring for a loved one with dementia, families may be at increased risk for demoralization, depression, and anxiety. Education and guidance may help families. Recommendation of a book such as *The 36-Hour Day* or a support group may provide supplemental education. Family members with particular difficulty coping may need encouragement to seek treatment or to simply take a reprieve. CBT has been shown to improve caregiver anxiety.

e. Medications are generally indicated for patients in whom the interventions mentioned in the preceding text have proved ineffective or only partially effective, or for whom anxiety is severe. There are no FDA-approved medications for anxiety in patients with AD. We recommend *citalopram* 20 mg per day, based on its safety, limited drug interactions, and the results of a randomized controlled trial. *Propranolol* at mean doses of 100 mg per day has led to reductions of neuropsychiatric inventory (NPI) anxiety scores in patients with AD and behavioral disruption. An industry-sponsored post hoc analysis of *olanzapine* in the treatment of anxiety symptoms in AD showed a modest improvement of anxiety symptoms in the low dose (5 mg per day) group; however, atypical antipsychotics should be used with caution in this population given the increased risk of mortality and cerebrovascular events. Case series suggest a benefit of *mirtazapine* in patients with AD and depression, anxiety, weight loss, and insomnia.

f. *Benzodiazepines* are not considered a first-line treatment of anxiety in dementia because of their adverse effect on cognition and propensity to induce delirium. Benzodiazepine use should generally be reserved for short term, low dose use in patients with acute anxiety, under close observation.

References

1. Ballard CD, Neill D, O'Brien J, et al. Anxiety, depression and psychosis in vascular dementia: Prevalence and associations. *J Affect Disord.* 2000;59(2):97–106.
2. Lyketsos CG, Lopez O, Jones B, et al. Prevalence of neuropsychiatric symptoms in dementia and mild cognitive impairment: Results from the cardiovascular health study. *JAMA.* 2002;288(12):1475–1483.
3. Mace NL, Rabins PV. *The 36-hour day: A family guide to caring for persons with Alzheimer disease, related dementing illnesses, and memory loss in later life.* Warner Books; 2001.
4. Nyth AI, Gottfries CG. The clinical efficacy of citalopram in the treatment of emotional disturbances in dementia

disorders. A nordic multicentre study. *Br J Psychiatry.* 1990;167:894–901.
5. Porter VR, Buxton WG, Fairbanks LA, et al. Frequency and characteristics of anxiety among patients with Alzheimer's disease and related dementias. *J Neuropsychiatry Clin Neurosci.* 2003;15(2):180–186.
6. Trinh NH, Hoblyn J, Mohanty S, et al. Efficacy of cholinesterase inhibitors in the treatment of neuropsychiatric symptoms and functional impairment in Alzheimer disease: A meta-analysis. *JAMA.* 2003;289(2): 210–216.

D. Generalized anxiety in patients with Parkinson disease
  1. **Clinical background**
      a. Major depression, apathetic syndromes, and anxiety disorders are commonly encountered in Parkinson disease (PD). Anxiety syndromes occur in up to 40% of patients with PD. Subjective anxiety may also be experienced with fluctuations in levels of levodopa and as a response to functional impairment. Anxiety usually appears after the diagnosis of PD although it can also present before the onset of motor symptoms.
      b. Anxiety in PD may be associated with autonomic dysfunction and predominantly left-sided symptoms. Anxiety levels have also been found to be higher in patients with a short allele of the promoter region for the serotonin transporter. There does not appear to be an association between anxiety and disability ratings.
      c. Patients with PD may experience greater fluctuations in the intensity of anxiety over the course of the day than patients with primary GAD.
  2. **Pathogenesis of anxiety in Parkinson disease.** The *pathogenesis* of psychiatric disturbances in PD is thought to be largely a consequence of the neurodegenerative disorder, including decreased pallidal inhibition of thalamofrontotemporal projections. This postulation does not ignore the clear psychological impact of the illness and its functional impairments. The destruction of dopamine-producing neurons in the substantia nigra exerts downstream effects on the caudate, putamen, frontal cortex, and cingulate cortex. PD is further associated with degradation of cholinergic, noradrenergic, and serotonergic systems. Alterations in noradrenergic output from the locus ceruleus have been suggested as a potential etiology of anxiety syndromes. This may occur as a consequence of the loss of dopaminergic inhibition of the locus ceruleus.
  3. **Diagnosis.** As in primary anxiety disorders, the diagnosis is clinical. A thoughtful and comprehensive evaluation is critical to consider the broad differential diagnoses of anxiety in this population. Anxiety syndromes can be difficult to diagnose because of the aforementioned association of subjective anxiety with fluctuations in levodopa levels. Further complicating the issue,

symptoms related to autonomic dysfunction such as racing heart or dizziness may be mistakenly attributed to anxiety.

4. **Treatment**

   a.   The clinician should optimize treatment of the PD, provide adequate pain management, and treat any underlying medical conditions.

   b.   Optimal treatment of the anxiety includes behavioral, psychosocial, and potentially pharmacologic modalities.

   c.   *Environmental interventions* such as home care for observation and therapy, support groups, and prescribed exercise may be helpful.

   d.   Relaxation training, physical therapy, and occupational therapy may be of benefit.

   e.   *Education* regarding the relationship between the patient's PD and their anxiety may be beneficial to patients and families. Supportive *psychotherapy* and counseling may assist patients and family in dealing with the current life changes and future expectations.

   f.   Medications are generally indicated for patients in whom the interventions mentioned in the preceding text have proved ineffective or only partially effective. There and no FDA-approved medications for the treatment of anxiety in patients with PD. Patients with PD may be particularly sensitive to the adverse effects of psychiatric medications, especially antipsychotics given their dopamine antagonism and subsequent propensity to induce parkinsonism. Antidepressants with demonstrated effectiveness for generalized anxiety may be considered first-line treatments. We recommend *escitalopram* 10 mg per day or *venlafaxine* 150 to 225 mg per day based on safety profile and efficacy in primary anxiety disorders. Benzodiazepines may increase fall risk and impair cognition and should therefore be avoided. As needed, low-dose trazodone (25 to 150 mg qhs) may help with insomnia. *Nortriptyline* has been studied in the treatment of depression in PD and may benefit anxiety symptoms.

   References

   1.   Andersen J, Aabro E, Gulmann N, et al. Antidepressant treatment in Parkinson's disease: A controlled trial of the effect of nortriptyline in patients with Parkinson's disease treated with L-Dopa. *Acta Neurol Scand.* 1980;62:210–219.

   2.   Marsh L. Neuropsychiatric aspects of Parkinson's disease. *Psychosomatics.* 2000;41(1):15–23.

   3.   Richard JH, Schiffer RB, Kurlan R. Anxiety and Parkinson's disease. *J Neuropscyhiatr Clin Neurosci.* 1996;8: 383–393.

E.   **Generalized anxiety in patients with Huntington disease**

   1.   **Clinical background**

      a.   Neuropsychiatric symptoms, including anxiety, are common in Huntington disease (HD) and may be the presenting symptoms in >75% of patients. Psychiatric symptoms may predate motor symptoms by more than a decade and over 75% of patients may require psychiatric hospitalization. NPI anxiety measures are elevated in >50% of cases.

  b. Psychiatric symptoms do not appear to be correlated with cognitive deterioration, the severity of motor symptoms, or the CAG repeat length.

  c. Chorea may worsen with anxiety.

2. **Pathogenesis of anxiety in Huntington disease.** The pathogenesis of neuropsychiatric symptoms in patients with HD is poorly understood. Circuits projecting to the orbitofrontal and dorsal regions of the prefrontal cortex may be involved in agitation, anxiety, and irritability.

3. **Diagnosis**

  a. As in primary anxiety disorders, the diagnosis is clinical. The diagnosis may be more difficult to make in later stages of the illness because of impaired cognitive function and apathy.

  b. The differential diagnosis includes vague paranoia, irritability, personality changes, and akathisia secondary to antipsychotic medications, which may be used to treat dyskinesia or psychosis. Chorea may also be misinterpreted as restlessness.

4. **Treatment**

  a. Optimal treatment often involves a combination of counseling, psychotherapy, and pharmacotherapy.

  b. Pretest and posttest *counseling* is necessary for genetic testing, which should only occur in the context of a physician–patient relationship and a genetic counseling program. Given the autosomal dominant inheritance of this illness, it is important to assess family supports and attend to the needs of family members.

  c. Brief structured psychotherapy (e.g., CBT) may be beneficial, although there are no controlled data on this issue. Unique *psychotherapeutic issues* may include blaming of parents, jealousy toward unaffected family members, and family planning issues.

  d. Medication is indicated if the anxiety is severe or if the interventions mentioned in the preceding text have not been sufficiently successful. There are no FDA-approved medications for the treatment of anxiety in patients with HD. We recommend *escitalopram* 10 mg per day or *venlafaxine* 150 to 225 mg per day based on safety profile and efficacy in primary GAD. On the basis of the results of an open label study, olanzapine may be considered as an adjunct, particularly if psychotic symptoms are present.

References

1. Leroi I, Michalon M. Treatment of the psychiatric manifestations of Huntington's disease: A review of the literature. *Can J Psychiatry.* 1998;43(9):933–940.

2. Paulsen JS, Ready RE, Hamilton JM, et al. Neuropsychi-
    atric aspects of Huntington's disease. *J Neurol Neurosurg
    Psychiatry*. 2001;71(3):310–314.

F. **Generalized anxiety in patients with traumatic brain injury**
    1. **Clinical background**
        a. Traumatic brain injury (TBI) results in a high frequency of
            anxiety disorders associated with demographic, personality,
            and other variables. Rates of anxiety disorders in TBI are
            elevated preinjury and rise significantly after injury to ap-
            proximately 25% of patients with a relative risk of 2.3 in
            some studies. These rates decrease as time from injury in-
            creases.
        b. It is unclear if the phenomenology of anxiety in TBI differs
            in any fundamental way from primary anxiety disorders.
    2. **Pathogenesis of anxiety in traumatic brain injury.** The *pathogenesis*
        of anxiety secondary to TBI is likely multifactorial and depen-
        dent on the degree and relative location of focal brain damage
        and diffuse axonal injury. Right hemispheric lesions are most
        often associated with anxiety.
    3. **Diagnosis**
        a. The diagnosis of GAD in patients with TBI is a clinical one.
        b. In addition to the general differential diagnosis for anx-
            iety, the differential diagnosis of anxiety symptoms in
            patients with TBI includes adrenal insufficiency, syn-
            drome of inappropriate antidiuretic hormone (SIADH),
            diabetes insipidus, and anterior hypopituitarism (panhy-
            popituitarism).
    4. **Treatment**
        a. Optimal treatment often involves a combination of psy-
            chotherapeutic, behavior modification, and pharmacologic
            approaches in addition to often intensive rehabilitation and
            pain management.
        b. *Psychotherapy* requires a strong working relationship and
            an appreciation of the patient's premorbid characteristics.
            Behavioral approaches with reinforcement contingent on
            target behaviors, including avoidance, poor compliance
            with treatment, and maladaptive behaviors, may be helpful
            when indicated.
        c. Medication is indicated if the anxiety is severe or if the in-
            terventions mentioned in the preceding text have not been
            sufficiently successful. There are no FDA-approved med-
            ications for the treatment of anxiety in patients with TBI.
            We recommend *sertraline* starting at low doses (25 mg per
            day) and with slow titration to 100 to 200 mg per day to
            minimize adverse events.
        d. According to a recent Cochrane review, β-blockers such
            as *propranolol* or *pindolol* may be effective for the treatment
            of agitation or aggression (which is sometimes associated
            with anxiety) in patients with TBI.

e. Benzodiazepines should be avoided given TBI patients' increased susceptibility to adverse effects and propensity for paradoxical agitation.

References

1. Borgaro S, Caples H, Prigatano GP. Non-pharmacological management of psychiatric disturbances after traumatic brain injury. *Int Rev Psychiatry.* 2003;15(4): 371–379.
2. Jorge RE, Robinson RG, Starkstein SE, et al. Depression and anxiety following traumatic brain injury. *J Neuropsychiatry Clin Neurosci.* 1993;5(4):369–374.
3. Lee HB, Lyketsos CG, Rao V. Pharmacological management of the psychiatric aspects of traumatic brain injury. *Int Rev Psychiatry.* 2003;15(4):359–370.

G. **Generalized anxiety in patients with multiple sclerosis**

1. **Clinical background**
   a. Approximately 33% of patients with multiple sclerosis (MS) report anxiety as measured by the NPI.
   b. Anxiety in MS has not been found to correlate with clinical variables or any regional or total lesion volume on structural imaging. Conflicting reports exist regarding an association between anxiety and physical impairment. Anxiety has been associated with a perceived high risk of wheelchair dependence. Additionally, corticosteroid use may result in anxiety.
   c. There are no reported differences in the *phenomenology* of anxiety compared with primary anxiety disorders.

2. **Pathogenesis of anxiety in multiple sclerosis.** Controversy exists as to whether the *pathogenesis* of anxiety in MS is related to underlying brain injury. Some have speculated that the paucity of associations to structural abnormalities or clinical variables supports the formulation of anxiety as a psychological reaction in MS; however, this remains an understudied topic.

3. **Diagnosis**
   a. The diagnosis of GAD in patients with MS is clinical.
   b. The differential diagnosis of anxiety in patients with MS includes anxiety secondary to corticosteroids or glatiramer (Copaxone). Anxiety secondary to chronic administration of interferon β-1b (Betaseron) has been described, although it is not supported by longitudinal studies.

4. **Treatment**
   a. Optimal treatment often involves a combination of psychotherapy and pharmacotherapy.
   b. *Coping skills* training and *support groups* may be helpful.
   c. *Psychotherapy* may address demoralization, functional losses, and living with a progressive demyelinating illness. A variety of psychotherapeutic modalities may be helpful, particularly CBT.
   d. Medication is indicated if the anxiety is severe or if the interventions mentioned in the preceding text have not been sufficiently successful. There are no FDA-approved

medications for the treatment of anxiety in patients with MS. We recommend *escitalopram* 10 mg per day or *venlafaxine* 150 to 225 mg per day based on safety profile and efficacy in primary anxiety disorders.

References

1. Diaz-Olavarrieta C, Cummings JL, Velazquez J, et al. Neuropsychiatric manifestations of multiple sclerosis. *J Neuropsychiatry Clin Neurosci.* 1999;11(1):51–57.
2. Zorzon M, deMasi R, Nasuelli D, et al. Depression and anxiety in multiple sclerosis. A clinical and MRI study of 95 subjects. *J Neurol.* 2001;248:416–421.

H. **Generalized anxiety in patients with epilepsy**
   1. **Clinical background**
      a. Nearly 50% of epilepsy patients have disturbances of mood, anxiety, or psychotic symptoms. Fear and anxiety are often associated with the ictal state. As many as 33% of patients with partial seizures report anxiety as part of their aura. Interictal anxiety is more common than anxiety in the general population.
      b. Interictal anxiety has been associated with depression and particularly left-sided temporal lobe epilepsy. Anxiety disorders may be more common in those with fear auras and persistent seizures. Anxiety may occur in the setting of withdrawal of antiepileptic drugs, notably phenobarbital, and phenytoin.
      c. Anxiety in epilepsy may involve concentration impairments, fatigue, insomnia, irritability, restlessness, and tension.
   2. **Pathogenesis of anxiety in epilepsy.** The *pathogenesis* of anxiety in epilepsy is not well understood. Ictal fear is associated with right temporal seizure foci. Postictal anxiety is not thought to be simply a psychological reaction to the seizure although social stressors and the unpredictability of seizures may contribute to anxiety.
   3. **Diagnosis**
      a. An attempt should be made to temporally link the psychiatric disturbance to the seizure. Anxiety often occurs as a preictal, postictal, or interictal phenomenon. In such cases, treatment of anxiety requires optimal seizure control.
      b. Rule out anxiety secondary to anticonvulsant medication withdrawal, which has been described with phenobarbital and phenytoin.
      c. Rule out anxiety as a side effect of anticonvulsant medications, particularly lamotrigine and felbamate.
   4. **Treatment**
      a. Optimal treatment often involves a combination of psychotherapy and pharmacotherapy.
      b. Biofeedback, relaxation training, and stress management may alleviate anxiety.

c. *Psychotherapy* may address stigma of the illness and demoralization. A variety of psychotherapeutic modalities may be helpful, especially CBT, which may be helpful for patients whose anxiety persists despite good seizure control.

d. Medication is indicated if the anxiety is severe or if the interventions mentioned in the preceding text have not been sufficiently successful. There are no FDA-approved medications for the treatment of anxiety in patients with epilepsy. We recommend *escitalopram* 10 mg per day or *venlafaxine* 150 to 225 mg per day based on safety profile and efficacy in primary anxiety disorders. Carbamazepine may decrease the clearance of escitalopram and stiripentol may decrease the metabolism of venlafaxine to its active metabolite, O-desmethylvenlafaxine; however, dosage adjustments are seldom necessary for these specific drug interactions.

e. *Benzodiazepines* should be used with caution and only over a short period of time. Benzodiazepine tapers should be gradual given the increased risk of seizures during withdrawal.

f. Use of *buspirone* is contraindicated given its propensity to lower seizure threshold. Caution should be exercised regarding drug interactions with anticonvulsants. Phenobarbital, primidone, phenytoin, and carbamazepine may decrease TCA levels, whereas valproic acid levels may increase TCA levels. TCAs may further increase the levels of many antiepileptic medications. Fluoxetine may increase levels of carbamazepine, phenytoin, and valproic acid.

g. Carbamazepine, gabapentin, tiagabine, valproate, and vigabatrin may improve anxiety. If clinically appropriate, these agents may be used preferentially.

References
1. Marsh L, Rao V. Psychiatric complications in patients with epilepsy: A review. *Epilepsy Research.* 2002;49: 11–33.

V. OBSESSIVE-COMPULSIVE DISORDER IN PATIENTS WITH NEUROLOGIC ILLNESS

A. **Obsessive-compulsive disorder general treatment pearls**

1. Exposure and response prevention (ERP), a type of behavioral therapy, is strongly recommended. Cognitive therapy is often included with this behavioral therapy. The relapse rate following discontinuation of CBT is lower than following discontinuation of an antidepressant.

2. Medications generally recommended for primary OCD include fluoxetine, fluvoxamine, sertraline, paroxetine, citalopram, clomipramine, and venlafaxine. Monoamine oxidase inhibitors may be considered for resistant cases. Starting and target doses are detailed in Table 6.4. Higher doses of

TABLE 6.4   Selected Psychiatric Medications for Treatment of Obsessive-Compulsive Disorder

Medication	Starting Dose	Usual Dosing Range
Tricyclic Antidepressants		
Clomipramine[a] (Anafranil)	10–25 mg/d	150–250 mg/d
Selective Serotonin Reuptake Inhibitors		
Fluoxetine[a] (Prozac)	20 mg/d	60–80 mg/d
Fluvoxamine[a] (Luvox)	50 mg/d	200–300 mg/d
Sertraline[a] (Zoloft)	25–50 mg/d	150–225 mg/d
Paroxetine[a] (Paxil)	10–20 mg/d	50–60 mg/d
Citalopram (Celexa)	10–20 mg/d	40–80 mg/d
Serotonin and Norepinephrine Reputake Inhibitors		
Venlafaxine (Effexor XR)	75 mg/d	225–375 mg/d

[a]U.S. Food and Drug Administration indication for obsessive-compulsive disorder.

antidepressant medications are typically required for treatment of OCD compared with depression. In addition, medication trials are typically of longer duration (i.e., 12 weeks).

B. **Poststroke obsessive-compulsive disorder**
1. **Clinical background.** Obsessive-compulsive behavior is rare following stroke.
2. **Pathogenesis of poststroke obsessive-compulsive disorder.** Poststroke OCD appears to occur primarily with basal ganglia infarcts.
3. **Diagnosis**
   a. The diagnosis is clinical and based on the presence of consensus criteria.
   b. The differential diagnosis includes temporal lobe epilepsy, tic disorders, and depression. OCD symptoms have been reported with psychostimulant use.
4. **Treatment**
   a. In addition to treatment and rehabilitation of the stroke, optimal treatment includes psychotherapy and medications.
   b. *ERP*, a type of behavioral therapy, is strongly recommended and often combined with cognitive therapy.
   c. Medication is indicated if the anxiety is severe or if the interventions mentioned in the preceding text have not been sufficiently successful. There are no FDA-approved medications for the treatment of poststroke OCD. We recommend *citalopram* 40 to 80 mg per day or *sertraline* 150 to 225 mg per day, based on their safety profile and efficacy in primary anxiety disorders. For nonresponders, we recommend *clomipramine* 150 to 250 mg per day, based on efficacy in primary anxiety disorders.

References
1. Carmin CN, Wiegartz PS, Yunus U, et al. Treatment of late-onset OCD following basal ganglia infarct. *Depress Anxiety*. 2002;15:87–90.

C. **Obsessive-compulsive disorder in patients with Parkinson disease**
1. **Clinical background**
   a. Obsessive-compulsive behavior is rare in patients with PD.
   b. Obsessive-compulsive symptoms in PD may be more common in patients with more severe left-sided motor symptoms.
   c. Ordering symptoms may be more common in patients with PD.
2. **Pathogenesis of obsessive-compulsive disorder in Parkinson disease** The *pathophysiology* of both PD and OCD, is thought to be related to dysfunction in the circuitry between frontal cortex and basal ganglia. Cases have been reported of improvement in both parkinsonian and obsessive-compulsive symptoms in patients with PD and OCD treated with subthalamic nucleus stimulation.
3. **Diagnosis**
   a. As in primary anxiety disorders, the diagnosis is clinical.
   b. The differential diagnosis includes obsessive-compulsive symptoms secondary to a depressive disorder or stimulant use.
4. **Treatment**
   a. Optimal treatment includes psychotherapy and medications.
   b. *ERP,* a type of behavioral therapy, is strongly recommended and often combined with cognitive therapy.
   c. Medication is indicated if the anxiety is severe or if the interventions mentioned in the preceding text have not been sufficiently successful. There are no FDA-approved medications for the treatment of OCD in patients with PD. We recommend *sertraline* 150 to 225 mg per day, based on its safety profile and efficacy in primary anxiety disorders. For nonresponders, we recommend *clomipramine* 150 to 250 mg per day, based on efficacy in primary anxiety disorders. Some patients with PD may be sensitive to side effects and require lower doses and slower titration.

References
1. Harbishettar V, Pal PK, Janardhan Reddy YC, et al. Is there a relationship between Parkinson's disease and obsessive-compulsive disorder? *Parkinsonism Relat Disord*. 2005;11(2):85–88.
2. Maia AF, Pinto AS, Barbosa ER, et al. Obsessive-compulsive symptoms, obsessive-compulsive disorder, and related disorders in Parkinson's disease. *J Neuropsychiatry Clin Neurosci*. 2003;15(3):371–374.
3. Marsh L. Neuropsychiatric aspects of Parkinson's disease. *Psychosomatics*. 2000;41(1):15–23.

D. **Obsessive-compulsive disorder in patients with Huntington disease**

1. **Clinical background**
    a. There are only a few reports in the literature of OCD in patients with HD.
    b. One HD-affected family was found to have unusually high rates of OCD and pathologic gambling in only those with the HD mutation.
    c. Given limited reports, no distinction regarding the phenomenology of obsessive-compulsive symptoms in patients with HD can be made.

2. **Pathogenesis of obsessive-compulsive disorder in Huntington disease**
    a. The *pathophysiology* of both HD and OCD has been suggested to relate to dysfunction of circuits between the basal ganglia and orbitofrontal areas.

3. **Diagnosis**
    a. As in primary anxiety disorders, the diagnosis is clinical. Controversy regarding the existence of a relationship between HD and OCD may require a higher burden of evidence to make the diagnosis of OCD secondary to HD.
    b. The differential diagnosis includes obsessive-compulsive symptoms secondary to a depressive disorder.

4. **Treatment**
    a. Optimal treatment includes psychotherapy and medications.
    b. *ERP*, a type of behavioral therapy, is strongly recommended and often combined with cognitive therapy.
    c. Medication is indicated if the anxiety is severe or if the interventions mentioned in the preceding text have not been sufficiently successful. There are no FDA-approved medications for the treatment of OCD in patients with HD. We recommend *flouxetine* 40 to 80 mg per day, based on the results of a case series. For nonresponders, we recommend *clomipramine* 150 to 250 mg per day based on its efficacy in primary OCD.

    References
    1. De Marchi N, Mennella R. Huntington's disease and its association with psychopathology. *Harv Rev Psychiatry.* 2000;7(5):278–289.

E. **Obsessive-compulsive disorder in patients following traumatic brain injury**

1. **Clinical background**
    a. Most surveys of TBI patients report low rates of OCD following injury although many report higher rates of obsessive-compulsive personality changes. Reports of cases of OCD following TBI have been present for decades.
    b. The emergence of obsessive-compulsive symptoms following brain injury, is thought to be influenced by a preexisting diathesis and lesion location. There is a frequent

comorbidity of affective disorders in those with OCD following TBI.

c. Perseverative behaviors occur commonly after TBI and may or may not be related to obsessive-compulsive symptoms in a given patient.

2. **Pathogenesis of obsessive-compulsive disorder in traumatic brain injury**

a. The *pathophysiology* of obsessive-compulsive symptoms following TBI, is proposed to be related to damage to orbitofrontal, mesial prefrontal, and basal ganglia regions. When functionally intact, these regions are thought to play a role in inhibiting obsessive experiences.

3. **Diagnosis**

a. As in primary anxiety disorders, the diagnosis is clinical. Onset of obsessive-compulsive symptoms following brain injury and lack of such symptoms preceding injury may help solidify diagnosis of OCD secondary to TBI.

b. The differential diagnosis includes temporal lobe epilepsy, tic disorders, and depression. OCD symptoms have additionally been reported with psychostimulant use.

4. **Treatment**

a. In addition to rehabilitation for the sequelae of brain injury, optimal treatment includes psychotherapy and medications. Explicit efforts to prevent obsessive and compulsive symptoms from impeding functional rehabilitation should be employed.

b. ERP, a type of behavioral therapy, is strongly recommended. Cognitive therapy is often included with this behavioral therapy.

c. Medication is indicated if the anxiety is severe or if the interventions mentioned in the preceding text have not been sufficiently successful. There are no FDA-approved medications for the treatment of OCD in patients with TBI. We recommend *citalopram* 40 to 80 mg per day or *sertraline* 150 to 225 mg per day, based on their safety profile and efficacy in primary OCD. For nonresponders, we recommend *clomipramine* 150 to 250 mg per day, based on efficacy in primary OCD.

References

1. Grados MA. Obsessive-compulsive disorder after traumatic brain injury. *Int Rev Psychiatry.* 2003;15(4):350–358.

F. **Obsessive-compulsive disorder in patients with Tourette syndrome**

1. **Clinical background**

a. Strong evidence supports an association between Tourette syndrome (TS) and OCD, including evidence of a genetic relationship between the two disorders. In addition, tics are commonly seen in 7% to 37% of OCD patients without TS.

b. Early onset OCD patients may share certain features with TS patients with OCD.

   c. In patients with TS and OCD, repetitive behaviors may be less likely preceded by obsessions and less likely associated with anxiety. They may have an increased likelyhood of having unusual sensations such as feelings of discomfort preceding these acts.

2. **Pathogenesis of obsessive-compulsive disorder in Tourette syndrome**

   a. The *pathophysiology* of OCD in TS remains to be elucidated. In addition to a genetic role, some have suggested that autoimmunity may play a role in a subset of patients. The association of OCD with Sydenham chorea, considered a complication of rheumatic fever, has further suggested a potential autoimmune role in a subset of patients.

3. **Diagnosis**

   a. As in primary anxiety disorders, the diagnosis of OCD is clinical.

   b. Motor tics should be carefully distinguished from compulsions to prevent misdiagnosis.

4. **Treatment**

   a. Optimal treatment includes psychotherapy and medications.

   b. *ERP*, a type of behavioral therapy, is strongly recommended. Cognitive therapy is often included with this behavioral therapy.

   c. Medication is indicated if the anxiety is severe or if the interventions mentioned in the preceding text have not been sufficiently successful. There are no FDA-approved medications for the treatment of OCD in patients with TS. We recommend *citalopram* 40 to 80 mg per day or *sertraline* 150 to 225 mg per day, based on their safety profile and efficacy in primary anxiety disorders. For nonresponders, we recommend *clomipramine* 150 to 250 mg per day, based on efficacy in primary anxiety disorders. Patients with OCD and TS may be less likely to respond to treatment with an SSRI alone and more likely to benefit from use of an *SSRI with an antipsychotic*. Antipsychotic augmentation of antidepressant treatment should therefore be initiated early. Case reports have shown favorable results from electroconvulsive therapy (ECT) in those with OCD and TS.

References

1. Maia AS, Barbosa ER, Menezes PR, et al. Relationship between obsessive-compulsive disorders and diseases affecting primarily the basal ganglia. *Rev Hosp Clin Fac Med Sao Paulo.* 1999;54(6):213–221.

2. Miguel EC, Shavitt RG, Ferrao YA, et al. How to treat OCD in patients with Tourette syndrome. *J Psychosom Res.* 2003;55(1):49–57.

3. McDougle CG, Goodman WK, Leckman JF, et al. Haloperidol addition in fluvoxamine-refractory obsessive compulsive disorder: A double-blind

placebo-controlled study in patients with and without tics. *Arch Gen Psychiatry.* 1994;51:302–308.

VI. PANIC DISORDER IN PATIENTS WITH NEUROLOGIC ILLNESS

A. **Panic disorder general treatment pearls**
1. CBT and/or SSRI are generally considered first-line treatments, based on their efficacy and safety in patients with primary panic disorder.
2. CBT may incorporate systematic desensitization for anxiety-provoking situations, especially if agoraphobia is present.
3. SSRIs and TCAs are generally considered to be equally effective in the treatment of panic disorder. Starting and target doses of selected medications for the treatment of panic disorder are detailed in Table 6.5. Monoamine oxidase inhibitors (MAOIs) are also effective in the treatment of panic disorder. Antidepressants are typically maintained for at least 1 year.
4. Benzodiazepines such as clonazepam are effective in reducing panic symptoms and frequency of attacks. Benzodiazepines have a relatively rapid onset of action that can be advantageous. The increased susceptibility in the elderly and those with neurologic conditions to adverse events and the limited long-term effectiveness of benzodiazepines limits their utility. Given concerns about long-term use of benzodiazepines, they should generally be used only in conjunction with an antidepressant, such as paroxetine 20 mg per day during the initiation phase of an antidepressant.

TABLE 6.5   Selected Psychiatric Medications for Treatment of Panic Disorder

Medication	Starting Dose	Usual Dosing Range
Benzodiazepines		
Clonazepam (Klonopin)	0.25 mg PO q.d.–b.i.d.	0.25–1 mg PO b.i.d.–t.i.d.
Tricyclic Antidepressants		
Clomipramine (Anafranil)	25 mg PO qhs	75–150 mg PO qhs
Imipramine (Tofranil)	25 mg PO qhs	75–150 mg PO qhs
Selective Serotonin Reuptake Inhibitors		
Fluoxetine[a] (Prozac)	20 mg/d	20–60 mg/d
Fluvoxamine (Luvox)	50 mg/d	50–200 mg/d
Sertraline[a] (Zoloft)	25–50 mg/d	50–200 mg/d
Paroxetine[a] (Paxil)	10–20 mg/d	20–40 mg/d
Citalopram (Celexa)	10–20 mg/d	20–60 mg/d
Other Antidepressants		
Venlafaxine[a] (Effexor XR)	75 mg/d	75–225 mg/d

[a]U.S. Food and Drug Administration indication for panic disorder.

B. **Panic disorder in Parkinson disease**
   1. **Clinical background**
      a. The prevalence of panic disorder in patients with PD may be as high as 25% although it has been estimated at 8% by studies using more stringent criteria.
      b. Panic attacks in PD are associated with an early age of PD onset, the presence of depression, need for higher doses of levodopa, and the "off" phase of levodopa fluctuations. Panic attacks in patients with PD are a not infrequent source of emergency department visits.
   2. **Pathogenesis of panic disorder in Parkinson disease.** Panic attacks in PD, are thought to be related to alterations in noradrenergic systems secondary to dysfunction of the locus ceruleus. This dysfunction may occur secondary to a decrease in dopaminergic inhibition of the locus ceruleus.
   3. **Diagnosis**
      a. Given the broad differential diagnosis of anxiety symptoms in PD, that includes medication effects, a careful history is required detailing the temporal relationship between panic disorder onset and the course of illness as well as between panic attack occurrence and medication administration. Having the patient complete a journal or timeline of panic attacks and medications administered may be helpful in delineating this relationship.
      b. The differential diagnosis for panic attacks in PD should additionally include hyperthyroidism, myocardial infarction, pheochromocytoma, specific phobia, and substance-induced.
   4. **Treatment**
      a. Optimal treatment includes psychotherapy and/or medications.
      b. CBT may be an effective treatment, based on efficacy in primary panic disorder.
      c. Medication is indicated if the anxiety is severe or if the interventions mentioned in the preceding text have not been sufficiently successful. There are no FDA-approved medications for the treatment of panic symptoms in patients with PD. If patients experience panic attacks primarily during off periods, adjustments in the dosage and timing of PD medications may be helpful. Additionally, we recommend the following agents with demonstrated efficacy in primary panic disorder and specific studies in PD: *Flouxetine* 20 to 60 mg per day based on retrospective study, *sertraline* 50 to 200 mg per day based on the results of a small open label study or *imipramine* 75 to 150 mg per day based on a small controlled study.
      References
      1. Lauterbach EC, Freeman A, Vogel RL. Correlates of generalized anxiety and panic attacks in dystonia and

Parkinson disease. *Cogn Behav Neurol.* 2003;16(4): 225–233.

2. Marsh L. Neuropsychiatric aspects of Parkinson's disease. *Psychosomatics.* 2000;41(1):15–23.

3. Walsh K, Bennett G. Parkinson's disease and anxiety. *Postgrad Med J.* 2001;77:89–93.

C. **Panic disorder in traumatic brain injury**

    1. **Clinical background**

       a. The prevalence of panic disorder in TBI has been estimated at 8% to 9%.

       b. Panic attacks in TBI have not been studied enough to warrant a discussion of associated factors or distinct phenomenologic characteristics.

    2. **Pathogenesis of panic disorder in traumatic brain injury.** Limited data exists to support a specific pathogenic hypothesis of panic disorder with TBI although evidence for causation secondary to TBI exists.

    3. **Diagnosis**

       a. A temporal relationship with brain injury is critical to the delineation of a panic disorder secondary to TBI.

       b. The differential diagnosis includes panic secondary to use of substances such as alcohol, caffeine, nicotine, and stimulants. Hypopituitarism may occur with even mild TBI although it is more likely to present with general anxiety.

    4. **Treatment**

       a. In addition to rehabilitation from the TBI, optimal treatment includes psychotherapy and/or medications.

       b. When expertise is available, CBT may be an effective first-line or adjunct treatment of panic disorder for patients with mild TBI or without significant cognitive decline.

       c. Medication is indicated if the anxiety is severe or if the interventions mentioned in the preceding text have not been sufficiently successful. There are no FDA-approved medications for the treatment of anxiety in patients with TBI. We recommend *sertraline* 50 to 200 mg per day (starting at 25 mg per day) or *paroxetine* 20 mg per day (starting at 10 mg per day), based on safety profile and efficacy in panic disorder. Benzodiazepines should generally be avoided given their negative impact on cognitive and physical performance.

    References

    1. Lee HB, Lyketsos CG, Rao V. Pharmacological management of the psychiatric aspects of traumatic brain injury. *Int Rev Psychiatry.* 2003;15(4):359–370.

    2. vanReekum R, Cohen T, Wong J. Can traumatic brain injury cause psychiatric disorders? *J Neuropsychiatry Clin Neurosci.* 2000;12(3):316–327.

D. **Panic disorder in patients with epilepsy**

    1. **Clinical background**

       a. Panic disorder may affect approximately 20% of epilepsy patients.

b.   Panic disorder appears to be associated with epilepsy with ictal fear.

c.   Brief panic sensations lasting <1 to 2 minutes during epileptic seizures are common and should be distinguished from overt panic attacks. Simple partial seizures may manifest as panic attacks.

2.   **Pathogenesis of anxiety in epilepsy.** The *pathogenesis* of panic attacks in epilepsy is not well understood. The high prevalence compared with the general population (approximately 20% vs. 1% to 2%) and temporal relationship to seizure activity provides strong evidence for causality.

3.   **Diagnosis**

a.   An attempt should be made to temporally link the psychiatric disturbance to the seizure. Experiences akin to panic attacks can occur during partial seizures or as an interictal phenomenon. Some argue that when associated with epileptic consciousness or aura, panic attacks should be diagnosed as epilepsy rather than panic disorder. Further complicating diagnosis, panic attacks in patients with epilepsy may be misdiagnosed as seizure activity.

b.   The differential diagnosis for panic attacks includes hyperthyroidism, specific phobia, substance-induced, and pheochromocytoma.

4.   **Treatment**

a.   Optimal treatment includes psychotherapy and/or medications.

b.   When expertise is available, CBT may be an effective first-line or adjunct treatment for panic disorder, particularly when the panic attacks are thought to be not related to seizure activity.

c.   Medication is indicated if the anxiety is severe or if the interventions mentioned in the preceding text have not been sufficiently successful. There are no FDA-approved medications for the treatment of panic in patients with epilepsy. We recommend *fluoxetine* as first-line pharmacologic treatment of panic disorder in patients with epilepsy, based on limited effects on seizure threshold and demonstrated effectiveness in panic disorder. Fluoxetine should be initiated at a low dose of 10 mg per day and titrated slowly with the dose increased to 20 mg after 1 week of treatment. Fluoxetine may increase levels of carbamazepine, phenytoin, valproic acid, and other antiepileptic drugs. Alternatively, *sertraline* 100 to 200 mg per day may be considered for the treatment of panic disorder in patients with epilepsy.

References

1.   Alvarez-Silva S, Alvarez-Rodriguez J, Perez-Echeverria MJ, et al. Panic and epilepsy. *J Anxiety Disord.* 2006;20(3): 353–362.

2.   Marsh L, Rao V. Psychiatric complications in patients with epilepsy: A review. *Epilepsy Res.* 2002;49:11–33.

E. Panic disorder in patients with migraine headache
1. **Clinical background**
   a. Panic disorder has been associated with migraine headache in population-based studies with a prevalence rate near 16%.
   b. Migraine or severe nonmigraine headache increases the risk of developing panic disorder. Panic disorder increases the risk of developing migraine headaches but not severe nonmigraine headache. Patients with panic disorder and migraine headache tend to have a longer duration of panic disorder and more frequent attacks. Patients with migraine and with panic attacks may face more frequent and more severe migraine attacks.
   c. Panic symptoms may occur at the peak of a migraine attack.
2. **Pathogenesis of panic disorder in migraine headache**
   a. Some authors have hypothesized that the relationship between panic attacks and migraine may be because of autonomic dysregulation. The relationship between panic attacks and migraine is thought to be noncausal.
3. **Diagnosis**
   a. The diagnosis of panic disorder in migraine headache is a clinical one. The distinction of panic disorder secondary to migraine may be difficult to substantiate without a predominance of panic attacks occurring at the peak of a migraine attack.
   b. The differential diagnosis includes though is not limited to panic secondary to the use of substances such as alcohol, caffeine, nicotine, and stimulants.
4. **Treatment**
   a. Optimal treatment includes psychotherapy and/or medications.
   b. CBT should be considered as a treatment option when expertise is available.
   c. Medication is indicated if the anxiety is severe or if the interventions mentioned in the preceding text have not been sufficiently successful. There are no FDA-approved medications for the treatment of panic in patients with migraine. We recommend *clomipramine* 75 to 150 mg per day or *imipramine* 75 to 50 mg per day, based on demonstrated effectiveness in the treatment of both migraine headache and panic disorder.

   References
   1. Breslau N, Schultz LR, Stewart WF, et al. Headache types and panic disorder: Directionality and specificity. *Neurology.* 2001;56(3):350–354.
   2. Ossipova VV, Kolosova OA, Vein AM. Migraine associated with panic attacks. *Cephalalgia.* 1999;19(8):728–731.
   3. Torelli P, D'Amico D. An updated review of migraine and co-morbid psychiatric disorders. *Neurol Sci.* 2004;25:S234–S235.

VII. POST-TRAUMATIC STRESS DISORDER IN PATIENTS WITH NEUROLOGIC ILLNESS

A. Post-traumatic stress disorder in traumatic brain injury
  1. Clinical background
     a. The prevalence of moderate to severe PTSD symptoms in TBI has been estimated at <20% although rates between studies vary widely from 1% to 50%.
     b. PTSD symptoms tend to diminish over time following TBI. PTSD negatively effects functioning and quality of life.
  2. Pathogenesis of panic disorder in traumatic brain injury
     a. Controversy exists as to whether loss of consciousness with TBI prevents encoding of the experience into memory and should subsequently preclude the development of PTSD.
  3. Diagnosis
     a. The diagnosis is clinical and is based on consensus criteria, which are detailed in the section entitled "Classification and Epidemiology of Anxiety Syndromes."
     b. The differential diagnosis should include depressive disorders, other anxiety disorders, personality disorders, and substance abuse/dependence.
  4. Treatment
     a. There is some evidence that CBT may improve acute psychological recovery from trauma and possibly diminish the probability of PTSD symptom development. Evidence for the prophylactic use of antidepressants after trauma to prevent PTSD does not currently justify this practice.
     b. CBT, supportive psychotherapy, and psychoeducation appear to be helpful in general populations with PTSD and may be useful in patients with TBI who are able to participate in such therapies. Resuming participation in valued activities and behavioral approaches to avoidance are important aspects to treatment.
     c. Medication is indicated if the anxiety is severe or if the interventions mentioned in the preceding text have not been sufficiently successful. There are no FDA-approved medications for the treatment of PTSD in patients with TBI. We recommend *sertraline* beginning at 25 mg per day with titration to 75 to 150 mg per day based on its safety profile and efficacy in PTSD. *Risperidone* 1 to 3 mg qhs may be considered for psychotic symptoms or treatment-refractory cases, based on the results of an open trial and a randomized controlled trial in patients with combat-related PTSD.
     d. Benzodiazepines are not recommended as monotherapy for PTSD and should generally be avoided in the treatment of patients with TBI.
     References
     1. Ursano RJ, Bell C, Eth S, et al. Practice guideline for the treatment of patients with acute stress disorder and posttraumatic stress disorder. *Am J Psychiatry.* 2004;161(Suppl 11):3–31.

Chapter 7

PSYCHOSIS IN NEUROPSYCHIATRIC DISORDERS

Laura A. Flashman, Thomas W. McAllister

I. BACKGROUND

A. **Definitions**

1. *Psychosis* is a term that has been defined in a number of ways, and no definition has achieved universal acceptance. Early classifications of psychosis (e.g., Diagnostic and Statistical Manual of Mental Disorders [DSM]-III and ICD-9) focused on the severity of functional impairment rather than specific symptoms; a mental disorder was referred to as "psychotic" if it resulted in impairment that grossly interfered with the capacity to meet the ordinary demands of life.

2. In its narrowest contemporary definition, the term "psychotic" is restricted to a syndrome characterized by the presence of delusions or prominent hallucinations, with the hallucinations occurring in the absence of insight into their pathologic nature. A slightly less restrictive definition would also include prominent hallucinations that the individual realizes are hallucinatory experiences.

3. Broader definitions of *psychosis* include other signs, such as disorganized speech and disorganized, or catatonic behavior. *Positive symptoms* appear to reflect an excess or distortion of normal functions; in contrast, *negative symptoms* appear to reflect a diminution or loss of normal functions (e.g., reduced range of affect). Psychosis is usually not diagnosed in the presence of negative symptoms alone.

4. *Disorganized speech* typically reflects distortions or exaggerations of language and communication. A person may lose track of

what he or she is saying, moving from one topic to another, circle around a question without ever directly addressing it, or answer questions in a way that is only obliquely related, or even in an unrelated manner.

5. *Grossly disorganized or catatonic behavior* can manifest itself in a number of ways, and ranges from silly, childlike behavior to unpredictable agitation. Problems can be seen in goal-directed behavior, or may be manifested by an unusual appearance (e.g., wearing several layers of clothing in the summer) or inappropriate anger (e.g., giving a harangue on a street corner).

B. **Classification of psychotic syndromes and disorders.** The Diagnostic and Statistical Manual of Mental Disorders, 4th edition (American Psychiatric Association, 1994) identifies a number of disorders that are characterized by having psychotic symptoms as the defining feature (schizophrenia spectrum disorders). It should be noted that there are other disorders that may present with psychotic symptoms, which are not defining features (see Table 7.1).

1. **Schizophrenia.** Schizophrenia is defined by a combination of psychotic symptoms that significantly impact on major areas of functioning, including work, interpersonal relations, or self-care. Disturbances of emotional, behavioral, cognitive, and perceptual functioning can be observed. Specifically, to meet the DSM-IV criteria for schizophrenia, a person must have two (or more) symptoms (i.e., delusions, hallucinations, disorganized speech or behavior, affective flattening, alogia, or avolition) present for a significant portion of time during a 1-month period (or less if successfully treated), with continuous signs of the disturbance persisting for at least 6 months, which may include

TABLE 7.1   Classification of Psychotic Syndromes and Disorders

Psychosis as defining feature ("primary psychosis")
- Schizophrenia
- Schizophreniform disorder
- Schizoaffective disorder
- Delusional disorder
- Brief psychotic disorder
- Shared psychotic disorder
- Psychotic disorder due to a general medical condition
- Substance-induced psychotic disorder
- Psychotic disorder, not otherwise specified

Presence of psychotic symptoms, not defining features
- Dementia of the Alzheimer type
- Substance-induced delirium
- Major depressive episode, with psychotic features
- Manic episode, with psychotic features
- Mixed episode, with psychotic features

periods of prodromal or residual symptoms. The symptoms must cause clinically significant distress or impairment in social, occupational, self-care, or other important areas of functioning. The median age of onset for the first psychotic episode of schizophrenia is in the early to mid-twenties for men, and in the late twenties for women. The first degree biologic relatives of individuals with schizophrenia have a 10-fold greater risk of developing schizophrenia than the general population, but both genetic and environmental factors have been shown to play a role in the development of schizophrenia.

2. **Schizophreniform disorder.** When the duration of the illness has been at least 1 month, but <6 months, a diagnosis of *schizophreniform disorder* is given. The essential features of this disorder are identical to those of schizophrenia, with two exceptions: (a) The total duration of the illness (including prodromal, active, and residual phases), as noted in the preceding text; and (b) impaired social and/or occupational functioning during some part of the illness is not required, although most individuals do experience dysfunction in various areas of daily functioning (e.g., work or school, interpersonal relationships, or self-care). Approximately two thirds of individuals with an initial diagnosis of schizophreniform disorder will progress to the diagnoses of schizophrenia or schizoaffective disorder.

3. **Schizoaffective disorder.** The essential feature of *schizoaffective disorder* is an uninterrupted period of illness during which there are concurrent mood and psychotic symptoms so that the full criteria are met for both a major depressive, manic, or mixed episode (see Chapter 5), as well as the symptoms of schizophrenia (i.e., delusions, hallucinations, disorganized speech or behavior, affective flattening, alogia, or avolition). In addition, during the same period of illness, there must be delusions or hallucinations for at least 2 weeks in the absence of prominent mood symptoms. Disturbances of emotional, behavioral, cognitive, and perceptual functioning are observed. Detailed information is lacking, but schizoaffective disorder appears to be less prevalent than schizophrenia.

4. **Psychotic disorder not otherwise specified.** This diagnosis is used when psychotic symptomatology (i.e., delusions, hallucinations, disorganized speech, grossly disorganized, or catatonic behavior) is present in the context of inadequate information to make a specific diagnosis, or about which there is contradictory information. It can also be used to characterize disorders with psychotic symptoms that do not meet the criteria for any specific psychotic disorder.

C. **Epidemiology.** Psychotic symptoms and syndromes are reported to be much more common in patients with certain neurologic disorders than in control or reference populations (see Table 7.2). The precise prevalence rates are difficult to establish given wide methodologic variation in the published reports. The highest rates of psychosis have been reported in patients with Alzheimer disease (AD) (~50%),

TABLE 7.2   Prevalence of Psychosis in Patients with Neurologic Disease

Alzheimer disease	~10%−70%; 50% estimates common
Lewy body dementia	Up to 80% have complex visual hallucinations
Parkinson disease	~20%−25%
Epilepsy	0%−27%; 2.8%−7.1% in larger, more rigorous studies
Traumatic brain injury	~0.7%−9.8%
Intellectual disability	~2%−8%; higher in selective ID syndromes
Huntington disease	~0.5%−8%
Multiple sclerosis	0%−5%
Poststroke	Rare

ID, intellectual disability.

dementia with Lewy bodies (DLB) (up to 80%), Parkinson disease (PD)(~20% to 25%), and epilepsy (2.8% to 27%). Nevertheless, even in those disorders in which it occurs with lower frequency, psychosis poses a significant complication, and results in significant distress to both individuals and their caregivers, decreases quality of life, and increases likelihood of nursing home placement.

D. **Prognosis.** A much smaller literature exists on the course and prognosis of psychosis associated with a neuropsychiatric illness. These limited data suggest that psychosis in the context of a neuropsychiatric illness may persist for months and even years after onset and its presence may increase both the morbidity and mortality of the illness (see discussion of specific illness in subsequent text).

II. NEUROBIOLOGY AND PATHOPHYSIOLOGY OF PSYCHOSIS

A. **Schizophrenia spectrum disorders.** The pathophysiology of schizophrenia spectrum disorders is not fully understood. Several regions in the brain appear to play important roles in the genesis and phenomenology of schizophrenia. The temporal lobes, particularly the left temporal lobe, including the hippocampal formation, appear to play a role in auditory hallucinations and some delusions. Abnormalities of right hemispheric function, particularly in parietal and frontal cortices, have also been associated with delusions of misidentification. Delusions of passivity and control have been linked to abnormalities of left temporal cortex. Several lines of evidence from neuropathologic studies and functional imaging studies suggest that dorsolateral prefrontal cortex is disordered in individuals with schizophrenia and probably accounts for observed cognitive deficits associated with the illness (e.g., working memory deficits) as well as problems in motivated behavior (e.g., apathy). Psychosis may be the result of genetically determined defects in neurotransmitter function, which may occur *de novo* or in response to psychosocial stress (the *stress-diathesis model*).

1. **Psychosis in patients with a neurologic illness.** The pathophysiology of psychosis in patients with neurologic illness is not known, but is likely to be heterogeneous. In terms of DSM-IV diagnoses, psychosis in the context of these neurologic disorders is referred to as "Psychosis due to a General Medical Condition," with the specific disorder identified as the medical condition. Psychosis in patients with a neurologic illness may reflect some combination of a recurrence of a preexisting psychiatric disorder, a result of other neurologic or general medical problems, a direct effect of the neurologic illness on particular brain systems (*endogenous* factor), or be related to the therapeutic interventions being used to treat the primary disorder (*exogenous* factor).

   Studies in patients with neuropsychiatric disease suggest a relation between psychosis and lesions of particular brain regions including frontal lobe dysfunction (cerebrovascular disease, AD, traumatic brain injury [TBI]), the temporal lobes including the hippocampus (TBI, epilepsy), and the basal ganglia and thalamus (TBI). Abnormalities in neurotransmitter and other receptors have also been implicated in some of these disorders (AD, PD), and other brain and genetic factors, such as density of neurofibrillary tangles (AD, Lewy body dementia [LBD]), demyelination (multiple sclerosis [MS]) and CAG repeat length (Huntington disease[HD]) have also been implicated (see subsequent text).

III. MANAGEMENT

A. **Principles of management.** The literature on the treatment of psychosis associated with neurologic disorders is quite sparse and does not rise to the level that would permit illness-specific practice guidelines. There are no medications with U.S. Food Drug Administration (FDA) indications for the treatment of psychosis associated with any given neurologic disorder. On the other hand, numerous case reports, small case series, and our clinical experience suggest that these individuals will respond to treatment approaches similar to those that have evolved for the treatment of schizophrenia spectrum disorders. Therefore, in general, the management of psychosis in patients with neurologic illness (regardless of whether the psychosis is considered to be "secondary" to the neurologic illness) should follow the Practice Guidelines for the Treatment of Patients with Schizophrenia, Second Edition by the American Psychiatric Association.

   1. **Perform a diagnostic evaluation**
      a. The diagnosis of a psychosis in patients with neurologic illness can be challenging. Some controversy exists about the most appropriate method for diagnosing psychosis in patients with neurologic or medical conditions, because some of the signs or symptoms (e.g., confusion, illusions) may result from the medical or neurologic illness. Further, medications used to treat these disorders may themselves result in psychotic symptoms. An additional diagnostic challenge relates to the assessment of symptoms that require

verbal expression (e.g., hallucinations, delusions, etc.) in patients who cannot speak (e.g., due to an aphasia) or clearly express themselves (e.g., due to an intellectual disability [ID] with limited vocabulary). In such cases, it may be necessary to give greater weight to clearly manifest *signs* of the psychotic disorder such as consistent misinterpretation of events in the environment in a paranoid fashion or apparent repetitive responses to internal stimuli.

Psychosis in individuals with neurologic disorders can be seen in several different settings. The first can be attributed to the neurologic disorder itself and is thought to occur when the illness involves or spreads to the brain regions critical in the genesis of psychotic symptoms that have already been described. The second context is psychosis occurring as part of a delirium or metabolic encephalopathy. This occurrence is typically seen in neurologic disorders occurring in the elderly or those that have common medical comorbidities. Iatrogenic causes, often related to medications used to treat the underlying illness, is another common cause of delirium. A third context is the development of a mood disorder with psychotic features. Most disorders of the central nervous system (CNS) have markedly increased rates of mood disorders (see Chapter 5). Both depression and mania can present with psychotic features. The fourth context is psychotic symptoms precipitated by substance use or abuse. Psychotic symptoms can also be seen in individuals with seizure disorders. Most commonly this occurs in the context of complex partial seizures, particularly when the seizure focus is in the temporal or frontal lobes. Psychotic symptoms can be seen ictally, postictally, or interictally (usually after many years of having a seizure disorder).

The diagnosis of new psychotic symptoms in the individual with neurologic disease should involve determining which of the "causes" mentioned in the preceding text are responsible. A neurologic examination and perhaps other neurodiagnostic studies like (electroencephalography [EEG], repeat neuroimaging) should be considered to ascertain whether the underlying neurologic disorder has progressed. A careful cognitive examination and history should be taken to determine whether the individual is delirious. If there is any suggestion of a delirium, screening laboratory studies (complete blood count [CBC], serum electrolytes, blood urea nitrogen [BUN], Cre, Ca++) should be done to determine the cause of the delirium. A careful history from the individual and reliable informants should be taken looking for indicators of a mood disorder. A urine toxicology screen should be done if there is any possibility of substance use. Psychotic symptoms of paroxysmal onset with brief duration, especially in the context of a

TABLE 7.3   Selected Medications for Treatment of Psychotic Symptoms

Medication	Starting Dose per Day	Dosing Range per Day
Typical antipsychotics		
Haloperidol	0.25–0.5 mg	0.25–4 mg
Atypical antipsychotics		
Risperidone	0.25 mg	0.25–4 mg
Aripiprazole	5 mg	5–15 mg
Clozapine	12.5 mg	12.5–300 mg
Quetiapine	12.5–25 mg	12.5–300 mg

known or suspected seizure disorder should prompt strong consideration of an EEG.

The judgment that the psychosis is secondary to the neurologic illness requires confirmation of a neurologic illness, evidence that the psychosis is a "direct physiological consequence" of that illness, and evidence that the psychosis is not better accounted for by another mental disorder. Determining whether the psychotic symptoms are "a direct physiological consequence" of the neurologic illness may be very challenging indeed, as there are no clear rules for establishing such an association. A potential relation is suggested by a temporal association between the neurologic illness's onset, exacerbation, or remission and that of the psychotic disorder (e.g., the psychosis begins shortly after the stroke); atypical features of a psychotic disorder; or a well-established relation between the psychotic disorder and the neurologic illness (e.g., as in the conditions listed in Table 7.2). However, certain disorders such as epilepsy and TBI can have lengthy latencies between onset of the disease and emergence of psychotic symptoms (often several years for both disorders). The absence of any premorbid indicators of psychotic symptoms or related prodrome, as well as the absence of family history of psychotic disorders, are also supportive evidence of an etiologic connection between the neurologic disorder and the psychosis.

2. **Implement a biopsychosocial treatment plan.** We discuss in the subsequent text specific recommendations for treatment of psychosis in patients with some of the more common neurologic illnesses.

    a. **Development of a therapeutic alliance and promotion of treatment adherence.** It is important to develop an alliance in a patient with psychosis. Many individuals, especially those with neurologic disorders, are resistant to being labeled as having a psychiatric disorder, especially a psychosis. This resistance can take the form of both a "psychological" denial (not wanting to be labeled as "crazy") as well as a deficit in self-monitoring and awareness of illness behavior. The latter shares many features with lack of awareness of neurologic symptoms, often referred to as anosognosia.

b. **Patient and family education and therapies.** Helping patients and families recognize early symptoms of relapse to prevent full-blown illness exacerbations is critical. Further, education to the family and caregivers about the nature of the illness and possible psychiatric symptoms, as well as coping strategies to diminish relapses and improve quality of life of patients is an important component of successful treatment.

c. **Treat comorbid conditions.** These comorbidities might include major depression, substance use disorders, or even physical discomfort or pain. Impaired processing of perceptual information is often a prominent aspect of psychotic disorders. Physical symptoms such as pain or discomfort may be either incorrectly perceived or misinterpreted by the affected individual. Somatic symptoms may occur in patients with psychosis and worsen their psychotic states, but may only be recognized later as physical problems. Patients with psychosis may be unable to comprehend or describe their physical symptoms adequately. Physical disorders of patients with psychosis may be overlooked if clinicians are not vigilant and thorough in assessing the patients' complaints, especially if such complaints sound delusional or bizarre. Problems with speech and language function are an important component of many brain disorders and can limit the individual's capacity to accurately report or describe physical symptoms that would ordinarily tip-off the alert clinician to the presence of significant medical disorders.

d. **Attend to patient's social circumstances and functioning.** An important goal is to work with team members, the individual, and the family to ensure that services are coordinated and that referrals for additional services are made when appropriate. This component is also often overlooked. Individuals with neuropsychiatric disorders frequently do not fit easily into standard systems of medical care (they are often perceived as "bad patients" or "acting out" in some willful fashion), nor community mental health systems or related agencies (behaviors often overattributed to the "medical issues" or "medical involvement").

e. **Integrate treatment from multiple clinicians.** This issue is important in patients with a neurologic illness, who are likely being followed by a primary care physician and a neurologist in addition to other specialists.

f. **Document treatment.** Documentation of treatment is also very important, because patients may have different practitioners over the course of their illness. Information about successful and unsuccessful therapies is very helpful to minimize multiple trials of medications, and detail clearly the interventions that have and have not worked in the past.

g. Finally, it is important to recognize that for all individuals with neuropsychiatric illness and psychotic symptoms, *psychiatric hospitalization* may be needed in the acute stages.

B. **Psychosis in individuals with particular neurologic disorders**

1. **Psychosis in Alzheimer disease**

a. **Clinical background**

(1) The reported *prevalence* of psychotic symptoms in patients with AD varies, but has been reported to be as low as 10% to 15% and as high as 50% to 70%. The incidence of new onset psychosis in AD has been reported to be approximately 30% over the course of 2 years.

(2) Several *identified risk factors* have been associated with psychosis in AD. These include gender, education, and race. Women have been reported to have a higher risk of developing psychosis within 2 years than men. Education has been associated with psychosis in mild or moderate stages of the dementia, whereas race has been associated with psychosis in moderate or severe stages. Psychotic symptoms, such as delusions and hallucinations may occur with increased frequency in individuals with certain genotypes. Candidate genes and related polymorphic alleles that have been identified as increasing the risk of psychotic symptoms include the long allele of an insertion or deletion polymorphism in the promoter region of the serotonin transporter (5-HTTPR), the 102C allele in the serotonin 2A receptor, and selected polymorphisms in the dopamine receptor genes DRD1 (B2 allele) and DRD3 (1 allele). In addition linkage signals on chromosome 2p (near marker D2S1356), chromosome 6 (near marker D6S1021) and chromosome 21 (near D21S1440) have also been identified. The apolipoprotein (APOE) and α_1-antichymotrypsin (ACT) genotypes do not appear to contribute to the risk of development of psychotic symptoms in AD. The presence of psychotic symptoms in AD confers increased risk of similar symptoms to affected siblings.

(3) The *phenomenology* of psychosis in patients with AD is associated with more severe cognitive deficits and a more rapidly deteriorating course. Two subtypes of psychosis in AD have been proposed: One involving misidentification and hallucinations, and the other involving persecutory delusions. Agitation has been associated with aggression and psychosis in mild or moderate stages, and psychosis was associated with aggression in moderate or severe stages of AD. Further, a constellation of psychiatric symptoms (e.g.,

anxiety, wandering, irritability, inappropriate behavior, uncooperativeness, emotional lability) has been associated with agitation, aggression, and psychosis, and reportedly varies according to the severity of the dementia, suggesting a progressive deterioration of frontal-temporal limbic structures.

(4) The *longitudinal course* of psychosis in AD is not fully known, although it has been noted that agitation, aggression, and psychosis are more frequently seen in the later stages of the disease.

b. **Pathogenesis**

(1) The *pathophysiology* of psychosis in patients with AD is not completely understood, but an association between psychosis and neurofibrillary tangle density has been inconsistently reported.

(2) Increased frontal lobe dysfunction (on the basis of neurobehavioral, cognitive, and single photon emission computed tomography [SPECT] measures) has been reported in patients with AD and psychosis. Quantitative EEG results indicate that patients with psychosis have greater overall absolute and relative delta power, and a concomitant decrease in relative α-power, with no regional predominance of slowing compared with those patients with AD and no psychosis.

(3) Functional neuroimaging data suggests increased orbitofrontal and midtemporal cholinergic M2 receptors with psychosis and hallucinations. Paranoid delusions have been associated with left dorsolateral prefrontal and left medial temporal decreases in activation on positron emission tomography.

(4) Patients with AD and psychosis have also been found to demonstrate significant elevations of glycerophosphoethanolamine and significant reductions of N-acetyl-L-aspartate, suggesting that excess impairment of neocortical, neuronal, and synaptic integrity may provide the structural substrate underlying psychosis in AD.

c. **Diagnosis.** The diagnosis is clinical and is based upon the presence of psychotic symptoms. However, if the dementing process impairs speech and language function, the individual may not be able to articulate or describe the symptoms and they may have to be inferred from the individual's behavior, as described under general principles. It is critical to determine what the underlying cause of the psychosis is. As with other neurologic disorders, psychosis in dementing disorders can be seen in several different settings including (1) as part of a delirium or metabolic encephalopathy, (2) as a component of a mood disorder, (3) as part of a seizure disorder or (4) related to substance use or abuse (less common in this context). Given that dementing disorders occur most commonly in the elderly with associated medical disorders, iatrogenic causes, often related to medications used to treat the underlying illness, is a common cause of delirium with associated psychotic symptoms.

The evaluation of new psychotic symptoms in the individual with dementia should involve determining which of the "causes" mentioned in the preceding text are responsible. A careful cognitive examination and history should be taken to determine whether the individual is delirious. If there is any suggestion of delirium, screening laboratory studies (CBC, serum electrolytes, BUN, Cre, Ca++, urinalysis and culture) should be done to determine the cause. A careful history from the individual and reliable informants should be taken looking for indicators of a mood disorder. A urine toxicology screen should be done if there is any possibility of substance use. Psychotic symptoms of paroxysmal onset with brief duration, especially in the context of a known or suspected seizure disorder should prompt strong consideration of an EEG.

d. **Treatment**
(1) *Optimize the physical health of the patient* and ensure that all underlying general medical disorders have been optimally treated, including pain management.
(2) Optimize the patient's *environment and lifestyle,* including the provision of a safe situation that minimizes the person's acting on delusions or hallucinations in a dangerous or violent manner. This type of behavior can put patients at risk for being overmedicated or restrained. Those living at home or in assisted living facilities are at increased risk for institutionalization.
(3) In addition to environmental modification, *behavioral management techniques* could include optimization of socialization and functional status, and education and support of caregivers. Caregivers of patients with psychosis and AD can experience considerable adversity, including increased physical demands involved in constant supervision of the patient, the emotional stress of caring for a loved one who is experiencing these symptoms, physical illness, and depression.
(4) *Medication approaches*—The use of medications to treat psychosis in dementia varies according to what is "causing" the psychosis.
(a) **Delirium.** Determine cause; treat accordingly (e.g., correct electrolyte imbalances, discontinue causative medications etc.). Use low-dose antipsychotic agents (see subsequent text).
(b) **Mood disorder.** Treat depression with antidepressants or mania with anticycling agents (see Chapter 5). If psychosis is endangering health and

well-being of the patient, family or caregiver, add low-dose antipsychotic agents (see subsequent text).

(c) **Seizure disorder.** In this context the usual seizure disorder is a complex partial seizure. Therefore, management of the seizure disorder becomes the primary concern. Management suggestions are beyond the scope of this chapter. The paramount treatment objective is control of the seizure frequency. If psychosis is endangering health and well-being of the patient, family or caregiver, add low-dose antipsychotic agents (see subsequent text).

(d) **Substance use or abuse.** In this context, the treatment objective becomes the identification and removal of the offending drug of abuse. If psychosis is endangering health and well-being of the patient, family or caregiver, add low-dose antipsychotic agents (see subsequent text).

(e) **Use of cholinesterase inhibitors.** When the psychosis is considered to be caused by the underlying dementing disorder, or when caused by one of the conditions mentioned in the preceding text in a circumstance in which the symptoms are endangering the health and well-being of the patient, family or caregiver, the use of medications is warranted. There are no FDA-approved medications for the treatment of psychosis in patients with AD. There is evidence, however, from controlled trials suggesting that neuropsychiatric symptoms, including psychotic symptoms can be improved with the use of cholinesterase inhibitors (see Chapter 4). If the symptoms are subacute and nonthreatening, these agents should be tried first. We suggest starting with donepezil 5 mg daily. The dose may be raised to 10 mg daily if the lower dose is ineffective but well tolerated for at least 4 weeks. Treatment-emergent side effects may include gastrointestinal symptoms, muscle cramping, frequent urination, and sleep disturbance (i.e., vivid dreams or nightmares). These side effects may respond to dose reduction and/or a slower dose titration schedule. Baseline and periodic liver function tests should be done. If there is no response to this regimen or side effects preclude its use, then we suggest rivastigmine 3 to 9 mg per day in divided doses.

(f) **Use of antipsychotic medication.** If the symptoms are endangering the health and well-being of the patient, family or caregiver the use of antipsychotic medication is warranted. There are important issues to consider with both the typical and atypical antipsychotics. The typical antipsychotics tend to cause more extrapyramidal effects and carry a higher risk of tardive dyskinesia, probably related to the degree of D2 receptor blockade. The associated psychomotor slowing, tremor, motor rigidity, cognitive slowing, and abulia associated with these medicines may exacerbate some challenging behaviors already present because of the stroke.

The atypical antipsychotics generally have less D2 receptor blockade and more 5HT1 antagonism relative to the typical antipsychotics. They are felt to carry less risk of extrapyramidal symptoms (EPS) and tardive dyskinesia. On the other hand, there is significant risk of weight gain, diabetes, and metabolic syndrome. There have been several published reports of increased risk of stroke and related cerebrovascular events in the elderly associated with these medicines. This risk has resulted in a recent, highly publicized "black box" warning and a concern about their use in individuals already predisposed to stroke. However, two recent studies have failed to find an increased risk of stroke in the elderly associated with the use of atypical antipsychotics, and raise the possibility that the earlier findings might be attributable to increased percentages of individuals with vascular dementia (and therefore at increased risk for cerebrovascular disease) in the risperidone group. Furthermore, some studies suggest that the risk of cerebrovascular events may be increased for all individuals on antipsychotic medications, regardless of the typical or atypical designation.

The case report and small case series literature is flawed but does suggest that both classes of agents can be effective. However, atypical antipsychotics have been examined in large randomized placebo-controlled trials and found effective (e.g., low-dose risperidone [0.95 to 2 mg per day] and olanzapine [2.5 mg starting dose, with a significant decrease in psychosis at 5 to 7.5 mg per day]). We suggest the following although the level of evidence to support it is weak.

Assuming little risk of metabolic syndrome or diabetes in these individuals, we will start with an atypical agent. We use risperidone, 0.25 mg or 0.5 mg per day and titrate slowly upward, rarely going >4 mg per day. If weight gain or other signs of metabolic syndrome emerge we cross taper to aripiprazole, 5 mg per day and titrate slowly to 15 mg per day as tolerated. If psychotic symptoms do not abate after 1 month we then consider another atypical, or use a typical agent such as haloperidol starting at 0.5 mg per day, titrating upward as needed and tolerated to 2 to 4 mg per day. If an effective treatment is found, we continue it for 6 to 12 months as tolerated and then attempt to slowly (2 months) taper off the medications.

References
1. Assal F, Cummings JL. Neuropsychiatric symptoms in the dementias. *Curr Opin Neurol.* 2002;15:445–450.
2. Bacanu SA, Devlin B, Chowdari KV, et al. Linkage analysis of Alzheimer disease with psychosis. *Neurology.* 2002;59:118–120.
3. Reeves RR, Torres RA. Orally disintegrating olanzapine for the treatment of psychotic and behavioral disturbances associated with dementia. *South Med J.* 2003;96:699–701.
4. Sultzer DL. Psychosis and antipsychotic medications in Alzheimer's disease: Clinical management and research perspectives. *Dement Geriatr Cogn Disord.* 2004;17: 78–90.

2. **Other dementing disorders—overview.** Many of the principles and specific treatments described in the preceding text are applicable to other dementing disorders including vascular dementia and the reader is referred to the preceding section and to Chapter 4. Psychotic symptoms in two other common dementing disorders—DLB and PD—are worth commenting specifically upon.

3. **Dementia with Lewy bodies**
   a. **Clinical background**
      (1) **Prevalence and occurrence.** DLB is in some series second only to AD as the most prevalent cause of dementia.
      (2) **Phenomenology.** Individuals with DLB may present fairly early in the course of illness with psychotic symptoms, particularly visual hallucinations. Up to 80% of individuals with DLB will have complex visual hallucinations, often associated with a variety of illusions and misidentification syndromes.
      (3) **Course and prognosis.** The Consortium on Dementia with Lewy Bodies describe DLB as a progressive and often rapidly disabling dementia in which attentional impairment, executive dysfunction, and visuospatial difficulties occur early and prominently. Fluctuating cognitive function, persistent well-formed visual hallucinations, and spontaneous motor features of parkinsonism are also core elements of DLB. The average age of onset is in the seventh decade, and the average life span after diagnosis is 6 to 7 years. There are no known disease-altering treatments.

b. **Pathogenesis**

(1) DLB is a dementing disorder characterized patho-logically by the presence of clumps of α-synuclein protein, identified microscopically as Lewy bodies. The abnormal clusters of protein in turn trigger an inflammatory response, impairment of the ubiquitin proteasome catabolic system, and triggering of the apoptotic cascade resulting in cell death.

(2) In addition to the widespread distribution of Lewy bodies, there are characteristic deficits in certain neu-rotransmitter systems including loss of cholinergic tone because of damage to cholinergic neurons in the basal forebrain nuclei, and indications of dysregulation of catecholaminergic and indolaminergic systems.

(3) A significant inverse correlation between persistent visual hallucinations and tangles has been reported (i.e., visual hallucinations were associated with the presence of less severe tangle pathology), although there was no significant association between tangle pathology and persistent delusions. Severity of illness has also been significantly correlated with the presence of persistent visual hallucinations and persistent delu-sions. Baseline psychotic features are reported to be significantly more frequent in DLB than in AD.

c. **Diagnosis.** This disorder is often mistaken for PD because of overlapping clinical and neuropathologic features between the two disorders. The diagnosis of psychosis in DLB is clin-ical and is based on the presence of symptoms that meet the criteria for a psychotic disorder. However, visual hallucina-tions are relatively more common in this context than other psychotic syndromes. It is critical to determine what the underlying cause of the psychosis is; in addition to being a symptom of the disorder itself, psychotic symptoms can be seen (1) as part of a delirium or metabolic encephalopathy, or (2) as a component of a mood disorder. Other causes are less likely in this context. Given that DLB occurs most commonly in the elderly with associated medical disorders, iatrogenic causes (often related to medications used to treat the underlying illness) are a common cause of delirium with associated psychotic symptoms.

The diagnosis of new psychotic symptoms in the indi-vidual with DLB should involve determining which of the "causes" mentioned in the preceding text are responsi-ble. A careful cognitive examination and history should be taken to determine whether the individual is delirious and if so screening laboratory studies (CBC, serum electrolytes, BUN, Cre, Ca++, urinalyis and urine culture if indicated) should be done to determine the cause. A careful history from the individual and reliable informants should be taken looking for indicators of a mood disorder.

d. **Treatment**

(1) *Optimize the physical health of the patient* and ensure that all underlying general medical disorders have been optimally treated, including pain management. It is also important to ensure that the altered behavior truly represents psychosis, and not disorders of vision causing illusions recorded as hallucinations, or misplacement of objects secondary to memory problems presenting as paranoia.

(2) Optimize the patient's *environment and lifestyle*, including the provision of a safe situation that minimizes the person's agitation and/or acting on their delusions or hallucinations in a dangerous or violent manner. Hallucinations and delusions are important contributors to patient and caregiver distress, and are often important risk factors for nursing home placement.

(3) *Treatment strategies* should include ruling out reversible causes of cognitive decline unrelated to the primary illness, implementing appropriate psychosocial strategies (see subsequent text), reduction of antiparkinsonian treatment, and judicious use of atypical antipsychotics.

(4) *Psychosocial strategies* might include additional support for the patient with DLB, increased light during the day and decreased light at night (that may improve orientation and minimize excessive sensory stimulation), education for the caregiver(s), and support for the family in their decisions regarding treatments, hospitalization, and long-term placement.

(5) *Medication approaches* to treat psychosis in DLB vary according to what is "causing" the psychosis.

   (a) **Delirium.** Determine the cause, and treat accordingly (e.g., correct electrolyte imbalances, discontinue causative medications).

   (b) **Mood disorder.** Treat depression with antidepressants or mania with anticycling agents (see Chapter 5).

   (c) **Use of cholinesterase inhibitors.** When the psychosis is considered to be caused by the underlying dementing disorder, or when caused by one of the conditions mentioned earlier, in a circumstance where the symptoms are endangering the health and well-being of the patient, family or caregiver, the use of medications is warranted. There are no FDA-approved medications for the treatment of psychosis in patients with DLB. There is evidence, however, from one controlled trial suggesting that neuropsychiatric symptoms, including psychotic symptoms can be improved with the use of cholinesterase inhibitors (see Chapter 4). The use of either typical or atypical antipsychotics in individuals with DLB is problematic because of a significantly increased sensitivity to the side effects (up to 50% of treated individuals in some studies). We therefore recommend initial treatment with cholinesterase inhibitors, and suggest starting with donepezil 5 mg daily. The dose may be raised to 10 mg daily if the lower dose is ineffective but well tolerated for at least 4 weeks. Treatment-emergent side effects may include gastrointestinal symptoms, muscle cramping, frequent urination, and sleep disturbance (i.e., vivid dreams or nightmares). These side effects may respond to dose reduction and/or a slower dose titration schedule. Baseline and periodic liver function tests should be done. If there is no response to this regimen or side effects preclude its use, then we suggest rivastigmine 3 to 9 mg per day in divided doses.

(d) **Use of antipsychotic medication.** In the event that the recommendations mentioned in the preceding text are not effective and the symptoms are endangering the health and well-being of the patient, family or caregiver, then the use of antipsychotics can be considered, weighing carefully the aforementioned increased rate of side effects associated with their use in the DLB population. There is no data suggesting that the atypical agents differ with respect to increased side effects in this population and Therefore, the important consideration is to start with very low doses and proceed cautiously. On the basis of the side effect profile and efficacy in other dementing disorders we use risperidone 0.25 mg or 0.5 mg per day and titrate slowly upward, rarely going >4 mg per day. If weight gain or other signs of metabolic syndrome emerge we cross taper to aripiprazole, 5 mg per day and titrate slowly to 15 mg per day as tolerated. If an effective treatment is found, we continue it for 6 to 12 months as tolerated and then attempt to slowly (2 month) taper off the medications.

References
1. Ballard CG, Jacoby R, Del Ser T, et al. Neuropathological substrates of psychiatric symptoms in prospectively studied patients with autopsy-confirmed dementia with lewy bodies. *Am J Psychiatry*. 2004;161:843–849.
2. McKeith I, Del Ser T, Spano PF, et al. Efficacy of rivastigmine in dementia with lewy bodies: A randomised, double-blind, placebo-controlled international study. *Lancet*. 2000; 356:2031–2036.

4. **Psychosis in patients with Parkinson disease**
   a. **Clinical background**
      (1) Psychosis is a common neuropsychiatric disturbance in PD, although a precise *prevalence* rate has been difficult to establish. In general, estimates range from 3% for delusions to 40% for visual hallucinations, with higher estimates (5% to 62%) in studies that include unselected patients with varied psychotic symptoms such as agitated confusion, reversible psychosis, and hallucinosis.
      (2) The *phenomenology* of psychosis in patients with PD is similar to that in patients with schizophrenia, with visual hallucinations and paranoid delusions being the most prominent symptoms. Visual hallucinations are more common in PD than in schizophrenia.
      (3) The most significant *risk factors* for developing psychosis in PD include coexistence of dementia, protracted sleep disturbances, and nighttime use of dopaminergic agonists. Other identified risk factors include age, stage and severity of PD, and depression.
      (4) The *cause* of psychosis in PD is usually multifactorial, but often involves the agents used to treat the motor symptoms of the disease. However, the precise relationship between dopaminergic medications and psychosis has not been clearly delineated. The dose and duration of dopaminergic therapy are not considered risk factors for hallucinations. However, early drug-induced psychosis (observed in up to 16% of patients treated with dopamine agonists) is associated with increased risk for the development of dementia later in the course of the disorder, and drug-induced psychosis may be a limiting factor of the therapeutic potential of pallidotomy in patients with PD.
      (5) The *longitudinal course* of psychosis in PD is unknown.
   b. **Pathogenesis**
      (1) The *mechanisms* that underlie psychosis in patients with PD remain to be determined. The most frequently proposed hypothesis is that denervation hypersensitivity of mesolimbic and mesocortical dopamine receptors occurs, and that dopaminergic medication stimulates these receptors, which results in psychosis. However, nondopaminergic systems are likely to be involved as well, and it has been proposed that a combination (or combinations) of neurotransmitter systems (e.g., a serotinergic or dopaminergic imbalance, or acetylcholine involvement) may play a role in the development of psychosis in PD. Promising reports of the use of cholinesterase inhibitors to treat psychotic symptoms in PD suggest that lowered cholinergic tone may also play a role in the development of psychotic symptoms in this disorder.

c. **Diagnosis.** The diagnosis of psychosis in PD is clinical and is based on the presence of symptoms that meet the criteria for a psychotic disorder. As with other conditions, it is critical to determine what the underlying cause of the psychosis is; in addition to being a symptom of the disorder itself, psychotic symptoms can be seen in several contexts including (1) as part of a delirium or metabolic encephalopathy, and (2) as a component of a mood disorder. The diagnosis of new psychotic symptoms in the individual with PD should involve determining which of the "causes" mentioned in the preceding text are responsible. A careful cognitive examination and history should be taken to determine whether the individual is delirious. If there is a suggestion of a delirium, screening laboratory studies (CBC, serum electrolytes, BUN, Cre, Ca++, urinalysis and urine culture) should be done to determine the cause. A careful history from the individual and reliable informants should be taken looking for indicators of a mood disorder.

d. **Treatment**

(1) It is important to keep in mind that both *exogenous* (related to therapeutic interventions) factors and *endogenous* (related to the disease process itself) factors can contribute to the development of psychotic symptoms in PD.

(2) *Optimize the physical health of the patient* and ensure that all underlying general medical disorders have been optimally treated, including pain management. It is also important to ensure that the altered behavior truly represents psychosis, and not disorders of vision causing illusions recorded as hallucinations, or misplacement of objects secondary to memory problems presenting as paranoia.

(3) Optimize the patient's *environment and lifestyle*, including the provision of a safe situation that minimizes the person's agitation and/or acting on their delusions or hallucinations in a dangerous or violent manner. Hallucinations and delusions are important contributors to patient and caregiver distress, and are often important risk factors for nursing home placement.

(4) *Treatment strategies* should include ruling out reversible causes of cognitive decline unrelated to the primary illness, implementing appropriate psychosocial strategies (see subsequent text), reduction of antiparkinsonian treatment, and judicious use of atypical antipsychotics.

(5) *Psychosocial strategies* might include additional support for the patient with PD, increased light during the day and decreased light at night (that may improve

orientation and minimize excessive sensory stimulation), education for the caregiver(s), and support for the family in their decisions regarding treatments, hospitalization, and long-term placement.

(6) *Treatment of the movement disorder should be optimized,* which will involve finding a balance between the doses of medication needed to alleviate the motor symptoms while not promoting psychotic symptoms. Initial treatment of psychotic symptoms involves dose reduction of antiparkinsonian agents. If this strategy is unsuccessful in alleviating the psychotic symptoms or results in unacceptable worsening of the movement disorder, one should consider adding an antipsychotic agent to the regimen.

(7) *Medication approaches* to treat psychosis in PD vary according to what is "causing" the psychosis.

(a) **Delirium.** Determine the cause, and treat accordingly (e.g., correct electrolyte imbalances, discontinue causative medications). Use of low-dose antipsychotic agents (see subsequent text) may be warranted.

(b) **Mood disorder.** Treat depression with antidepressants or mania with anticycling agents (see Chapter 5). If psychosis is endangering health and well-being of the patient, family or caregiver, add low-dose antipsychotic agents (see subsequent text).

(c) **Use of cholinesterase inhibitors.** As with DLB, individuals with PD are sensitive to the side effects of typical and atypical antipsychotic medications. Furthermore there is promising evidence that the neuropsychiatric symptoms associated with PD, including psychotic symptoms can be improved with cholinesterase inhibitors. Therefore, in the nonurgent situation, the initial treatment intervention is a trial of a cholinesterase inhibitor. We suggest starting with donepezil 5 mg daily. The dose may be raised to 10 mg daily if the lower dose is ineffective but well tolerated for at least 4 weeks. Treatment-emergent side effects may include gastrointestinal symptoms, muscle cramping, frequent urination, and sleep disturbance (i.e., vivid dreams or nightmares). These side effects may respond to dose reduction and/or a slower dose titration schedule. Baseline and periodic liver function tests should be done. If there is no response to this regimen or side effects preclude its use, then we suggest rivastigmine 3 to 9 mg per day in divided doses.

(d) **Use of antipsychotic medication.** In the event that the recommendations mentioned in the preceding text are not effective and the symptoms are endangering the health and well-being of the patient, family or caregiver, then the use of antipsychotics can be considered, weighing carefully the increased rate of side effects associated with their use in the PD population. None of the medications has specific FDA indications for the treatment of psychosis in PD. The case report and small case series literature is flawed but does suggest that both typical and atypical antipsychotic agents can be effective. However, the atypical antipsychotics are felt to carry less risk of EPS and tardive dyskinesia. This is a particular advantage in this context especially when the initial intervention is to attempt to lower the dopaminergic agonists. The evidence for efficacy of atypical antipsychotics is somewhat equivocal, however. Several case studies have supported the use of quetiapine in patients with PD and psychosis with and without dementia with minimal side effects. Two small placebo-controlled, double-blind studies of olanzapine (vs. placebo) for treatment of drug-induced psychosis in PD failed to show superior efficacy for olanzapine, whereas one open-label trial showed improvement in hallucinations and delusions.

Clozapine is the only atypical antipsychotic agent to be tested in a large-scale, placebo-controlled clinical trial in patients with PD and psychosis; whereas the use of clozapine is less frequently recommended because of its anticholinergic activity for psychosis associated with AD and Lewy body dementia, Clozapine appears to be the atypical antipsychotic drug of choice in patients with PD, at daily doses of 50 mg or less. Careful monitoring of labs as described in the subsequent text occurs for patients on a clozapine protocol.

Medications with other mechanisms of action have been considered, including agents that have primary effects on the neurotransmission of serotonin (e.g., ondansetron) and acetylcholine (e.g., acetyl cholinesterase inhibitors), although results have been mixed. Ondansetron (a 5HT3 antagonist) showed partial or complete improvement in open-label studies of patients with PD and psychosis in two studies, but not in a third study. The efficacy and tolerability of acetylcholinesterase inhibitors in patients with PD and psychosis remains to be determined.

We start with aripiprazole, on the basis of its safety profile and relative ease of use compared with the weekly blood draws and potential marrow toxicity associated with clozapine. We start with 5 mg per day and titrate slowly to 15 mg per day as tolerated. If psychotic symptoms do not abate after 1 month we then consider another atypical, or use a combination of aripiprazole and haloperidol. If there is no response to the recommendations mentioned in the preceding text, we then go to a trial of low-dose clozapine. The initial work-up includes and electrocardiogram (EKG), EEG, and CBC. The absolute neutrophil count must be over 2,000. We start with a dose of 12.5 mg per day and titrate upwards in 12.5 mg per day increments weekly as tolerated until achieving a dose of 50 mg per day. The use of clozapine is complicated by the increased risk of agranulocytosis and the need for weekly monitoring of white blood counts, at least for the first 6 months after which it can be monitored every alternate week. Additional side effects include sedation and drooling. If an effective treatment is found, we continue it for 1 year as tolerated and then attempt to slowly (2 months) taper off the medications.

(8) *Electroconvulsive therapy (ECT)* has occasionally been used to treat patients with PD and psychosis, especially those who are unable to tolerate medications, although there have been no controlled trials. The use of ECT followed by maintenance with low-dose clozapine has been reported to be effective and well tolerated in PD and drug-induced psychosis. The cognitive risks include disorientation, delirium, and amnesia.

References

1. Breier A, Sutton VK, Feldman PD, et al. Olanzapine in the treatment of dopamimetic-induced psychosis in patients with Parkinson's disease. *Biol Psychiatry.* 2002;52:438–445.
2. Dewey RB Jr, O'Suilleabhain PE. Treatment of drug-induced psychosis with quetiapine and clozapine in Parkinson's disease. *Neurology.* 2000;55:1753–1754.
3. Factor SA, Molho ES, Brown DL. Combined clozapine and electroconvulsive therapy for the treatment of drug induced psychosis in Parkinson's disease. *J Neuropsychiatr.* 1995;7:304–307.
4. Ismail MS, Richard IH. A reality test: How well do we understand psychosis in Parkinson's disease? *J Neuropsychiatry Clin Neurosci.* 2004;16:8–18.

5. Melamed E, Zoldan J, Freidberg G. Is hallucinosis in Parkinson's disease due to central serotonergic hyperactivity? *Mov Disord*. 1993;8:406–407.

5. **Psychosis in patients with epilepsy**
    a. **Clinical background**
        (1) *Prevalence rates* of between 0% and 27% have been reported in small clinic-based studies of psychosis in individuals with epilepsy; more rigorous and larger studies report rates of approximately 3% to 7%.
        (2) Psychosis and other psychiatric symptoms may occur peri- or interictally. Peri-ictal psychotic symptoms may occur before, during, or after the ictus. Typically these symptoms are brief and do not require treatment per se, as their frequency will diminish with improvement in seizure control. Patients with epilepsy may also experience psychosis during the interictal phase, in which the symptoms are more commonly chronic than episodic. Clinical presentation varies according to the temporal relation of the symptoms relative to seizure occurrence.
        (3) The *phenomenology* of peri-ictal psychosis (i.e., postictal acute confusional state) is characterized by generalized confusion, fluctuating sensorium, agitation, hallucinations, and delusions. Paranoia and referential delusions are common. This condition generally resolves within a few hours after the seizure, although it may persist in rare instances for several days.
        (4) The *phenomenology* of interictal or chronic psychosis can be characterized as paranoia, with hypervigilance, hostility, suspiciousness, and systematized persecutory delusions, or as a schizophrenia-like syndrome, with hallucinations, delusions, ideas of passivity and control, ideas of reference, and thought broadcasting and insertion. It is associated with impaired function and quality of life.
        (5) The *longitudinal course* of psychosis in patients with epilepsy is notable for a variable interval between onset of epilepsy and onset of psychosis; reports indicate this can be as much as 9 to 14 years. Further, there is evidence to suggest that there can be a progression from peri-ictal psychosis to interictal psychosis in some individuals.
        (6) Potential *risk factors* for epileptic psychosis (either interictal or peri-ictal) include ID, family history of psychosis or mood disorders, increased seizure frequency (especially with generalized tonic-clonic seizures), and greater resistance to epilepsy treatment. In contrast, age of epilepsy onset, age at onset of psychosis, and presence of generalized tonic-clonic seizures differs between those with interictal psychosis and those with peri-ictal psychosis. Histories of prolonged febrile

episodes have also been associated with interictal psychosis. Individuals with both interictal and peri-ictal psychosis (bimodal psychosis) show characteristics associated with both peri-ictal and interictal psychosis.

b. **Pathogenesis**

(1) Although the *pathophysiology* of epileptic psychosis is not fully known, it generally appears to be associated with complex partial seizures, especially with temporal lobe foci. However, psychotic symptoms are also reported with regularity in patients with frontal lobe epilepsy. Psychotic syndromes are more likely to occur in conjunction with left-sided temporal lobe lesions.

(2) Mixed findings related to hippocampus and amygdala volume reductions have been reported in patients with epileptic psychosis, as have seizure discharges in the left amygdala on EEG; both left and bilateral reductions have been reported in both regions.

(3) SPECT scan results have suggested that postictal psychosis in patients with temporal lobe epilepsy is associated with hyperactivation of both temporal and frontal lobe structures, which may reflect ongoing subcortical discharges, active inhibitory mechanisms that terminate the seizure, or simply a dysregulation of cerebral blood flow. Temporal lobectomy for medically intractable epilepsy may precipitate a schizophrenia-like psychosis. Potential risk factors include bilateral functional (EEG) and structural abnormalities, particularly of the amygdala, pathology other than mesial temporal sclerosis in the excised lobe, and recurrence of seizures contralateral to the resection. A correlation has also been reported between presurgical acute interictal psychosis and postsurgical psychotic disorder. In addition, there have been reports of psychotic symptoms occurring in individuals with refractory epilepsy following implantation of a vagus nerve stimulator (VNS) to control seizures. On the other hand, it is also the case that improved seizure control can have a dramatic effect on psychotic symptoms associated with epilepsy, even when the exact relationship between the seizure and the psychotic symptoms is not entirely clear cut. Therefore, in our view, the presence of psychosis is not an absolute contraindication to invasive interventions designed to improve seizure control.

(4) Research on autosomal dominant nocturnal frontal lobe epilepsy (ADNFLE) indicates that a mutation in a gene coding for the nicotinic acetylcholine receptor CHRNA4 (776ins3) may be associated with psychotic symptoms.

c. **Diagnosis.** The diagnosis is clinical and is based on the presence of psychotic symptoms. However, it is critical to determine the underlying cause of the psychosis. The first step is to clarify whether the psychotic symptoms are best categorized as peri-ictal or interictal. If it is the former, then the treatment is best directed toward improved seizure control. If it is the latter, then the treatment more closely follows the algorithm for management of other chronic psychotic conditions. If it is not clear whether the psychotic symptoms are peri- or interictal, consideration of 24-hour ambulatory EEG or in-hospital EEG video monitoring for clarification is given. As with other neurologic disorders, psychosis in epilepsy can also be seen in different settings including (1) as part of a delirium or metabolic encephalopathy, (2) as a component of a mood disorder, or (3) related to substance use or abuse. More rarely psychotic symptoms have been associated with use of some of the newer antiepileptic medications such as Kepra. The diagnosis of new psychotic symptoms in the individual with epilepsy should involve determining which of the "causes" mentioned in the preceding text are responsible. A neurologic examination and perhaps other neurodiagnostic studies (EEG, repeat neuroimaging etc.) should be considered. A careful cognitive examination and history should be taken to determine whether the individual is delirious. Screening laboratory studies (CBC, serum electrolytes, BUN, Cre, Ca++, and serum anticonvulsant levels) should be done if a delirium is suspected. A careful history from the individual and reliable informants should be taken looking for indicators of a mood disorder. A urine toxicology screen should be done if there is any possibility of substance use.

d. **Treatment**
(1) As a first step, the clinician should *optimize the physical health of the patient* and ensure that all underlying general medical disorders have been optimally treated.
(2) The patient's *environment and lifestyle should be optimized*, including the promotion of exercise and a regular sleep–wake cycle.
(3) *Biopsychosocial treatment of the epilepsy* should be optimized, including minimization of anticonvulsant polypharmacy. Improved seizure control is the most important step in the management of psychotic syndromes associated with epilepsy. Although changes in behavior including psychotic symptoms have been linked to improved seizure control ("forced normalization") this should not prevent aggressive attempts to reduce the frequency of seizures as most commonly, this will alleviate psychotic symptoms or at least make them easier to treat. Although psychosis has been considered by some neurologists to be a contraindication for epilepsy surgery, with appropriate psychiatric

intervention, patients with refractory epilepsy and chronic interictal psychosis can successfully undergo surgical evaluation and interventions.

(4) *Psychotherapeutic interventions* should also be considered, including disease education, as well as individual (particularly cognitive-behavioral therapy), group (including formal support groups), and family therapy, although the efficacy of such interventions has not been formally studied.

(5) *Medication approaches.* It is important to consider the *anticonvulsant medications* the person has been prescribed, as some of the newer antiepileptic drugs have been associated with side effects including psychosis. Lamotrigine, tiagabine, and levetiracetam seem to be associated with improvement or little change in mood and behavior. Vigabatrin has been associated with both psychosis and depression. Gabapentin appears to have little effect on behavior but may exacerbate behavioral problems, at least in children with preexisting difficulties. Topiramate has been reported to precipitate both psychosis and depression, but this is less likely to occur if the currently recommended lower starting doses, escalation rates, and target doses are used. There are some reported cases of psychosis and other behavioral disturbances with felbamate. There is some evidence for psychosis with zonisamide, but there is also a suggestion that this drug may be of benefit in treating psychiatric disorders. Careful assessment of each individual should enable the clinician to determine whether the medication or some other factor is responsible for the psychotic symptom(s). If other factors are likely contributing, the following algorithms are considered.

  (a) **Delirium.** Determine the cause, and treat accordingly (e.g., correct electrolyte imbalances, discontinue causative medications). Use of low-dose antipsychotic agents (see subsequent text) may be warranted.

  (b) **Mood disorder.** Treat depression with antidepressants or mania with anticycling agents (see Chapter 5). If psychosis is endangering health and well-being of the patient, family or caregiver, add low-dose antipsychotic agents (see subsequent text).

  (c) **Substance use or abuse.** In this context, the treatment objective becomes the identification and removal of the offending drug of abuse. If psychosis is endangering health and well-being of the patient, family or caregiver, add low-dose antipsychotic agents (see subsequent text).

(d) **Use of antipsychotic medication.** There are important issues to consider with both the typical and
atypical antipsychotics. None of the medications
have specific FDA indications for the treatment of
psychosis in epilepsy. The case report and small
case series literature is flawed but does suggest
that both classes of agents can be effective. The
atypical antipsychotics generally have less D2 receptor blockade and more 5HT1 antagonism relative to the typicals. They are felt to carry less risk
of EPS and tardive dyskinesia. On the other hand
there is significant risk of weight gain, diabetes,
and metabolic syndrome. The following is our approach, but the level of evidence to support it is
weak.

   We use risperidone based on its safety profile
and demonstrated efficacy in trials of psychosis
associated with other brain disorders such as AD.
We use 0.25 mg or 0.5 mg per day to start and titrate
upward slowly. We rarely go over 4 mg per day,
and most individuals are treated with 2.0 to 3.0 mg
per day. If weight gain or other signs of metabolic
syndrome emerge we cross taper to aripiprazole,
5 mg per day and titrate slowly to 15 mg per day as
tolerated. If psychotic symptoms do not abate after
1 month we then consider another atypical, or use
a combination of aripiprazole and haloperidol. We
start with haloperidol 0.5 mg per day and titrate
upward slowly as needed and tolerated. We rarely
go >5 mg per day. If all of these regimens are ineffective we initiate a trial of clozapine, starting with
12.5 mg per day and titrating upwards in 12.5 mg
increments weekly as tolerated and carefully monitoring CBC and absolute neutrophil counts on a
weekly basis. The use of clozapine is complicated
by the increased risk of agranulocytosis and the
need for weekly monitoring of white blood counts,
at least for the first 6 months after which every
other week monitoring can be used. Additional
side effects include sedation and drooling. Clozapine has been used to successfully treat severe psychosis in at least one case series, despite concerns
related to its increased risk of seizures. In fact,
none of the patients in this series had an increase
in their seizure frequency and half of the patients
had a substantial reduction in number of seizures.

(6) Although there is no literature on this, we generally
continue successful therapy for 1 year and then attempt
a slow taper off of the antipsychotic regimen.

References
1. Besag FM. Behavioural effects of the newer antiepi-leptic drugs: An update. *Expert Opin Drug Saf.* 2004;3:1–8.
2. Devinsky O. Psychiatric comorbidity in patients with epilepsy: Implications for diagnosis and treatment. *Epilepsy Behav.* 2003;4:S2–S10.
3. Langosch JM, Trimble MR. Epilepsy, psychosis and clozapine. *Hum Psychopharmacol.* 2002;17:115–119.
4. Liu HC, Chen CH, Yeh IJ, et al. Characteristics of postictal psychosis in a psychiatric center. *Psychiatry Clin Neurosci.* 2001;55:635–639.
5. Marchetti RL, Azevedo D Jr., de Campos Bottino CM, et al. Volumetric evidence of a left laterality effect in epileptic psychosis. *Epilepsy Behav.* 2003;4:234–240.

6. **Psychosis in patients with traumatic brain injury**
   a. **Clinical background**
      (1) *Occurrence and prevalence.* Whereas psychosis is a relatively rare complication of TBI, psychotic syndromes occur 2 to 3 times more frequently in individuals who have sustained a TBI than in the general population.
      (2) The *phenomenology* of psychosis in patients with TBI varies according to the injury severity. The more mild the injury, the more closely the symptoms resemble those seen in individuals with schizophrenia. Positive symptoms are more common than negative symptoms, and delusions (often persecutory) are the most common symptom of psychosis following TBI. In individuals with more severe injuries, psychotic symptoms can be more difficult to identify related to injury-induced speech and language difficulties as well as cognitive impairment.
      (3) Potential *risk factors* for psychosis in patients with TBI can be divided into preinjury factors, injury factors, and postinjury factors. *Preinjury risk factors* include male gender, neurodevelopmental disorders, prior history of TBI, substance disorders, and positive family history of schizophrenia. *Injury risk factors* include left hemisphere, particularly temporal lobe lesions, increased severity of injury with more diffuse brain damage, and coma of >24 hours. *Postinjury risk factors* include EEG abnormalities including asymmetric temporal slowing and intermittent spikes, posttraumatic epilepsy, substance abuse disorders and other posttraumatic psychiatric disorders. Greater degrees of cognitive impairment have also been associated with psychotic symptoms.
      (4) *Onset and longitudinal course.* In the initial period after injury, during the period of posttraumatic amnesia, visual hallucinations, and delusions may occur, although

the delusions are not usually well organized. More frequently, the onset of the psychosis in TBI is delayed relative to the injury. In many series, psychotic symptoms have not become evident until 5 to 10 years after the injury. Localized brain damage (particularly involving the temporal lobe) and posttraumatic epilepsy have been associated with delayed, rather than immediate, onset of psychosis. When onset is delayed, individuals are more likely to experience hallucinations (auditory greater than visual) than those with earlier onset. Onset may be gradual, and depression may occur before onset of psychosis. In such cases, it is important to determine if the psychosis is related to an underlying mood disorder, as this will alter the treatment approach.

b. **Pathophysiology**
   (1) The *neural substrate* of psychosis in patients with TBI is not known, but many of the brain regions implicated in schizophrenia overlap with those vulnerable to injury in the typical TBI. For example, frontal lobe regions, including dorsolateral and orbitofrontal cortex, temporal lobes (particularly the hippocampal formation), basal ganglia, and thalamus are commonly affected in TBI.
   (2) There is evidence to suggest that *genetic vulnerability* can interact with TBI to increase the risk of developing schizophrenia.

c. **Diagnosis.** The diagnosis is clinical and is based on the presence of psychotic symptoms. However, as with other neurologic disorders psychosis after TBI can be seen in several different settings including (1) as part of a delirium or metabolic encephalopathy during the period of posttraumatic amnesia, (2) as a component of a post-TBI mood disorder, (3) as part of a post-TBI seizure disorder or (4) related to substance use or abuse.

   The diagnosis of new psychotic symptoms in the individual with TBI should involve determining which of the "causes" mentioned in the preceding text are responsible. A neurologic examination and perhaps other neurodiagnostic studies (EEG, repeat neuroimaging, etc.) should be considered to ascertain whether there is another CNS process at work or if there is a late complication of the TBI (e.g., development of normal pressure hydrocephalus or posttraumatic epilepsy). A careful cognitive examination and history should be taken to determine whether the individual is delirious and screening laboratory studies (CBC, serum electrolytes, BUN, Cre, Ca++) should be done to determine the cause if this is suspected. A careful history from the individual and reliable informants should be taken looking for indicators of a mood disorder. A urine toxicology screen should be done if there is any possibility of substance use. Psychotic symptoms of paroxysmal onset with brief duration, especially in the context of a known or suspected seizure disorder should prompt strong consideration of an EEG.

d. **Treatment**

(1) *Optimize the physical health of the patient.* As a first step, the clinician must make an accurate *diagnosis and determination of the etiology* of the psychosis. This requires distinguishing psychotic symptoms from other brain injury–related symptoms including confabulation, misidentification syndromes, and illusions, and treatment of any comorbid or contributing general medical conditions have been optimally treated. The list of current medications must be carefully scrutinized and those that are not necessary discontinued or the minimum effective dose determined.

(2) Optimize the patient's *environment and lifestyle,* including the provision of a safe situation that minimizes the person's acting on their delusions or hallucinations in a dangerous or violent manner. This type of behavior can put patients at risk for being overmedicated or restrained. Those living at home or in assisted living facilities are at increased risk for institutionalization.

(3) In addition to environmental modification, *behavioral management techniques* could include optimization of socialization and functional status, and education and support of caregivers. Caregivers of patients with psychosis and TBI can experience considerable adversity, including increased physical demands involved in constant supervision of the patient, the emotional stress of caring for a loved one who is experiencing these symptoms, physical illness, and depression.

(4) *Medication approaches* to treat psychosis in TBI vary according to what is "causing" the psychosis.

(a) **Delirium.** Determine the cause, and treat accordingly (e.g., correct electrolyte imbalances, discontinue causative medications). Use of low-dose antipsychotic agents (see subsequent text) may be warranted.

(b) **Mood disorder.** Treat depression with antidepressants or mania with anticycling agents (see Chapter 5). If psychosis is endangering the health and well-being of the patient, family or caregiver, add low-dose antipsychotic agents (see subsequent text).

(c) **Seizure disorder.** In this context the usual seizure disorder is a complex partial seizure. Therefore, management of the seizure disorder becomes the primary concern. Management suggestions are beyond the scope of this chapter. The paramount treatment objective is control of the seizure frequency. If psychosis is endangering health the and well-being of the patient, family or caregiver, add low-dose antipsychotic agents (see subsequent text).

(d) **Substance use or abuse.** In this context, the treatment objective becomes the identification and removal of the offending drug of abuse. If psychosis is endangering the health and well-being of the patient, family or caregiver, add low-dose antipsychotic agents (see subsequent text).

(e) **Use of antipsychotic medication.** When the psychosis is considered to be caused by the TBI, or when caused by the conditions mentioned in the preceding text, but endangering the health and well-being of the patient, or family or caregiver, the use of antipsychotic medications is warranted. There are important issues to consider with both the typical and atypical antipsychotics. None of the medications have specific FDA indications for the treatment of psychosis following TBI. Whereas a variety of case reports and small case series suggest that most of the atypical antipsychotics are effective in treating psychosis in individuals with TBI, no randomized placebo-controlled trials have been completed.

We use risperidone, based on its safety profile and demonstrated efficacy in trials of psychosis associated with other brain disorders such as AD. We begin with 0.25 mg or 0.5 mg per day to start and titrate upward slowly. We rarely go over 4 mg per day, and most individuals are treated with 2.0 to 3.0 mg per day. If weight gain or other signs of metabolic syndrome emerge we cross taper to aripiprazole, 5 mg per day and titrate slowly to 15 mg per day as tolerated. If psychotic symptoms do not abate after 1 month we then consider another atypical, or use a combination of aripiprazole and haloperidol. We start with haloperidol 0.5 mg per day and titrate upward slowly as needed and tolerated. We rarely go >5 mg per day. If all of these regimens are ineffective, we initiate a trial of clozapine, starting with 12.5 mg per day and titrating upwards in 12.5 mg increments weekly as tolerated and carefully monitoring CBC and absolute neutrophil counts on a weekly basis, as described in the preceding text. If an effective treatment is found, we continue it for 1 year as tolerated and then attempt to slowly (2 months) taper off the medications.

References

1. Arciniegas DB, Harris SN, Brousseau KM. Psychosis following traumatic brain injury. *Int Rev Psychiatry.* 2003;15:328–340.

2. Malaspina D, Goetz RR, Friedman JH, et al. Traumatic brain injury and schizophrenia in members of schizophrenia and bipolar disorder pedigrees. *Am J Psychiatry.* 2001;158:440–446.
3. McAllister TW, Ferrell RB. Evaluation and treatment of psychosis after traumatic brain injury. *Neurorehabilitation.* 2002;17:357–368.
4. Sachdev P, Smith JS, Cathcart S. Schizophrenia-like psychosis following traumatic brain injury: A chart-based descriptive and case-control study. *Psychol Med.* 2001;31:231–239.

7. **Psychosis in patients with intellectual disability**
   a. **Clinical background**
      (1) Schizophrenia-like syndromes have a prevalence rate of approximately 2% to 8% in individuals with ID. There is a broad range, however, and at least one report suggests a 30% rate of psychotic disorder in individuals with velo-cardio-facial syndrome.
      (2) A major *complicating factor* that can impede the accurate diagnosis of psychotic syndromes in the intellectually disabled is related to the baseline frequency of psychotic-like behaviors often observed in this population, including audible self-talk, imaginary friends, and repetitive overvalued ideas.
      (3) The *longitudinal course* of psychosis in ID is unknown.
   b. **Pathogenesis**
      (1) The *pathophysiology* of psychosis in ID is unknown.
   c. **Diagnosis.** The diagnosis is clinical and is based on the presence of criteria for a psychotic disorder. However, several indicators predictive of response to antipsychotic medications have been identified, including a change in the frequency and/or intensity of these otherwise possibly normal behaviors, an increase in the frequency and/or intensity of unpredictable aggression related to these behaviors, and the consistent misinterpretation of events in the immediate environment in a paranoid-like fashion. It is critical to determine the underlying cause of the psychosis. As with other disorders, psychosis in individuals with ID can be seen in several different settings including (1) as part of a delirium or metabolic encephalopathy, (2) as a component of a mood disorder, (3) as part of a seizure disorder or (4) related to substance use or abuse (less common in this context), or (5) as a schizophrenia-like illness. The diagnosis of new psychotic symptoms in the individual with ID should involve determining which of the "causes" mentioned in the preceding text are responsible. A neurologic examination and perhaps other neurodiagnostic studies (EEG, repeat neuroimaging, etc.) should be considered to ascertain whether the heretofore presumed static cause of the ID is actually a progressive neurodegenerative disorder (e.g., a mitochondrial or related metabolic storage disorder) that

has begun to progress. A careful cognitive examination and
history should be taken to determine whether the individual is delirious and if so, screening laboratory studies (CBC,
serum electrolytes, BUN, Cre, Ca++) should be done to
determine the cause. A careful history from the individual
and reliable informants should be taken looking for indicators of a mood disorder. A urine toxicology screen should
be done if there is any possibility of substance use. Psychotic symptoms of paroxysmal onset with brief duration,
especially in the context of a known or suspected seizure
disorder, should prompt strong consideration of an EEG.

d. **Treatment**

(1) As a first step, the clinician should *optimize the physical health of the patient* and ensure that all underlying
general medical disorders have been optimally treated,
including pain management. It is quite common to have
medical disorders (e.g., urinary tract infections, sinusi-
tis, abscessed teeth, pain, etc.) present as psychotic-like
symptoms in individuals with ID who are unable to
express themselves verbally. As noted in the preceding
text, it is also important to ensure that the altered behavior truly represents psychosis, and not normal but
psychotic-like behaviors often observed in this population (e.g., audible self-talk, imaginary friends, and
repetitive over-valued ideas).

(2) The patient's *environment and lifestyle should be optimized*, including the provision of a safe situation that
minimizes the person's agitation and/or acting on their
delusions or hallucinations in a dangerous or violent
manner. Hallucinations and delusions are important
contributors to patient and caregiver distress, and are
often important risk factors for institutional placement.

(3) *Treatment strategies* often include a combination of some
form of psychological treatment plus pharmacologic
treatment. Usually, a psychological approach aimed
at changing specific undesirable behaviors is tried.
Because the causes of neurobehavioral dyscontrol in
the intellectually disabled are multifactorial, multiple
treatment approaches must be considered.

(4) No *pharmacologic treatment* is approved by the FDA for
treatment of behavioral disturbance associated with ID.
There are few evidence-based reports in the form of
controlled, randomized drug trials concerning pharmacotherapy of neuropsychiatric illness in the context of
ID. Most of the literature on treatment of behavioral disturbance in individuals with ID consists of individual
case reports or reports of small series of patients; an extensive computer literature search for evidence of efficacy for any antipsychotic drug for treatment of people

with a dual diagnosis of schizophrenia and ID indicated "no trial evidence to guide the use of antipsychotic medication for those with both ID and schizophrenia." Except in emergencies, we recommend a conservative approach to pharmacotherapy in individuals with ID. The main points of this approach are starting with single agents in low doses, followed by slow up-titration of dosage, with sufficient time between dose changes to observe both positive and negative effects. We recommend beginning with single agents and using augmentation strategies or adding more drugs only when monotherapy has clearly failed. The use of medications to treat psychosis in individuals with ID varies according to what is "causing" the psychosis.

(a) **Delirium.** Determine the cause, and treat accordingly (e.g., correct electrolyte imbalances, discontinue causative medications). Use of low-dose antipsychotic agents (see subsequent text) may be warranted.

(b) **Mood disorder.** Treat depression with antidepressants or mania with anticycling agents (see Chapter 5). If psychosis is endangering the health and well-being of the patient, family or caregiver, add low-dose antipsychotic agents (see subsequent text).

(c) **Seizure disorder.** In this context, the usual seizure disorder is a complex partial seizure. Therefore, management of the seizure disorder becomes the primary concern. Management suggestions are beyond the scope of this chapter. The paramount treatment objective is control of the seizure frequency. If psychosis is endangering health and well-being of the patient, or family or caregiver, add low-dose antipsychotic agents (see subsequent text).

(d) **Substance use or abuse.** In this context, the treatment objective becomes the identification and removal of the offending drug of abuse. If psychosis is endangering the health and well-being of the patient, family or caregiver, add low-dose antipsychotic agents (see subsequent text).

(e) **Use of antipsychotic medication.** When the psychotic symptoms are endangering the health and well-being of the patient, family or caregiver, the use of antipsychotic medications is warranted. We use risperidone based on its safety profile and demonstrated efficacy in trials of psychosis associated with other brain disorders such as AD. We use 0.25 mg or 0.5 mg per day to start and titrate upward slowly. We rarely go over 4 mg per day, and most individuals are treated with 2.0 to 3.0 mg per day. If weight gain or other signs of metabolic syndrome emerge we cross taper to aripiprazole, 5 mg per day and titrate slowly to 15 mg per day as tolerated. If psychotic symptoms do not abate after 1 month we then consider another atypical, or use a combination of aripiprazole and haloperidol. We start with haloperidol 0.5 mg per day and titrate upward slowly as needed and tolerated. We rarely go >5 mg per day. If all of these regimens are ineffective we initiate a trial of clozapine, starting with 12.5 mg per day and titrating upwards in 12.5 mg increments weekly as tolerated and carefully monitoring CBC and absolute neutrophil counts on a weekly basis. Careful monitoring of patients taking clozapine was described in the preceding text. If an effective treatment is found, we continue it for 6 to 12 months as tolerated and then attempt to slowly (2 month) taper off the medications.

(5) Literature about *use of ECT* in the treatment of psychiatric disorders in persons with ID is not extensive. The sense of this case-report literature is that ECT is a safe and effective treatment for persons with ID and psychiatric syndromes that are indications for ECT. Our view is that ECT should be considered for individuals with ID and psychiatric symptoms that are very severe and that are refractory to vigorous pharmacotherapy. Affective syndromes may be more responsive. A careful risk–benefit analysis is essential.

References

1. Duggan L, Brylewski J. Effectiveness of antipsychotic medication in people with intellectual disability and schizophrenia: A systematic review. *J Intellect Disabil Res.* 1999;43:94–104.
2. Ferrell RB, Wolinsky EJ, Kauffman CI, et al. Neuropsychiatric syndromes in adults with intellectual disability: Issues in assessment and treatment. *Curr Psychiatry Rep.* 2004;6:380–390.
3. Murphy KC, Jones LA, Owen MJ. High rates of schizophrenia in adults with velo-cardio-facial syndrome. *Arch Gen Psychiatry.* 1999;56:940–950.

8. **Psychosis in patients with Huntington disease**
    a. **Clinical background**
        (1) The *prevalence* of psychotic symptoms in HD is higher than in the general population.
        (2) The *phenomenology* of psychosis in HD is similar to that of primary psychosis. In general, psychosis presents after the full clinical syndrome of HD is manifest. Rarely psychosis is the presenting symptom, preceding the

motor manifestations of HD by several years, or occurring in patients with minimal motor symptoms who are unaware they are affected.

(3) *Risk factors* for psychosis in patients with HD include family history of psychosis.

(4) There are no studies of the *longitudinal course* of psychosis in HD.

b. **Pathogenesis.** The *neurobiology* of psychosis in patients with HD is not known. Symptoms of psychosis apparently do not correlate with CAG repeat length, although one study suggested an inverse correlation between earlier age of onset of psychosis and higher number of CAG repeats.

c. **Diagnosis.** The diagnosis is clinical and is based on the presence of symptoms that meet criteria for a psychotic disorder. However, it is critical to determine what the underlying cause of the psychosis is. As with other neurologic disorders, psychosis in HD can be seen in several different settings including (1) as part of a delirium or metabolic encephalopathy, (2) as a component of a HD-related mood disorder, (3) as part of a HD-related seizure disorder or (4) related to substance use or abuse (less common in this context).

The diagnosis of new psychotic symptoms in the individual with HD should involve determining which of the "causes" mentioned in the preceding text are responsible. A careful cognitive examination and history should be taken to determine whether the individual is delirious. Screening laboratory studies (CBC, serum electrolytes, BUN, Cre, Ca++) should be done if delirium is suspected, to determine the cause. A careful history from the individual and reliable informants should be taken looking for indicators of a mood disorder. A urine toxicology screen should be done if there is any possibility of substance use. Psychotic symptoms of paroxysmal onset with brief duration, especially in the context of a known or suspected seizure disorder, should prompt strong consideration of an EEG.

d. **Treatment**

(1) It is important to keep in mind that both *exogenous* (related to therapeutic interventions) factors and *endogenous* (related to the disease process itself) factors can contribute to the development of psychotic symptoms in HD.

(2) *Optimize the physical health of the patient* and ensure that all underlying general medical disorders have been optimally treated, including pain management. It is also important to ensure that the altered behavior truly represents psychosis, and not disorders of vision causing illusions recorded as hallucinations, or misplacement of objects secondary to memory problems presenting as paranoia.

(3) Optimize the patient's *environment and lifestyle*, including the provision of a safe situation that minimizes the person's agitation and/or acting on their delusions or hallucinations in a dangerous or violent manner. Hallucinations and delusions are important contributors to patient and caregiver distress, and are often important risk factors for nursing home placement.

(4) *Treatment strategies* should include ruling out reversible causes of psychosis unrelated to the primary illness, implementing appropriate psychosocial strategies (see subsequent text), reduction of unnecessary medications, and judicious use of atypical antipsychotics.

(5) *Psychosocial strategies* might include additional support for the patient with HD, increased light during the day and decreased light at night (that may improve orientation and minimize excessive sensory stimulation), education for the caregiver(s), and support for the family in their decisions regarding treatments, hospitalization, and long-term placement.

(6) *Medication approaches.* In general, the use of medications to treat psychosis in HD varies according to what is "causing" the psychosis.

 (a) **Delirium.** Determine the cause, and treat accordingly (e.g., correct electrolyte imbalances, discontinue causative medications). Use of low-dose antipsychotic agents (see subsequent text) may be warranted.

 (b) **Mood disorder.** Treat depression with antidepressants or mania with anticycling agents (see Chapter 5). If psychosis is endangering the health and well-being of the patient, family or caregiver, add low-dose antipsychotic agents (see subsequent text).

 (c) **Seizure disorder.** In this context, the usual seizure disorder is a complex partial seizure. Therefore, management of the seizure disorder becomes the primary concern. Management suggestions are beyond the scope of this chapter. The paramount treatment objective is control of the seizure frequency. If psychosis is endangering the health and well-being of the patient, family or caregiver, add low-dose antipsychotic agents (see subsequent text).

 (d) **Substance use or abuse.** When applicable, the treatment objective becomes the identification and removal of the offending drug of abuse. If psychosis is endangering the health and well-being of the patient, family or caregiver, add low-dose antipsychotic agents (see subsequent text).

(e) **Use of antipsychotic medication.** When the psychosis is considered to be caused by the underlying disorder, or when caused by the conditions mentioned in the preceding text, in the circumstance where the symptoms are endangering the health and well-being of the patient, family or caregiver, the use of antipsychotic medications is warranted. There are no FDA-approved agents for the specific treatment of psychosis associated with HD. Therefore, treatment is modeled on approaches to primary psychotic disorders. There are important issues to consider with both the typical and atypical antipsychotics, as has been previously discussed. The following is our approach, but the level of evidence to support it is weak.

In individuals with little known risk for metabolic syndrome or diabetes, we will start with an atypical agent. We use risperidone, based on its safety profile and demonstrated efficacy in trials of psychosis associated with other brain disorders such as AD. We start with 0.25 mg or 0.5 mg per day and titrate slowly upward, rarely going >4 mg per day. If weight gain or other signs of metabolic syndrome emerge we cross taper to aripiprazole, 5 mg per day and titrate slowly to 15 mg per day as tolerated. If psychotic symptoms do not abate after 1 month we then consider another atypical, or use a combination of aripiprazole and haloperidol as described in the preceding text. When using a typical antipsychotic we use haloperidol 0.25 or 0.5 mg per day or b.i.d to start and slowly titrate upwards as tolerated. We rarely go beyond 4 mg per day total. If there is no response to two trials of an atypical antipsychotic and a trial of a typical antipsychotic then we move to a trial of low-dose clozapine. The initial workup includes and EKG, EEG, and CBC. The absolute neutrophil count must be over 2,000. We start with a dose of 12.5 mg per day and titrate upwards in 12.5 per day increments weekly as tolerated until achieving a dose of 50 mg per day. Careful monitoring of labs as described in the preceding text occurs for patients on a clozapine protocol. If an effective treatment is found, we continue it for 6 to 12 months as tolerated and then attempt to slowly (2 month) taper off the medications.

References

1. Bonelli RM, Hofmann P. A review of the treatment options for Huntington's disease. *Expert Opin Pharmacother*. 2004;5:767–776.
2. Tarsy D, Baldessarini RJ, Tarazi FI. Effects of newer antipsychotics on extrapyramidal function. *CNS Drugs*. 2002;16:23–45.
3. Tsuang D, Almqvist EW, Lipe H, et al. Familial aggregation of psychotic symptoms in Huntington's disease. *Am J Psychiatry*. 2000;157:1955–1959.

9. **Psychosis in patients with multiple sclerosis**
    a. **Clinical background**
        (1) Psychosis, although not a prominent feature of MS, has been reported to occur in approximately 5% of cases. One hypothesis that has been put forth to explain the relatively low frequency of psychosis in MS is that MS is predominately a white matter disease, whereas psychosis has more typically been linked to gray matter abnormalities
        (2) The *phenomenology* of psychosis in patients with MS appears similar to that of patients with primary schizophrenia spectrum disorders, although this issue has not been well studied. Primary symptoms include lack of insight, persecutory delusions, heightened or changed perception, and "minor" hallucinations (e.g., music, noises). MS-related psychosis has a later age of presentation, quicker resolution of symptoms, fewer psychotic relapses, better response to treatment, and a more favorable outcome than primary schizophrenia.
        (3) Identified potential *risk factors* for psychosis in patients with MS include male gender, and higher lesion load in the region of the temporal horns of the lateral ventricles.
        (4) The *longitudinal course* of psychosis in patients with MS has not been thoroughly studied, although research suggests that median duration of the first psychotic episode is approximately 5 weeks. In one case series, more than half of the patients experienced no further psychotic episodes, 30% had a single relapse, and only one patient (10%) had multiple recurrences.
    b. **Pathogenesis**
        (1) There is some speculation that demyelination and psychosis have a shared, viral *pathogenesis* in patients with MS.
        (2) The relationship between lesions of the CNS, as seen in MS, and psychiatric illness has not been established, although the temporal lobe in general, and temporal horn lesion load specifically, has been implicated. This is consistent with the literature suggesting a role for the temporal lobe in the pathogenesis of psychosis in general.
    c. **Diagnosis.** The diagnosis is clinical and is based on the presence of psychotic symptoms. However, it is critical to determine what the underlying cause of the psychosis is. As with other neurologic disorders, psychosis associated with MS can be seen in several different settings including (1) as part of a delirium or metabolic encephalopathy, (2) as a component of an MS-associated mood disorder, (3) as part of an MS-associated seizure disorder or, less often, (4) related to substance use or abuse.

The diagnosis of new psychotic symptoms in the individual with MS should involve determining which of the "causes" mentioned in the preceding text are responsible. A neurologic examination and perhaps other neurodiagnostic studies (EEG, repeat neuroimaging, etc.) should be considered to ascertain whether the underlying demyelinating disorder has progressed. A careful cognitive examination and history should be taken to determine whether the individual is delirious. Screening laboratory studies (CBC, serum electrolytes, BUN, Cre, Ca++) should be done if a delirium is suspected, to determine the cause. Immunotherapeutic agents are another potential cause of delirium in MS patients. These are more likely to occur in the context of higher dose regimens or combination regimens. A careful history from the individual and reliable informants should be taken looking for indicators of a mood disorder. A urine toxicology screen should be done if there is any possibility of substance use. Psychotic symptoms of paroxysmal onset with brief duration, especially in the context of a known or suspected seizure disorder, should prompt strong consideration of an EEG.

d. **Treatment**
  (1) *Optimize the physical health of the patient.* As a first step, the clinician must make an accurate *diagnosis and determination of the etiology* of the psychosis. The list of current medications must be carefully scrutinized and those that are not necessary discontinued or the minimum effective dose determined.
  (2) Optimize the patient's *environment and lifestyle,* including the provision of a safe situation that minimizes the person's acting on their delusions or hallucinations in a dangerous or violent manner. This type of behavior can put patients at risk for being overmedicated or restrained. Those living at home or in assisted living facilities are at increased risk for institutionalization.
  (3) In addition to environmental modification, *behavioral management techniques* could include optimization of socialization and functional status, and education and support of caregivers. Caregivers of patients with psychosis and MS can experience considerable adversity, including increased physical demands involved in constant supervision of the patient, the emotional stress of caring for a loved one who is experiencing these symptoms, physical illness, and depression.
  (4) *Medication approaches* to treat psychosis in MS vary according to what is "causing" the psychosis.
    (a) **Delirium.** Determine the cause, and treat accordingly (e.g., correct electrolyte imbalances, discontinue causative medications). Use of low-dose

antipsychotic agents (see subsequent text) may be warranted.

(b) **Mood disorder.** Treat depression with antidepressants or mania with anticycling agents (see Chapter 5). If psychosis is endangering the health and well-being of the patient, family or caregiver, add low-dose antipsychotic agents (see subsequent text).

(c) **Seizure disorder.** In this context, the usual seizure disorder is a complex partial seizure. Therefore, management of the seizure disorder becomes the primary concern. Management suggestions are beyond the scope of this chapter. The paramount treatment objective is control of the seizure frequency. If psychosis is endangering the health and well-being of the patient, family or caregiver, add low-dose antipsychotic agents (see subsequent text).

(d) **Substance use or abuse.** The treatment objective becomes the identification and removal of the offending drug of abuse. If psychosis is endangering the health and well-being of the patient, family or caregiver, add low-dose antipsychotic agents (see subsequent text).

(e) **Use of antipsychotic medication.** When the psychosis is considered to be caused by the MS, or when caused by the conditions mentioned in the preceding text but endangering the health and well being of the patient, family or caregiver, the use of antipsychotic medications is warranted. There are important issues to consider with both the typical and atypical antipsychotics. None of the medications have specific FDA indications for the treatment of psychosis in MS. The atypical antipsychotics generally have less D2 receptor blockade and more 5HT1 antagonism relative to the typicals. They are felt to carry less risk of EPS and tardive dyskinesia. On the other hand, there is significant risk of weight gain, diabetes, and metabolic syndrome. The following is our approach, but the level of evidence to support it is weak.

We use risperidone based on its safety profile and demonstrated efficacy in trials of psychosis associated with other brain disorders such as AD. We start with 0.25 mg or 0.5 mg per day to start and titrate upward slowly. We rarely go over 4 mg per day, and most individuals are treated with 2.0 to 3.0 mg per day. If weight gain or other signs of metabolic syndrome emerge we cross taper to aripiprazole, 5 mg per day and titrate slowly to 15 mg per day as tolerated. If psychotic symptoms do not abate after 1 month we then consider another atypical antipsychotic, or use a combination of aripiprazole and haloperidol. We start with haloperidol 0.5 mg per day and titrate upward slowly as needed and tolerated. We rarely go >5 mg per day. If all of these regimens are ineffective, we initiate a trial of clozapine, starting with 12.5 mg per day and titrating upwards in 12.5 mg increments weekly as tolerated and carefully monitoring CBC and absolute neutrophil counts on a weekly basis, as described in the preceding text. If an effective treatment is found, we continue it for 1 year as tolerated and then attempt to slowly (2 months) taper off the medications.

References

1. Davison K, Bagley CR. Schizophrenia-like psychosis associated with organic disorders of the central nervous system. A review of the literature. In: Herrington RN, ed. *Current problems in neuropsychiatry*. Ashford, Kent: Hedley; 1969:113–184.
2. Feinstein A. The neuropsychiatry of multiple sclerosis. *Can J Psychiatry*. 2004;49:157–163.
3. Feinstein A. *The clinical neuropsychiatry of multiple sclerosis*. Cambridge, MA: Cambridge University Press; 1999.
4. Stevens JR. Schizophrenia and multiple sclerosis. *Schizophr Bull*. 1988;14:231–241.

10. Poststroke psychosis
  a. Clinical background
    (1) The *prevalence* of psychosis in patients with stroke is not known, but it appears to be relatively rare compared with other neuropsychiatric complications such as poststroke depression or anxiety.
    (2) The *occurrence* of psychosis appears to be related to stroke location (right frontoparietal lesions). In addition, there is some suggestion that individuals with other preexisting neurologic disease (e.g., earlier strokes, cerebral atrophy, or seizure disorder) may be at greater risk.
    (3) The *phenomenology* of poststroke psychosis is similar to that of a primary psychosis, with hallucinations, and delusions being the most prominent symptoms. However, if the stroke impairs speech and language function, the individual may not be able to articulate or describe the symptoms and they may have to be inferred from the individual's behavior, as described under general principles.
    (4) The *longitudinal course* of psychosis after stroke is unknown. It is our experience that psychotic symptoms can occur immediately after the stroke in which case the syndrome may be short lived, or occur months to years after the event in which case it seems to have a more protracted course.

b. **Pathogenesis of poststroke depression**
   (1) The *pathophysiology* of psychosis in patients with stroke is not fully understood. However, as noted, right frontoparietal lesions, a significantly greater degree of subcortical atrophy, and increased incidence of seizures have been reported in patients with psychosis relative to those without psychosis.
c. **Diagnosis.** The diagnosis is clinical and is based on the presence of psychotic symptoms. However, it is critical to determine the underlying cause of the psychosis. As with other neurologic disorders, psychosis after stroke can be seen in several different settings including (1) as part of a delirium, (2) as a component of a poststroke mood disorder, (3) as part of a poststroke seizure disorder or (4) related to substance use or abuse (less common in this context). Stroke occurs most commonly in elderly individuals who often have several other medical disorders. Iatrogenic etiologies, often related to medications used to treat these associated disorders, are a common cause of delirium with associated psychotic symptoms.

   The evaluation of new psychotic symptoms in an individual with stroke should involve determining which of the mentioned in the preceding text "causes" are responsible. A neurologic examination and perhaps other neurodiagnostic studies (EEG, repeat neuroimaging, etc.) should be considered to ascertain whether the underlying cerebrovascular disorder has progressed. A careful cognitive examination and history should be taken to determine whether the individual is delirious. Screening laboratory studies (CBC, serum electrolytes, BUN, Cre, Ca++, urinalysis) should be done. A careful history from the individual and reliable informants should be taken looking for indicators of a mood disorder. A urine toxicology screen should be done if there is any possibility of substance use. Psychotic symptoms of paroxysmal onset with brief duration, especially in the context of a known or suspected seizure disorder should prompt strong consideration of an EEG.
d. **Treatment**
   (1) *Optimize the physical health of the patient* and ensure that all underlying general medical disorders have been optimally treated, including pain management.
   (2) *Optimize the patient's environment and lifestyle*, including the provision of a safe situation that minimizes the person's acting on their delusions or hallucinations in a dangerous or violent manner. This type of behavior can put patients at risk for being overmedicated or restrained. Those living at home or in assisted living facilities are at increased risk for institutionalization.

(3) *Medication approaches.* The use of medications to treat psychosis after stroke varies according to what is "causing" the psychosis.
  (a) **Delirium.** Determine the cause, and treat accordingly (e.g., correct electrolyte imbalances, discontinue causative medications, treat infections). Use low-dose antipsychotic agents (see subsequent text) may be warranted.
  (b) **Poststroke mood disorder.** Treat depression with antidepressants or mania with anticycling agents (see Chapter 5). If psychosis is endangering the health and well-being of the patient, family or caregiver, add low-dose antipsychotic agents (see subsequent text).
  (c) **Poststroke seizure disorder.** In this context, the usual seizure disorder is a complex partial seizure. Therefore, management of the seizure disorder becomes the primary concern. Management suggestions are beyond the scope of this chapter. The paramount treatment objective is control of the seizure frequency. If psychosis is endangering, health and well-being of the patient, family or caregiver, add low-dose antipsychotic agents (see subsequent text).
  (d) **Substance use or abuse.** In this context, the treatment objective becomes the identification and removal of the offending drug of abuse. If psychosis is endangering, health and well-being of the patient, family or caregiver, add low-dose antipsychotic agents (see subsequent text).
  (e) **Use of antipsychotic medication.** When the psychosis is considered to be caused by the underlying cerebrovascular disorder, or when caused by one of the conditions mentioned in the preceding text in a circumstance where the symptoms are endangering the health and well-being of the patient, family or caregiver, the use of antipsychotic medications is warranted. There are important issues to consider with both the typical and atypical antipsychotics. None of the antipsychotic medications have specific FDA indications for the treatment of psychosis after stroke. Therefore, the choice of antipsychotic agent is governed by the safety profile.
We start with risperidone on the basis of its safety profile and demonstrated efficacy in trials of psychosis associated with other brain disorders such as AD. We begin with a dose of 0.25 mg or 0.5 mg per day and titrate slowly upward, rarely going >4 mg per day. If weight gain or other signs of metabolic syndrome emerge we cross taper to aripiprazole,

5 mg per day and titrate slowly to 15 mg per day as tolerated. If psychotic symptoms do not abate after 1 month, we then consider another atypical, or use a typical agent such as haloperidol, starting with 0.5 mg per day and titrating upward as tolerated or needed to 5 mg per day. If there is no response to the recommendations mentioned in the preceding text, and the psychosis is associated with a significant threat to the individual and or their caregivers, we consider a trial of low-dose clozapine analogous to the algorithm for treating other refractory psychoses. The initial workup includes an EKG, EEG, and CBC. The absolute neutrophil count must be >2,000. We start with a dose of 12.5 mg per day and titrate upward in 12.5 per day increments weekly as tolerated until achieving a dose of 50 mg per day. Careful monitoring of patients taking clozapine was described in the section on Psychosis in PD. If an effective treatment is found, we continue it for 6 to 12 months as tolerated and then attempt to slowly (2 month) taper off the medications.

References
1. Chemerinski E, Robinson RG. The neuropsychiatry of stroke. *Psychosomatics*. 2000;41:5–14.
2. Levin DN, Finkelstein S. Delayed psychosis after right temporoparietal stroke or trauma: Relation to epilepsy. *Neurology*. 1982;32:267–273.
3. Rabins PV, Starkstein SE, Robinson RG. Risk factors for developing atypical (schizophreniform) psychosis following stroke. *J Neuropsychiatry Clin Neurosci*. 1991;3: 6–9.

11. **Summary.** Psychosis in neuropsychiatric disorders is a growing concern because of its frequency, its negative effect on the quality of life of the individuals and its contribution to caregiver and family distress. It can often be the most disabling symptom of a disorder, posing a serious threat to an individual's ability to maintain independence; psychosis is the single greatest risk factor for nursing home placement. It is important to aggressively look for other medical and contributing factors that may be impacting an individual's presentation, and to work with the family, caregivers, and situational or lifestyle modifications to provide the safest and most manageable environment possible. Although nonpharmacologic treatments for the behavioral disturbances should be tried first, medications are often needed to enable the individual to be cared for adequately. To minimize side effects, these medications should be started at low dosages that are increased incrementally in small doses with longer intervals between increases. Clinicians should strive to make one change at a time when modifying medication regimens, and ineffective drugs should be discontinued. While pharmacologic interventions are often helpful for management of psychotic symptoms in these disorders, evidence to support the use of specific pharmacologic agents in patients with psychosis is limited

by the absence of randomized, placebo-controlled trials. Randomized controlled trails support the efficacy of risperidone and olanzapine in psychosis in AD, and the use of low-dose clozapine in psychosis in PD. Further work evaluating the efficacy of antipsychotic and other medication to manage psychotic symptoms in neuropsychiatric disorders is needed.

Chapter 8

NONEPILEPTIC SEIZURES

Karen E. Anderson

I. BACKGROUND

A. **Definition and terminology**

1. Nonepileptic seizures (NES) are defined as a conversion disorder manifested by paroxysmal changes in behavior that mimic epileptic seizures but which are not associated with electrographic ictal activity. The term *spells* is also used, meaning episodic phenomena with or without alteration of awareness. Other descriptives such as "psychogenic seizures" and "psuedoseizures" are also used, implying a conversion disorder causing a seizure; no single term completely encompasses the condition. NES will be used throughout this chapter in reference to this disorder.

2. Conversion disorders are classified by the Diagnostic and Statistical Manual of Mental Disorders, 4th edition (DSM-IV) as one of the somatoform disorders, which also include somatization disorder (previously termed *hysteria* or *Briquet syndrome*), undifferentiated somatoform disorder, pain disorder, hypochondriasis, body dysmorphic disorder, and somatoform disorder not otherwise specified. These conditions are all linked by the presence of physical symptoms that are suggestive of medical illness but are not explained by the presence of a medical disorder, effects of a substance, or symptoms of another psychiatric condition, such as loss of energy because of a current episode of major depression. The patient cannot produce them intentionally.

Other conditions such as factitious disorder and malingering, where symptoms are consciously produced (either for psychological gain in assuming the sick role, as in factitious disorder, or to avoid responsibilities or gain compensation of some sort in malingering) are considered to be separate entities by the DSM-IV. Attribution of intent and assessment of whether a symptom is consciously produced is a particularly difficult endeavor, and a definitive answer to this issue may not be possible in many cases.

B. Epidemiology

1. Clinicians who work with epilepsy will undoubtedly encounter patients whose symptoms appear to be non-neurologic in nature. Approximately one third of new patients seen by neurologists have symptoms that are described as "not at all" or only "somewhat" explained by disease; statistics that are similar to the incidence of somatoform disorders in primary and secondary care settings for other medical specialties (de Waal et al.).[1] In neurologic specialty clinics, psychogenic symptoms are common; nonepileptic seizures account for 10% to 20% of cases referred to epileptologists for lack of response to antiepileptic medications and 50% of status epilepticus admissions.

2. Risk factors for development of NES include female gender, lower socio-economic status, history of previously unexplained medical symptoms, history of other psychiatric conditions (including personality disorders); history or abuse or trauma may also increase risk of NES.[2]

3. The public health implications of somatoform or conversion disorders in general are known to be considerable although NES have received little study in particular. These patients use health care resources at high rates, including frequent office visits, demands for expensive evaluations, unneeded surgical interventions, and referrals for numerous consultations and second opinions. Niemark et al. using a conservative estimate that psychogenic symptoms of all types account for 10% of medical costs, calculated that the annual cost of these symptoms to the US health care system is over $100 billion.[3] The estimate does not include time spent on disability or compensation received because of psychogenic symptoms. NES have been shown to cause reduction in quality of life comparable to or exceeding that seen in epileptic seizures.

C. Phenomenology

1. Nonepileptic spells are often dramatic in nature, and can be extremely upsetting to those who witness them. Signs and symptoms, reviewed in Table 8.1, may include, but are not limited to thrashing, violent movements, side-to-side head movement, asynchronous eye movements, unresponsiveness, and episodes mimicking partial seizures.[2,4] Approximately two thirds of NES consist primarily of motor signs and symptoms. Commonly, the nonepileptic spells last for over 2 minutes; a fluctuating course of illness is often seen. Nonepileptic spells that are not explained by a medical condition such as syncope, migraine, or metabolic disorder may be a somatoform disorder, or may result from factitious disorder or malingering (see Table 8.2 for conditions to consider in evaluation of nonepileptic spells).

TABLE 8.1   Common Signs and Symptoms of Nonepileptic Seizures or Spells

Thrashing, violent movements of limbs or entire body
Side-to-side head movements
Asynchronous eye movements
Pelvic thrusting
Weeping
Out of phase movements of extremities
Unresponsiveness
Episodes mimicking partial epileptic seizures

D. **Comorbidity**
1. NES may occur in up to 50% of patients with epilepsy. NES may be particularly common in patients with treatment refractory epilepsy.
2. Other psychiatric conditions such as depression and affective disorders are commonly seen in somatoform disorders.[1] Personality disorders and somatization are also seen with high frequency, reflecting the abnormal coping skills these patients have learned in their development. History of abuse or trauma may increase risk of NES; therefore, patients should be queried about dissociative symptoms and post-traumatic stress disorder.
E. **Etiology.** The pathophysiology of psychogenic conditions in general, or of NES, in particular is not understood. Associations between psychogenic symptoms in general and head injury have been observed, suggesting a possible etiologic connection. Brain injury because of traumatic insult or disease processes may predispose patients to having psychogenic symptoms and may also provide a model for development of psychogenic symptoms. Brain injury early in life, especially if it leads to intellectual deficits, may increase vulnerability.

TABLE 8.2   Differential Diagnosis of Spells

Epileptic seizures
Nonepileptic seizures
Vasovagal episodes
Cardiac conditions
Endocrine and metabolic disorders (e.g., hypoglycemia, drugs, alcohol)
Migraines
Vestibular disorders
Dystonia, myoclonus, tics
Sleep disorders (e.g., rapid eye movement [REM] sleep disorders, narcolepsy)
Other psychiatric conditions (e.g., anxiety disorder, depressive fugues, schizophrenia, depersonalization disorder, attention deficit disorder)

F. Prognosis

1. Medical morbidity resulting from NES can be considerable. Patients are exposed to numerous procedures, often repeatedly, in search of a diagnosis. Medications used to treat epileptic seizures may be given erroneously, exposing patients to side effects. Dependence on benzodiazepines may occur in patients who receive large doses over long periods. Polypharmacy is common, again exposing patients to side effects, especially because of medication interactions.

2. Data on the natural history of NES suggests that in some, but not all individuals, symptoms develop in response to a specific stressor or situation. However, many patients do not have a particular event that triggers onset, but rather develop NES as part of poor general coping skills and to gain attention and support that are otherwise unavailable to them.

3. Approximately 40% of patients stop having NES once a diagnosis is reached. Most patients continue to have NES and experience considerable disability, including inability to fulfill obligations at work and at home. Up to half of patients who continue to have NES will remain on some form of public assistance for their financial support.

4. Prognostic features of good outcome include diagnosis of NES soon after symptom onset and acceptance of the NES diagnosis.

5. Indicators of poor prognosis include the presence of comorbid psychiatric disorders.

II. MANAGEMENT

A. Diagnosis

1. **Differential diagnosis.** As noted in Table 8.2, in addition to nonepileptic seizures many conditions can cause spells that resemble epileptic seizures.

   a. *Syncope* is the other most common medical disorder that is mistaken for epilepsy. The usual associated cardiac and other symptoms (e.g., nausea, lightheadedness) generally make syncopal episodes easily identifiable as such. It is not widely recognized that tonic and clonic movements may be seen during syncopal episodes, and this may be a cause of confusion with epileptic seizures.[5] *Transient ischemic attacks* may resemble partial seizures, but are not followed by typical sequelae of epileptic seizures. A long-time course for onset of symptoms is suggestive of *migraine, migraine equivalents, and vertigo.* Any *movement disorder* of a paroxysmal nature, such as tics or myoclonus, may be mistaken for epilepsy. Many *sleep disorders* have features that can cause them to be mistaken for epileptic seizures, for example, loss of tone in narcoleptic cataplexy. Metabolic disorders are usually of long duration and have distinctive characteristics that are evident on history (see reference,[2] for an excellent review).

b. *Psychiatric conditions* with paroxysmal signs and symptoms that may mimic epilepsy include anxiety disorders, especially panic attacks. There is considerable overlap between feelings of depersonalization, derealization, and tremulousness that may occur during a panic attack and the emotional and physical symptoms experienced by patients suffering from partial epileptic seizures. Panic attacks are generally longer in duration than epileptic seizures, and often have specific triggers such as the patients finding themselves in an enclosed space. Psychotic symptoms are sometimes mistaken for epilepsy, although they usually have a much longer time course and are more complex in nature than the stereotypical picture seen in epilepsy. Depersonalization disorder and attention deficit hyperactivity disorder are two other conditions mistaken for epilepsy in children because of resulting poor concentration and academic difficulties.

2. **Diagnosis of nonepileptic seizures.** This is based on the occurrence of a spell that is not associated with the electrophysiology of the brain, typical of a seizure.

3. **Clinical indicators.** Several clinical indicators can point to a diagnosis of NES; therefore it is critical to obtain a good history. The following suggestions can be helpful:

- Make a list of all symptoms early on in the interview to avoid devoting too much time on any one symptom.
- Ask about disability, detailing onset, and course.
- Ask about relationships with previous doctors, illness beliefs the patient may have, involvement in worker's compensation or legal proceedings, and marital relationships.
- Speak with a spouse or other caregiver, if present, to obtain additional history and assess how others view the symptoms.
- Inquire about physical or sexual abuse but not until later visits as revelation of abuse is unlikely to lead to a quick "cure," and may precipitate extreme distress in the patient.

There are several points in the patient's history that are suggestive (but not diagnostic) of a psychogenic disorder, as follows:

- Abrupt onset of the symptoms
- Occurrence of an event with high emotional valence, such as a death in the family or an assault, which occurred just before the onset of symptoms. Events surrounding symptom onset do not need to be particularly dramatic or life threatening in nature to trigger psychogenic symptoms, especially if the patient has poor premorbid coping skills.
- Symptoms that vary according to setting (public vs. home) or depending on who is accompanying the patient
- Multiple evaluations by other clinicians with a long list of negative diagnostic studies. Some patients may conceal prior evaluations and consultations with nonspecific results out of

fear they will not be taken seriously or that the physician will simply agree with prior opinions.

Psychogenic spells often change over time, and may later be accompanied by other complaints of memory loss, visual changes, or gastrointestinal symptoms. It is wise to ask if similar symptoms occurred in a family member or friend, or if the patient has worked in a health care setting where they have repeatedly observed epileptic seizures.

4. **General medical and neuropsychiatric examination.** The goal is to identify conditions (medical, neurologic, psychiatric) that require treatment including cardiac conditions, epileptic seizures, or axis I or II psychiatric disorders (Table 8.2). Particular studies chosen depend on the clinical picture.

5. **Laboratory investigations.** *Prolonged video electroencephalogram (EEG) monitoring* is indicated in patients suspected of having NES. This is done in an inpatient epilepsy monitoring unit (EMU) with the goal of capturing the patient's behavior during a typical spell on videotape, which is synchronized with continuous EEG monitoring for seizure activity. Most EMUs are experienced in aiding in diagnosis of NES. An EMU admission is especially indicated in cases in which there is reluctance on the part of the physician or patient to withdraw antiepileptic medications or where there is a question of whether a patient has both NES and epileptic seizures. The diagnosis of coexisting NES and epileptic seizures is established by capturing both during one or more video EEG monitoring sessions. The presence of interictal abnormalities in patients with NES makes the additional diagnosis of epilepsy "probable" but not conclusive. The main limitation of an EMU admission is that a patient may not have a typical spell during the monitoring. Some physicians will use induction techniques in these cases, for example, holding an alcohol swab to a patient's forehead and saying it contains a seizure inducing agent. The utility of these provocation maneuvers is highly questionable, as they will jeopardize the patient's trust in the treatment team when they are informed that the seizure induction was a sham. For patients who are unable or unwilling to undergo EMU admission, 24-hour ambulatory EEG monitoring is available at some centers. A patient is connected to EEG leads, then given a portable monitoring device. They are instructed to push a button when an episode occurs, indicating in the tracing where a spell has taken place. This option may be particularly useful in patients who have most of their spells outside a hospital or clinic setting.

"Invasive" EEG, which uses electrodes to directly contact the brain, is indicated only in very select cases where the differentiation of NES and epilepsy is extremely problematic and only after other monitoring techniques have failed. It involves placing electrodes inside the skull over a specific brain region. Various techniques are available, including depth electrodes (intracerebral), epidural and subdural electrodes, depending on clinical indications.

a. A *routine EEG* has limited value in patients with NES because of numerous pitfalls including muscle artifacts because of motion, the need to obtain the study during a spell, EEG changes caused by medications (especially withdrawal of antiepileptic medications). There is also a fairly high rate of "abnormal" EEG findings in all patients who undergo EEG studies, even when seizures are not found. An abnormal EEG report, even if not indicative of seizures, will not reassure the patient and may be taken as evidence that a neurologic disorder does exist. However, an NES is highly likely in the setting of a normal EEG with preserved alpha rhythm during a typical attack manifested by loss of consciousness.

b. *Serum prolactin levels* are not routinely indicated in patients with NES. Although serum prolactin levels are typically elevated after generalized seizures but not after NES, such elevations may not be seen following frontal lobe seizures, simple partial seizures, or simple epilepsy. In addition, elevated prolactin levels may be seen in patients experiencing stress or in those taking antipsychotic medications.

c. *Serum creatine kinase (CK)* levels are not routinely indicated in patients with NES. While serum CK may be elevated following generalized tonic clonic seizures, the same finding may occur in some patients with NES.

d. *Neuropsychological testing* is not routinely indicated. Although the Minnesota Multiphasic Personality Inventory (MMPI) may reveal psychopathology in many patients with NES, this finding is not diagnostic.

e. *Structural brain imaging* is not routinely indicated in patients with NES, as structural brain changes may be seen in a sizable proportion of such patients, as well as in those with other somatoform disorders.

f. *Metabolic brain imaging (single photon emission computed tomography [SPECT], positron emission tomography [PET], functional magnetic resonance imaging [fMRI])* is not routinely indicated, as a small number of patients with NES may demonstrate findings (hypoperfusion) typical of patients with epilepsy.

B. **Treatment**

1. Identify all medical and neuropsychiatric comorbidities, and ensure that all such conditions are optimally treated. The presence of mood or anxiety disorders should prompt treatment of such disorders as described in Chapters 5 and 6. The clinician should focus particularly on minimizing drug–drug interactions in patients receiving anticonvulsant medications.

2. Coordinate the care with other clinicians (neurologists, psychiatrists, therapists, etc.). This is critical to convey a consistent

message to the individual about diagnostic and treatment recommendations across what is often a complex array of care
providers. It is often helpful to facilitate a "team meeting" to
avoid splitting amongst the different providers.

3. Explain NES and conversion disorder to the patient and family
in a manner that educates, reduces shame, promotes understanding, and motivates the patient to undertake treatment.
When first discussing the diagnosis, it is helpful to explain why
symptoms do not fit into those of a recognizable disorder. This
information should be presented as "good news"—no progressive neurodegenerative condition or life-threatening disorder
has been found after thorough evaluation. It is helpful to tell the
patient that the medical professionals involved do not think the
patient is "crazy" and that these symptoms occur in many individuals. Assure the patient that these symptoms can get better
with time, although they may not resolve entirely in the near
future and may worsen at times, especially if a situation is
stressful. It is important to emphasize that that patient will not
be abandoned and that ongoing visits for care of the condition
will continue.

4. Explore with the patient the causes of the NES. Possible stressors
include anger at employers or family members, attempts to
obtain relief from a problematic situation, gain of support and
attention from others. As was discussed in the preceding text, a
clear precipitating event or extreme stressor will not be found
in all cases. Even when a particular event or situation appears
to be linked to NES, this identification usually does not resolve
the NES symptoms.

5. Provide psychotherapy. Although there are no controlled treatment studies of psychotherapy for patients with NES, psychotherapy may be extremely helpful in cases where the patient
is amenable to this mode of treatment and sufficiently psychologically minded to participate. Both psychoanalysis and
cognitive behavioral therapy (CBT) have been used to treat
various psychogenic conditions.[6] CBT has been widely studied specifically for treatment of psychogenic conditions and has
been shown to be beneficial in controlled trials of hypochondriasis and somatization.[6] On the basis of the limited data available,
CBT, with its pragmatic approach and focus on current issues,
is the psychotherapy of choice for NES.

6. Understand that treatment of nonepileptic spells is extremely
challenging. Even with proper diagnosis, many patients continue to have spells and are subject to ongoing disability.[7] The
guidelines mentioned in the subsequent text outline steps in
evaluation and treatment of NES.

a. **Referrals.** Once medical and neurologic disorders have been
ruled out by the evaluations described in the preceding text,
which may include referrals to a general neurologist or internist to address complex cases, the practitioner should

consider whether a referral to an epileptologist is warranted. An epilepsy specialist can be extremely helpful in determining the etiology of spells, especially when both epileptic seizure and NES coexist. Consultation with an epileptologist is also critical in determining which cases warrant EMU admission to clarify the diagnosis.

b. **Treatment team approach.** Evidence suggests that patients with NES benefit from structured treatment programs and extended support from epilepsy centers.[7] Many of these programs integrate treatment under several disciplines, including neurology, psychiatry, psychology, and physical therapy into a team approach. More frequent office visits with the primary clinician, to help reassure the patients that they are not being abandoned, are also recommended.

c. **Evaluation and treatment of comorbid psychiatric conditions.** The patient should receive treatment for any identified axis I disorder. Major depression and many anxiety disorders occur with high frequency in patients with NES. Substance abuse may also play a role. Aggressive and early treatment of underlying psychopathology may be helpful in improving the overall quality of life and in facilitation of participation in treatment for psychogenic symptoms of various types.[8–10] Patients with axis II pathology can benefit from insight-oriented psychotherapy to specifically address personality disorders. It should be remembered that even successful treatment of comorbid psychiatric illness may not ameliorate NES.

d. **Medications.** No medications are indicated specifically for the treatment of NES; rather, antidepressants, antianxiety agents and mood stabilizers should be used to treat comorbid psychiatric conditions. Treatment of insomnia with hypnotics and panic symptoms with judicious use of benzodiazepines can help ameliorate some symptoms in the early stages of treatment; patients should be weaned off these medications when possible. Antiepileptic medications, unless they are being used to treat another psychiatric disorder, should be tapered off gradually to prevent precipitation of an epileptic seizure. It is important to stop unnecessary antiepileptic agents as their use exposes patients to a high risk of side effects.

III. SUMMARY

Patients with NES represent some of the most challenging cases seen by any practitioner. Thorough medical and neurologic evaluation is indicated in many patients to rule out an organic cause of spells. Because of the high comorbidity of other psychiatric disorders in patients with NES, evaluation for psychopathology and aggressive treatment of symptoms are important components of treatment. Consultation with an epileptologist is indicated in more complex cases, especially if concurrent epileptic seizures are suspected or if EMU admission is being considered.

A treatment team approach, used by many epilepsy centers, is the most successful treatment strategy if available. Psychotherapy, especially CBT, can be helpful in addressing psychopathology related to NES. There is no medication indicated for NES. Psychopharmacologic interventions should focus on identified psychiatric symptoms. NES do not always respond to treatment, and even with successful treatment, many patients with NES will have residual symptoms.

References
1. de Waal MW, Arnold IA, Eekhof JA, et al. Somatoform disorders in general practice: Prevalence, functional impairment and comorbidity with anxiety and depressive disorders. *Br J Psychiatry.* 2004;184:470–476.
2. Mellers JDC. The approach to patients with "non-epileptic seizures". *Postgrad Med J.* 2005;81:498–504.
3. Neimark G, Caroff SN, Stinnett JL. Medically unexplained physical symptoms. *Psychiatr Ann.* 2005;35(4):298–305.
4. Lesser RP. Psychogenic seizures. *Psychosomatics.* 1986;27:823–829.
5. Lempert T, Bauer M, Schmidt D. Syncope: A videometric analysis of 56 episodes of transient cerebral hypoxia. *Ann Neurol.* 1994;36:233–237.
6. Kroenke K, Swindle R. Cognitive-behavioral therapy for somatization and symptom syndromes: A critical review of controlled clinical trials. *Psychother Psychosom.* 2000;69(4):205–215.
7. Krumholz A. Nonepileptic seizures: Diagnosis and management. *Neurology.* 1999;53(5 Suppl 2):S76–S83.
8. O'Malley PG, Jackson JL, Santro J, et al. Antidepressant therapy for unexplained symptoms and symptom syndromes. *J Fam Pract.* 1999;48(12):980–990.
9. Reuber M, Mitchell AJ, Howlett SJ, et al. Functional symptoms in neurology: Questions and answers. *J Neurol Neurosurg Psychiatry.* 2005;76(3):307–314.
10. Stone J, Carson A, Sharpe M. Functional symptoms and signs in neurology: Assessment and diagnosis. *J Neurol Neurosurg Psychiatry.* 2005;76(Suppl 1):i2–i12.

Chapter 9

PARKINSONIAN MOVEMENT DISORDERS

Edward C. Lauterbach

I. HYPOKINESIAS: THE PARKINSONISMS

A. Classification of hypokinetic parkinsonian disorders

1. Movement disorders present as *hypokinesias* and *hyperkinesias*. *Hypokinesias* are syndromes of reduced movement and refer to parkinsonian disorders (the parkinsonisms), including Parkinson disease (PD), progressive supranuclear palsy (PSP), multiple system atrophies (MSAs), including those with parkinsonism (MSA-P), dysautonomia (MSA-A), or cerebellar features (MSA-C), corticobasal degeneration ([CBD]), and other conditions. FTDP-17 is a parkinsonism associated with frontotemporal dementia and tau mutations and is discussed in the chapter on Dementia.

2. The most common movement disorder is PD, described by Parkinson in 1817. The disorder is characterized by disturbances in motor, cognitive, and emotional function. The motor disturbances include bradykinesia, rigidity, loss of postural reflexes, and a 3 to 8 Hz resting tremor. Many patients also develop dementia or depression.

3. Parkinsonism is also observed in other conditions. *Dementia with Lewy bodies* (DLB) presents with a dementia attended by features of PD. *Normal pressure hydrocephalus* (NPH) sometimes presents with rigidity, suggesting a parkinsonian disorder. *Drug-induced movement disorders* are considered briefly in terms of diagnosis and treatment rather than comprehensively, because they do not constitute the primary focus of this chapter. The reader is referred to the text edited by Watts and Kohler for a comprehensive treatment of this subject.[1]

TABLE 9.1   Prevalence of Parkinsonian Disorders

Disorder	Prevalence per 100,000 Population
Parkinson disease	168–300
Multiple system atrophy	4.4
Progressive supranuclear palsy	2–6.4
Corticobasal degeneration	4.9–7.3

B. **Epidemiology.** Known or estimated prevalences of these disorders are shown in Table 9.1. PD is an age-related illness, with a prevalence of 60 per 100,000 between the ages of 65 to 69, 270 between 75 to 79, and 350 between 85 and 90 determined in one study. Men are more often affected with PSP than women.

C. **Etiology and pathophysiology.** PD is believed to result from degeneration of nigrostriatal tracts projecting from the dopaminergic substantia nigra pars compacta to the striatum. Although the pathophysiology is quite complex, the loss of dopamine results in excessive activation of the inhibitory ("indirect") basal ganglia pathway, reducing activation of motor cortices. The cause of the dopaminergic degeneration is not known. Typical PD is not inherited, but there are single gene mutations that cause a form of parkinsonism (e.g., PARK1 to 10 mutations, Nurr1, several mitochondria genes, tyrosine hydroxylase, etc.). Oxidant stress and toxin exposure (1-methyl-4-phenyl-1,2,3,6-tetrahydro-pyridine [MPTP] and rotenone) have also been implicated in PD pathogenesis.

The pathophysiologies of the other parkinsonisms are less well established. MSA is related to nigral and putamenal degeneration, often with at least one other site involved. MSA-P (striatonigral degeneration [SND]) is thought to result from trans-synaptic degeneration of the putamen as a consequence of nigral disease. MSA-A (Shy-Drager syndrome [SDS]) is linked to degeneration of the autonomic nervous system, and MSA-C (olivopontocerebellar atrophy [OPCA]) to olivocerebellar and pontine degeneration.

PSP is associated with widespread neuronal loss and gliosis in the nucleus basalis of Meynert, globus pallidus, subthalamic nucleus, substantia nigra, pedunculopontine nucleus, intralaminar thalamic nuclei, red nucleus, reticular formation, locus coeruleus, superior colliculus, cranial nerve nuclei III and IV, vestibular nuclei, dentate nucleus, and pons, along with midbrain and frontotemporal atrophy.

CBD is associated with neuronal loss and gliosis and Pick pathology in the substantia nigra, frontoparietal cortex, thalamus, subthalamic nucleus, and red nucleus.

DLB is described in Chapter 4, but frontotemporal cortical degeneration and Lewy bodies are prominent features.

D. **Diagnosis and differential diagnosis**

1. The diagnosis of PD is based on clinical features including bradykinesia, rigidity (also called *extrapyramidal rigidity, plastic*

rigidity, lead pipe rigidity), loss of postural reflexes, and a 3 to 8 Hz alternating resting tremor.[2] PD is generally diagnosed by the presence of at least two of these four cardinal features. *Bradykinesia* refers to slowness in movement, such as gait, but is also manifest in slowed finger taps, rapid alternating movements, and foot taps. Unlike upper motor neuron spastic rigidity, the *rigidity* encountered in PD is not associated with upper motor neuron lesions or signs (e.g., hyperreflexia). The *loss of postural reflexes* leads to falls and contributes to *en bloc* turns, festinating gait, and retropulsion and propulsion on neurologic exam. The posture is generally forward flexed (stooped), with arms slightly flexed, diminished arm swing on gait, and small shuffling steps referred to as *march en petit pas*. *Akinesia* is hesitancy or inability to initiate a movement. In more advanced cases, akinesia delaying the initiation of gait (*start hesitancy*) and *freezing* (*motor blocks*) that slows or arrests gait in narrow confined passageways can be evident. The 3 to 8 Hz *resting tremor* (more usually, 4 to 6 Hz) is most apparent when the limb is at rest and diminishes on assuming postures or with activity. Patients with PD can often temporarily suppress their tremor by moving their limb, in contrast to most other types of tremor. The tremor also displays a side-to-side quality (produced by alternating firing of agonist and antagonist musculature), whereas most other tremors have an up-and-down motion when the arms are extended (caused by simultaneous firing of agonist and antagonist musculature). PD presents *unilaterally* in most cases, although in 20% it presents bilaterally. The *facies* display diminished expression resembling flattened affect referred to as a *poker face* or *hypomimia* and the nasolabial folds are diminished. There is a staring quality, usually with reduced blinking in the untreated state. In contrast to Parkinson-plus syndromes, a relatively good response to levodopa is usually maintained throughout the illness, despite treatment complexities and complications that evolve late in the disease.

2. The chief differential involves Parkinson-plus syndromes and secondary parkinsonism (symptomatic parkinsonism). In contrast to Parkinson-plus syndromes, PD usually lacks *additional neurologic signs* and has a good *response to levodopa*. Magnetic resonance imaging (MRI) is generally unrevealing except for sometimes-apparent midbrain nigral atrophy and *I-123 beta-CIT* single photon emission computed tomography (SPECT) *imaging* shows reduced striatal dopamine uptake. In Parkinson-plus syndromes (atypical parkinsonisms), there are additional signs, which may include supranuclear gaze palsy, falls occurring within the first 3 years of illness, autonomic dysfunction, cerebellar signs, other movement disorders including dystonia or myoclonus, apraxia, alien hand sign, and so on. These can define PSP, MSAs (including those with parkinsonism [MSA-P], dysautonomia [MSA-A], or cerebellar features [MSA-C]), CBD, and other conditions. DLB presents with a dementia attended

by early visual hallucinosis, delirial cognitive fluctuations, and one or more features of PD. A problem in considering the differential diagnosis is the capacity of one disorder to sometimes share clinical features of another disorder, and less than unitary correlations between clinical and histopathologic diagnoses. Clinically diagnosed disorders often result in surprises at autopsy, with pathologic findings not infrequently indicating a disease other than the presumed clinical diagnosis. Neuroimaging can at times be helpful in distinguishing these disorders.

a.   **Multiple system atrophies.** The mean age of onset is 53 years, much earlier than PD. Hence, early age of onset and presentation with a negligible levodopa response, significant dysautonomia (97% in one series) or cerebellar signs suggest MSA, of which there are three types: SND (MSA-P), SDS (MSA-A), and olivopontocerebellar atrophy (OCPA) [MSA-C].[2,3] The diagnosis is made by looking for the features of MSA-P, MSA-A, and MSA-C occurring in any combination, with a 9-year median survival. *REM behavior disorder* ([*RBD*]; see section **IE1j**) is often seen in these patients. The absence of supranuclear gaze palsy and cognitive impairment can help exclude PSP in many cases. The putamen in MSA may be hypointense but a hyperintense lateral putamenal border on T2-weighted MRI is specific for MSA and differentiates it from PD when this radiologic sign is present.

(1)   MSA-P usually presents with bradykinesia and rigidity but, in contrast with PD, is negligibly responsive to levodopa and early autonomic dysfunction is present. Hyperreflexia, anterocollic dystonia, various types of tremors, sleep apnea with respiratory stridor, and MSA radiologic findings can further distinguish MSA-P from PD.

(2)   Signs of dysautonomia are preeminent in MSA-A (SDS) (e.g., erectile dysfunction, orthostatic hypotension, sphincter dysfunction, incontinence, and constipation), unlike in PD. The presence of central and obstructive sleep apneas, especially the latter with vocal cord stridor, can help distinguish MSA-A from PD. Cerebellar or pyramidal signs are present in at least half of the cases, in contrast with PD.

(3)   MSA-C often initially presents as an ataxia with mild parkinsonian features. In contrast to PD, upper motor neuron (Babinski sign, hyperreflexia, clonus, spastic rigidity) and cerebellar signs (ataxia, rebound, terminal kinetic tremor (intention tremor), dysdiadochokinesia) may attend parkinsonian features, sometimes with dysautonomic signs. Eventually eye signs (horizontal nystagmus, impaired upgaze and convergence, loss of the vestibulo-ocular reflex), dysarthria, dysphagia, incontinence, upper motor neuron signs, lower motor neuron signs, cerebellar and brainstem atrophy, and

pontine demyelination on MRI T2-weighted images may be evident, distinguishing MSA-C from PD.

b. **Progressive supranuclear palsy.** The mean age of onset is 63, later than MSA but earlier than PD, with a 6 to 7 year survival. Diagnostic features include an early broad-based and stiff gait with backward falls and a supranuclear gaze palsy with slow vertical saccades and difficulty looking down.[2,4] The latter two features (prominent postural instability with falls within the first year and supranuclear gaze palsy) have the best diagnostic positive predictive value. Other features include axial rigidity (greater than limb rigidity, unlike PD), nuchal dystonia (often with the neck held in extension, contrasting with neck forward flexion in PD), exaggerated nasolabial folds (contrasting with diminished nasolabial folds in PD), dysarthria, dementia, and a poor response to levodopa. Dysarthria, dysphagia, and "emotional incontinence" are other signs common in PSP, usually occurring in late PD. Speech may be characteristically hypernasal, ataxic, and low-pitched, unlike PD. MRI evidence of midbrain and frontotemporal atrophy with third ventricle dilatation is supportive of the diagnosis, contrasting with the midbrain atrophy of PD. In contrast with PD, olfaction is spared.

c. **Corticobasal degeneration.** The mean age of onset is 63, with a 6- to 7-year course, like PSP. CBD is a gradually progressive condition recognized by unilateral akinesia and rigidity responding poorly to levodopa, along with apraxia (usually ideomotor apraxia).[5,6] The early onset, levodopa response, and apraxia distinguish CBD from PD. Apraxia of some type may occur in 70% of patients with CBD. Other features include cortical reflex myoclonus, limb dystonia, alien limb sign, and occasionally, a cortical sensory loss, none of which are characteristic of PD. A marked cortical asymmetry is apparent on MRI in most cases, and atrophy of the middle one third of the corpus callosum may be present, unlike PD.

3. Other conditions sometimes presenting with parkinsonism include normopressure hydrocephalus (NPH, characterized by a magnetic apractic gait, early incontinence, occasional rigidity or paratonia, and dementia), heredodegenerative disorders (see Table 9.2), vascular (multi-infarct, Binswanger disease), infectious (e.g., postencephalitic, AIDS, subacute sclerosing panencephalitis [SSPE], prionic), drug induced, toxic (e.g., MPTP, CO, Mn, Hg, carbon disulfide, cyanide, methanol, ethanol), traumatic (e.g., pugilistic), metabolic (e.g., hepatocerebral degeneration), endocrinologic (e.g., parathyroid, hypothyroidism), neoplastic (e.g., tumor, paraneoplastic), structural (e.g., NPH, noncommunicating hydrocephalus, syringomesencephalia), degenerative (hemiatrophy-hemiparkinsonism), and psychogenic disorders (e.g., severe psychomotor retardation, catatonia, conversional). *Drug-induced parkinsonism (DIP)*

TABLE 9.2   Heredodegenerative Disorders Associated with Secondary Parkinsonism

	D	P	C	M
X-Linked Recessive				
Lubag (DYT3 X-linked dystonia-parkinsonism)	D	P		
Autosomal Dominant				
Juvenile parkinsonism	D	P		
Autosomal dominant Lewy body disease		P		
Huntington disease	D	P	C	M
Dystonia	D	P		M
Machado-Joseph disease (SCA3)	D	P	C	
Other spinocerebellar degenerations	D	P	C	M
Familial Fahr syndrome (basal ganglia calcification)	D	P	C	
Familial parkinsonisms		P		
Disinhibition-dementia-parkinsonism-amyotrophy-complex (FTDP-17)		P		
Pallido-ponto-nigral degeneration (FTDP-17)		P		
Parkinsonism-depression-weight loss-central hypoventilation (Perry disease)		P		
Gerstmann-Strausler-Scheinker disease		P		
Familial progressive subcortical gliosis		P		
Autosomal Recessive				
Wilson disease	D	P	C	M
Juvenile neuronal ceroid-lipofuscinosis (Batten disease)	D	P	C	M
Hallervorden-Spatz disease (pantothenate kinase associated neurodegeneration)	D	P	C	M
Neuroacanthocytosis	D	P	C	
Olivopontocerebellar atrophies	D	P	C	M
Hereditary hemochromatosis		P		
Hereditary ceruloplasmin deficiency		P		
Mitochondrial				
Leber disease	D	P		
Other mitochondrial encephalopathies	D	P	C	M
Other				
Fragile X permutation (CGG repeat—X-linked)		P		M
Familial amyotrophy-dementia-parkinsonism		P		
Parkinsonian—pyramidal syndrome		P		

P, parkinsonism; D, dystonia; C, chorea; M, myoclonus. Appreciation is expressed to Dr. Linda R. Adkison, PhD for her help in the correct genetic classification of these disorders and to Gail Sheffield for assistance in preparing this table.

occurs with dopamine D_2 receptor antagonists (including metoclopramide) and, less commonly, with other agents (e.g., SSRIs, reserpine). A severe reaction necessitating emergency treatment, *neuroleptic malignant syndrome* (*NMS*), can develop with these drugs, and is generally recognized by fever attended by an extrapyramidal syndrome and delirium. Classic features include fever, leukocytosis, elevated creatine phosphokinase, autonomic instability, and parkinsonian rigidity and tremor, although other types of movement disorders may also occur.

E. **Neuropsychiatric features**

1. **Parkinson disease.** Neuropsychiatric features are common in PD, the best studied among the hypokinesias.[7,8] These include disorders that comorbidly occur in PD, and some that are related to dopaminergic function (i.e., *nonmotor offs*). Among these, cognitive impairment and depressive disorders are two of the strongest determinants of quality of life in PD.

   a. **On-off, nonmotor phenomena.** Some neuropsychiatric disorders are manifestations of *off-period phenomenon*, times at which there is a loss of response to levodopa. Such *nonmotor off* symptoms can include bouts of pain, akathisia, anergia, dysphoria, depression, anxiety, and panic.

   b. **Delirium.** Delirium is usually secondary to the complications of PD (aspiration, bowel obstruction, etc.), treatment (dopaminergic agents, anticholinegics, amantadine, deep brain stimulation [DBS], etc.), or withdrawal of dopaminergic agent (including a syndrome resembling NMS) or amantadine. Postoperative delirium can occur after pallidotomy or implantation of DBS leads.

   c. **Personality changes.** Apathy occurs in over 10% of patients with PD. Apathy and disinhibition are occasional complications of posteroventral pallidotomy and bilateral subthalamic DBS. The latter procedure has been associated with personality changes in one third of patients, including impulsivity, aggression, disinhibition, emotional hyperreactivity, and pathologic crying.

   d. **Dementia.** Dementia occurs in almost 30% of all patients with PD, but the risk grows with disease duration, among other factors, and prevalences of up to 80% have been reported in some longitudinal series. The dementia of PD is characterized by a progressive dysexecutive syndrome with attentional deficits and fluctuating cognition. Dementia in PD can therefore resemble DLB (see DLB in subsequent text) or Alzheimer disease (AD), and is called *PD dementia* (PDD) if the patient had diagnosable PD before the onset of DLB features, and DLB if DLB features preceded diagnosable PD. PDD is an important determinant of caregiver distress, quality of life, nursing home placement, and mortality. Mini-Mental State Examination (MMSE) scores decline about two points per year, not dissimilar to AD. Pathologic findings are usually consistent with DLB or AD. *Cognitive impairments* have been observed after pallidotomy, including attentional, executive, working memory, and fluency difficulties, and after subthalamic nucleus DBS, including dysexecution.

   e. **Psychosis.** Psychosis is a major determinant of quality of life, caregiver burden, and nursing home placement, occurring in approximately half the patients. Psychosis occurs more

frequently with direct dopamine agonists than with levodopa. Visual hallucinations and paranoia are more common than auditory hallucinations and delusions. Psychosis
and thought disorder sometimes have been encountered as
a complication of subthalamic nucleus DBS.

f. **Mania.** Mania is occasionally encountered and may be
a complication of treatment with dopaminergic agents,
anticholinergics, pallidotomy, and bilateral subthalamic
nucleus DBS.

g. **Depression.** Depression is a major determinant of quality
of life, mortality, caregiver burden, and spousal depression. Depressive disorders occur in approximately half the
patients, including major depression, atypical depression,
and dysthymia. Depression can also present as a prodrome
before the onset of PD. Major depression, occurring in approximately 20% of patients with PD, is characterized by
prominent anxiety and less proclivity toward self-punitive
ideation than in primary major depression. Suicide attempts
are infrequent, but may be quite common in patients undergoing subthalamic DBS. Depression is sometimes seen
as a complication of pallidotomy and DBS.

h. **Anxiety.** Anxiety disorders have been observed in up to 40%
of patients with PD, with panic disorder in 25% and panic
attacks in 32%. Simple phobia has also been seen in 36% of
patients with PD. Anxiety has occasionally been observed
as a complication of bilateral subthalamic nucleus DBS.

i. **Substance abuse.** Substance abuse is rare in PD, but occasionally patients abuse dopaminergic agents due to sedative,
analgesic, and euphoric effects. *Hedonistic homeostatic dysregulation* (HHD) involves dopaminergic therapy abuse and
dependence despite complications (e.g., severe dyskinesias,
mania, psychosis), seen especially in men and early onset
PD. Withdrawal dysphoria may attend dose reductions
to a more appropriate dose. *Dopamine dysregulation syndrome* involves HHD with behavioral complications such
as paraphilias, punding, and gambling. Occasionally, substance abuse has been reported as a complication of bilateral
subthalamic nucleus DBS.

j. **Sleep disorders.** These are quite common, reported in up to
94% of patients, and include frequent awakenings, excessive daytime sleepiness, nightmares, nocturnal cramps, and
RBD, which involves acting out one's dreams during rapid
eye movement (REM) sleep, indicating a disruption of the
usual mechanism that normally produces atonia while in
this stage of sleep

(1) **Insomnia.** Insomnia is common and related to dopaminergic agents, nocturnal PD motor symptoms, and
depression. PD nocturnal motor symptoms include
immobility, rest tremor, eye blinking, dyskinesias, periodic and nonperiodic limb movements in sleep, restless

legs syndrome, fragmentary myoclonus, and respiratory dysfunction in sleep.

(2) **Parasomnias.** Parasomnias include RBD, vivid dreams, and psychosis. RBD may occur in one third of patients. Injury can result from RBD in approximately 70% of cases. RBD may be more common in patients with Park2 mutation. Nightmares correlate with levodopa dosage.

(3) **Excessive daytime somnolence.** Excessive daytime somnolence (EDS) occurs in at least 15% to 47% of patients with PD and is variably associated with dopaminergic agents.

(4) Sleep attacks constitute a distinct problem in PD, with 43% of patients reporting sudden onsets of sleep, associated with sleep disturbances and dopamine agonists, especially nonergoline agonists (e.g., ropinirole, pramipexole).

k. **Sexual disorders.** Most patients with PD have sexual disorders, although these are far less robust than in MSA-A. These include low sexual desire and arousal difficulties in most patients, dysorgasmia, and premature ejaculation.

(1) **Paraphilias.** Dopamine agonist–related paraphilias have been reported in PD, including reversible transvestic fetishism. Penile erections and hypersexuality have also been reported.

2. **Dementia with Lewy bodies.** This is the second most common progressive dementia of old age after AD, usually attended by parkinsonism, well-formed visual hallucinations, and fluctuations in cognition, vigilance, and attention.[9] Other symptoms can include RBD and intolerance of neuroleptics due to extrapyramidal side effects, and a proclivity to syncope and falls. The usual age of onset of DLB is 60 to 68 years of age, the average duration of illness is 6 to 7 years, and men are affected more often than women. DLB diagnostic criteria provide a mean sensitivity of only 49% with a mean specificity of 92%[3] and better criteria are needed. Working memory and visuospatial impairments, visual hallucinations, depression, apathy, and anxiety are early indicators of DLB.

a. **Dementia.** DLB has been characterized as a visual-perceptual and attentional-executive dementia. Pathologic findings include cortical Lewy bodies and nigral degeneration. Cases of DLB with more significant Lewy body pathology present with classical DLB symptoms whereas those with more extensive neurofibrillary tangles tend toward an AD presentation.

b. **Psychosis.** The most common symptoms include auditory and visual hallucinations and paranoid and phantom boarder delusions (the delusion that someone is living in the house that does not belong there). Visual hallucinations may be well formed.

     c. **Depression.** Depression occurs in DLB, but its prevalence and features have not been clarified.

     d. **Sleep disorders.** RBD is common. Sleep disturbances and EDS are more common than in AD.

     e. **Other neuropsychiatric disorders.** These are yet to be clarified in DLB.[10]

3. **Multiple system atrophies.** [10] MSA-P (SND) has been associated with mild memory and frontal (executive, attention, verbal fluency) impairments and frontal lobe atrophy, and sleep apnea is common. MSA-A (SDS) has occasionally been associated with delirium with hallucinations (in the context of the ergot lisuride), emotional lability, depression, RBD, and sleep apneas, although impotence may constitute a presenting sign in one third of patients and eventually is almost ubiquitous. MSA-C (OPCA) has been linked to dementia, auditory hallucinations, paranoia, depression, RBD, and sleep apnea.[10]

4. **Progressive supranuclear palsy.** [10] *Dementia* is apparent in approximately half the patients, characterized by a frontal subcortical dementia with executive impairment, motor slowing, and impaired retrieval and procedural learning. Frontal release signs may be apparent, along with reduced verbal fluency and impaired imitation and utilization behavior. *Personality changes* include apathy, irritability, disinhibition, and labile mood and may be evident early in the disease. *Pseudobulbar affect* can be present in one third of patients, regardless of dementia. Studies are inconclusive as to whether psychosis, depression, or anxiety are features of PSP, but bipolar disorder has not been associated with the disease. *Insomnia* is extremely common and can be severe, especially late in the illness.

5. **Corticobasal degeneration.** [10] *Frontal cognitive impairment* occurs early in the disease, including attentional, executive, visuospatial, and semantic memory difficulties. Right parietal cortical involvement is associated with visuospatial dysfunction, constructional impairment, and dressing apraxia. Dyscalculia is common, and aphasia may occur in approximately one fifth of patients, often a transcortical motor aphasia with left hemispheric involvement. *Personality changes* include aggressive behavior, irritability, disinhibition, and Kluver-Bucy syndrome. Apathy has been seen in 40%. Dysphoric mood or depression is common and, in one study, helped differentiate CBD from PSP. Among *sleep disorders*, there have been single case reports of RBD and periodic leg movements in sleep.

F. **Treatment**

1. Look for typical Parkinson disease diagnostic features.

     a. Treatment in *early PD* is generally reserved until symptoms become problematic and involves the initiation of *levodopa* (levodopa/carbidopa [Sinemet, Madopar]) or *direct dopamine agonists*, including nonergot (ropinirole [Requip], pramipexole [Mirapex]) and ergot (bromocriptine [Parlodel], pergolide [Permax]).[11,12] *Anticholinergics* have been

used for PD presenting with prominent tremor, but may impair cognition. Some clinicians opt to use selegeline 5 mg b.i.d. or amantadine 100 mg b.i.d. (or, if other medical illnesses are present, starting at 100 mg q AM during the first week, then increasing to 100 mg b.i.d.) in early disease, but their antiparkinsonian effects are only mild and their heuristic neuroprotective properties are unproven.[11] *Selegeline should not be given to patients taking antidepressants.* Levodopa is generally the most effective agent once PD has progressed to moderate stages but has a higher risk of dyskinesia than dopamine agonists.[11] Carbidopa/levodopa is usually begun at 1/2 of a 25/100 mg pill t.i.d. during the first week and then advanced to 25/100 t.i.d. the second week. Thereafter, if needed, the dose may be escalated to 1/2 of 25/250 t.i.d. in the third week and then to 25/250 t.i.d. Usually, doses exceeding 25/250 q.i.d. are excessive in early disease. Direct acting dopamine agonists have their own unique titration schedules. For example, pramipexole is generally started at 0.125 mg t.i.d. in the first week and advanced to 0.25 mg t.i.d. the second week and advanced by 0.25 mg t.i.d. each week thereafter until a significant effect occurs. An average dose is 0.5 mg t.i.d. Ropinirole is begun at 0.25 mg t.i.d. in the first week and increased by 0.25 mg t.i.d. each week thereafter. Response generally occurs between 3 and 9 mg per day.

   b.   A full discussion of more advanced treatment approaches is beyond the scope of this manual, but a brief overview of principles follows. In more *advanced PD*, patients treated with levodopa often develop the *on-off syndrome* several years into treatment, characterized by a temporary sudden loss of response to the drug lasting minutes to hours before a sudden return of response. On-off is thought to be related to pharmacodynamic perturbations involving dopamine receptors. Although levodopa is associated with *end-of-dose wearing-off* (plasma trough at the end of a dose associated with an exacerbation of PD signs immediately before the onset of the next dose) and on-off phenomena, dopamine agonists carry a greater proclivity to *excessive daytime sleepiness, orthostatic hypotension, nausea, and edema.* Dopamine agonists, however, have a longer duration of action than levodopa and can minimize plasma peaks and troughs, thereby attenuating *dyskinesia* and reducing off-time, respectively. The end-of-dose wearing-off phenomenon is treated by increasing the dose of levodopa, or if dyskinesias ensue, giving smaller doses more frequently throughout the day; alternatively, a dopamine agonist is added, reducing troughs. There are reports of improvement in dyskinesia with buspirone (double-blind, crossover study), mirtazapine, fluoxetine, trazodone, and desipramine, but the conventional first-line treatment is to adjust the dopaminergic agent. Isolated *dyskinesia* is usually improved by reducing the corresponding dose; however, *dystonia* may occur at times during *peaking* (I-D-I [improvement-dystonia-improvement] pattern) or *troughing* (D-I-D pattern) and may therefore require either a dopamine agonist or a controlled-release preparation of levodopa to reduce plasma level fluctuations. *Controlled release levodopa* preparations (e.g., Sinemet CR) can reduce the amplitude of peaks and troughs. Evidence of delayed clinical progression, determined by slower advance to defined clinical endpoints than in patients who are placebo treated, has been documented with both levodopa and dopamine agonists, but this does not necessarily equate to true disease modification in a neuroprotective sense. Moreover, several functional imaging studies have found a faster rate of decline of presynaptic dopaminergic terminals in the striatum of patients treated with levodopa in comparison to either placebo or dopamine agonist. The use of *catechol-o-methyl-transferase (COMT) inhibitors* such as entacapone (Comtan) and tolcapone (Tasmar) can extend the life of a dose of levodopa as long as half an hour. For example, entacapone 200 mg can be added to each carbidopa/levodopa dose, but should not exceed 1,600 mg per day. Various combinations of these agents can therefore be applied to the PD patient with the aim of achieving optimal motility and function without excessive dyskinesia, end-of-dose wearing-off effects, and on-off phenomena. An agent that combines a controlled-release preparation of levodopa with entacapone is Stalevo. *Orthostatic hypotension* with levodopa and dopamine agonists can lead to falls, and patients should be monitored for this condition. Medication-refractory PD can be referred for subthalamic nucleus DBS. Older procedures include internal globus pallidus DBS and posteroventral pallidotomy. Some of the problems seen in Parkinson-plus syndromes (e.g., urinary, respiratory) occasionally develop in PD and can be treated in the same way as described below. Constipation is a not infrequent problem in PD. Orthostatic hypotension can be managed by dose reduction when possible and by conventional treatments (support hose, salt tablets, midodrine, fludrocortisone).

2. *Parkinson-Plus Syndromes* may be variably responsive to levodopa and deserve a trial. Sometimes there is a suitable initial response before loss of response. Dyskinesias will sometimes occur with levodopa or dopamine agonists despite a lack of therapeutic response.
   a. Dementia with Lewy bodies. See section **IF6**.
   b. Multiple system atrophies. In MSA-A, urinary incontinence has been treated with intermittent catheterization, anticholinergics, or desmopressin nasal spray. Support hose,

leg crossing, salt tablets, midodrine, and fludrocortisone can be used to manage orthostatic hypotension. In men with benign prostatic hypertrophy (BPH), tamsulosin may be preferred. Sildenafil has been used for erectile dysfunction, but it can precipitate or aggravate orthostatic hypotension in the patient with MSA and must be used with caution. Continuous positive airway pressure (CPAP) and tracheostomy have been used for obstructive apnea and laryngeal stridor.

   c. Progressive supranuclear palsy. Once the response to levodopa and dopamine agonists is lost, noradrenergic agents (e.g., idazoxan) have been found to improve motor function in progressive supranuclear palsy.

   d. Corticobasal degeneration. Myoclonus has been improved with clonazepam, and painful rigidity and dystonia sometimes responds to botulinum toxin in corticobasal degeneration.

   e. FTDP-17. There are no specific treatments for the FTD or the parkinsonism in FTDP-17, although there may be an initial response to levodopa.

  3. In *drug-induced parkinsonism*, the principle is to reduce or discontinue the offending agent. Residual DIP, particularly that engendered by antipsychotics, is generally treated by adding an anticholinergic, such as benztropine 0.5 to 2 mg PO b.i.d. NMS generally necessitates discontinuation of the offending agent and supportive management (rehydration, antipyretic, etc.). Some have advocated the use of anticholinergics to attempt reversal of rigidity rather than starting dantrolene; however, this might best be reserved for patients with negligible delirium. When fevers exceed 100°F, the patient should be transferred to the intensive care unit for close monitoring. Cooling blankets and other measures can be employed, and the administration of dantrolene (1 mg per kg by IV push and advancing the dose until symptoms resolve, usually before 10 mg per kg) or dopamine agonist should be considered to ameliorate the NMS process.

  4. In *nonmotor off neuropsychiatric features* it is advisable to determine if the pattern of the symptoms corresponds to off-periods, in which case the symptoms may be preempted by minimizing these periods (see section IF1b). If the symptoms correspond to wearing-off phenomenon, then increasing the dose or dosing frequency of levodopa may obviate the problem. If the symptoms result from true on-off phenomenon, then switching levodopa to a dopamine agonist, or adding a dopamine agonist to the regimen, may ameliorate the symptoms. Continuous duodenal levodopa infusion has been used for on-off fluctuations in extreme cases.

  5. **Neuropsychiatric disorders in PD.**[8] The treatment of these conditions in PD[10] depends on the neuropsychiatric disorder diagnosed. Psychotropics are administered as described elsewhere in this volume, and it is generally wise to employ time-honored

geropsychiatric principles, such as starting with half the dose and advancing the dose more slowly than in adults under the age of 65.

a. **Delirium.** The treatment of delirium is to find the etiologic cause (see section **IE1b**), treat it, provide supportive care (fluids, antipyretics, etc.), and, if needed, provide symptomatic treatment. The use of lorazepam and atypical antipsychotics for delirial behavior in PD has not been studied, so an extremely cautious approach is recommended before adding these agents, which can produce a delirium of their own accord. As of this writing, there are no reports of outcome in treating patients with lorazepam or antipsychotics in the specific context of delirium in PD. In the event of an *NMS-like syndrome*, the usual supportive treatment of the patients with NMS should be employed (see section **IF3**) and, assuming a correct diagnosis, the dopaminergic agent should be escalated back to previous levels, with a maintenance, or at least a much more gradual reduction, of dose once the patient has recovered.

b. **Personality change.** Apathy has been associated with low testosterone levels in PD. Apathy has been improved with bilateral subthalamic nucleus DBS. Other approaches to treating apathy, although not necessarily validated in PD, include dopamine agonists, amantadine, and cholinesterase inhibitors.

c. **Dementia.** Improvements in executive function have been reported with levodopa, fluoxetine, repetitive transcranial magnetic stimulation, and adjustment of stimulus parameters in the context of subthalamic nucleus DBS. Several double blind, placebo-controlled studies of donepezil and rivastigmine have demonstrated significant improvements in cognition without worsening of PD signs. Rivastigmine has specifically been associated with improvements in attention, verbal fluency, behaviors associated with dementia, and activities of daily living, but also with side effects including nausea, vomiting, and tremor.

d. **Psychosis.** In trying to minimize psychosis, drugs should be reduced according to a risk-to-benefit ratio, seeking to first minimize or eliminate anticholinergics, then selegiline, then dopamine agonists, then amantadine, then COMT inhibitors, then levodopa as clinical conditions permit, and then adding an antipsychotic. Delirial etiologies should also be excluded. Atypical antipsychotics should be used with vigilance for neuroleptic sensitivity reactions, occurring in one fourth of patients. Clozapine at doses of up to 50 mg per day is a well-established efficacious treatment, although the dose is best started at 12.5 mg per day and gradually titrated upward. The usual precautions regarding agranulocytosis are observed. Usually well tolerated, patients should be monitored for motor worsening. Sedation, increased sial-orrhea, and dizziness are other concerns. Quetiapine does not have established efficacy in PD, and other atypicals are likely more inclined to exacerbate PD signs.

e. **Depression.** Selegeline should be discontinued before attempting antidepressant treatment to avoid fatal reactions and serotonin syndrome. Nortriptyline demonstrated efficacy in a single double-blind, placebo-controlled trial, although orthostatic hypotension can be a concern. Well-controlled data, although limited, suggest the utility of amitriptyline with the same concern. Open label data suggest efficacy for SSRIs with only occasional worsening of PD signs. Antidepressant effects and efficacy against anhedonia have been demonstrated for pramipexole in patients with PD. An open trial of ECT showed improvements in mood after seven treatments and motor symptoms after two treatments, but delirium and other complications can occur, so some have recommended that ECT be given only once or twice a week to the patient with PD. A single case report indicated the safety and efficacy of ECT in a patient undergoing bilateral subthalamic DBS. A rater blind study indicated that repetitive transcranial magnetic stimulation was as effective as fluoxetine, but with faster cognitive improvement and less motor slowing in the stimulated group.

f. **Anxiety.** There are few data to guide treatment. Bromazepam, a benzodiazepine, was proved effective for anxiety in PD in a double-blind placebo-controlled study. Other benzodiazepines have been used in the clinical arena for anxiety in PD, but the usual caveats regarding cognition, gait, falls, and so on, should be carefully considered before prescribing these agents. Buspirone has only demonstrated improvements in dyskinesia to date.

g. **Sleep disorders.** Insomnia can be treated by lowering dopaminergic or anticholinergic agents when these drugs are culpable, increasing dopaminergic agents when PD symptoms lead to insomnia, adding an antidepressant when depression is the cause, instructing the patient in sleep hygiene, or prescribing a short half-lived hypnotic agent. Management of RBD involves counseling about taking preventive safety measures and the use of clonazepam or melatonin 1 to 3 mg PO h.s. When EDS persists and dopamine agonists cannot be reduced, several double blind, placebo-controlled, crossover studies have demonstrated the efficacy of modafinil 200 mg PO q AM. Patients should be warned in regard to sleep attacks while driving when dopaminergic agents are prescribed, especially with ropinirole and pramipexole.

h. **Sexual disorders.** Sildenafil has improved desire, erections, and orgasm for erectile dysfunction in men with PD, but can exacerbate hypotension.

    i.   **Paraphilias.** A reduction in dopaminergic dose may be helpful, when possible. Clozapine (see section **IF5d**) has been found to be useful for dopaminergic-induced paraphilias in PD.

    j.   **Other psychiatric disorders.** There are no data to guide treatment.

6.   **Neuropsychiatric disorders in dementia with Lewy bodies.**[9,10]

    a.   **Dementia.** Cholinesterase inhibitors have produced varying results. Tacrine led to deterioration in dementia and PD motor status. Rivastigmine did not improve MMSE scores but did improve attention, working memory, and episodic memory.

    b.   **Personality change.** Rivastigmine has led to improvement in apathy.

    c.   **Psychosis.** Delusions, hallucinations, and agitation have been reported to improve with rivastigmine. Quetiapine has improved psychosis and behavior in DLB, but has produced worsened PD signs and orthostatic hypotension in 30%. Olanzapine at 5 mg per day improved hallucinations and delusions but was less effective at higher doses. *Extreme caution should be used if antipsychotics are given in DLB because of reports in the literature of fatal neuroleptic intolerance.*

    d.   **Sleep disturbances.** Rivastigmine has been reported as useful for DLB sleep disturbances.

    e.   **Other neuropsychiatric disorders.** There are no data to inform treatment.

7.   **Neuropsychiatric disorders in multiple system atrophies**[10] These disorders have been understudied.

    a.   No information is available on MSA-P (SND).

    b.   In MSA-A (SDS) even mild obstructive sleep apnea can lead to sudden death and prophylactic tracheostomy has been recommended in the literature. *Sildenafil can significantly exacerbate hypotension in patients with MSA.*

    c.   There is a case report of treatment resistant depression in MSA-C responding to clozapine (see section **IF5d** for dosing) in a single patient.

8.   **Neuropsychiatric disorders in progressive supranuclear palsy.** citeref9.10 Controlled trials of cholinesterase inhibitors (donepezil) in PSP dementia have not yielded improvement, except on the Double Memory Test, and activities of daily living and motor scores have actually worsened. There are no other data to guide treatment.

9.   **Neuropsychiatric disorders in corticobasal degeneration.** [10] There is essentially no data to inform treatment. In a single patient, ideomotor and dressing apraxias improved with amantadine but not with levodopa.

References

1.   Watts RL, Koller WC, eds. *Movement disorders: Neurologic principles and practice,* 2nd ed. New York: McGraw-Hill, 2004:1–994.

2. Litvan J, Bhatia KP, Burn DJ, et al. SIC Task Force appraisal of clinical diagnostic criteria for Parkinsonian disorders. *Mov Disord.* 2003;18:467–486.
3. Gilman S, Low PA, Quinn N, et al. Consensus statement on the diagnosis of multiple system atrophy. *J Auton Nerv Syst.* 1998;74:189–192.
4. Kowalska A, Jamrozik Z, Kwiecinski H. Progressive supra-nuclear palsy–parkinsonian disorder with tau pathology. *Folia Neuropathol.* 2004;42:119–123.
5. Mahapatra RK, Edwards MJ, Schott JM, et al. Corticobasal degeneration. *Lancet Neurol.* 2004;3:736–743.
6. Dickson DW, Bergeron C, Chin SS, et al. Office of Rare Diseases neuropathologic criteria for corticobasal degeneration. *J Neuropathol Exp Neurol.* 2002;61:935–946.
7. Lauterbach EC. The neuropsychiatry of Parkinson's disease. *Minerva Med.* 2005;96:155–173.
8. Lauterbach EC, Freeman A, Vogel RL. Differential DSM-III psychiatric disorder prevalence profiles in dystonia and Parkinson disease. *J Neuropsychiatry Clin Neurosci.* 2004;16:29–36.
9. McKeith IG, Galasko D, Kosaka K, et al. Consensus guidelines for the clinical and pathologic diagnosis of dementia with Lewy bodies (DLB): Report of the consortium on DLB international workshop. *Neurology.* 1996;47:1113–1124.
10. Lauterbach EC. The neuropsychiatry of Parkinson's disease and related disorders. *Psychiatr Clin North Am.* 2004;27: 801–825.
11. Miyasaki JM, Martin W, Suchowersky O, et al. Practice parameter: Initiation of treatment for Parkinson's disease: An evidence-based review: Report of the Quality Standards Subcommittee of the American Academy of Neurology. *Neurology.* 2002;58:11–17.
12. Bhatia K, Brooks DJ, Burn DJ, et al. Updated guidelines for the management of Parkinson's disease. *Hosp Med.* 2001;62:456–470.

Chapter 10

HYPERKINETIC MOVEMENT DISORDERS

Edward C. Lauterbach

I. HYPERKINETIC MOVEMENT DISORDERS

A. **Classification of hyperkinetic movement disorders**
1. *Hyperkinetic movement disorders* (*hyperkinesias, hyperkinetic dyskinesias*) are characterized by excessive, unwanted, involuntary movements, and are classified according to their phenomenology. The *form* of the movement can assist in diagnosis and may be rhythmic or arrhythmic, generalized or focal, unilateral or bilateral, fast or slow, brief or sustained, repetitive or nonrepetitive, small or large in amplitude, proximal or distal, complex or simple, suppressible or nonsuppressible, positional or nonpositional, synchronous or asynchronous, paroxysmal or nonparoxysmal, and occurring while awake or asleep. Some movement disorders appear to be bizarre and are sometimes misdiagnosed as psychiatric disorders, for example, dystonia. Although an overgeneralization, Table 10.1 indicates candidate movement disorders based on their properties.
2. Hyperkinetic movement *forms* include *rhythmic* movements, which generally represent tremor, whereas most other movement disorders are nonrhythmic. *Generalized* movements usually suggest chorea, childhood-onset dystonia, myoclonus, tics, and akathisia, whereas more *focal* movements are typical of adult-onset dystonia and some types of myoclonus, tics, tremors, and hemifacial spasm (HFS). *Unilateral* movements may indicate parkinsonian tremor, secondary dystonia, or chorea due to a focal lesion, hemiballismus, and HFS. Most hyperkinesias

TABLE 10.1   Diagnosis of Hyperkinesias by Movement Form

Form of Movement	Movement Disorders
Rhythmic	Tremors of various types, some myoclonias
Nonrhythmic	Most other movement disorders
Generalized	Chorea, childhood-onset dystonia, tics, akathisia, some myoclonias
Focal	Adult-onset dystonia, tics, hemifacial spasm, task-specific tremors, some myoclonias
Unilateral	Most parkinsonian tremors, dystonias and tremors due to focal brain lesions, hemiballismus, hemifacial spasm
Bilateral	Most other movement disorders
Slow, sustained movements	Most dystonias, some tics
Fast, brief movements	Most other movement disorders
Repetitive	Dystonia, myoclonus, tics, akathisia, hemifacial spasm, tremor
Nonrepetitive	Chorea
Large amplitude	Ballismus, severe akathisia, some choreas, dystonias, and tics
Small amplitude	Chorea, dystonia, myoclonus, tremor, hemifacial spasm
Proximal movements	Ballismus, some dystonias
Distal movements	Tremor, chorea
Complex movements	Complex tics, dystonia
Simple movements	Chorea, myoclonus, simple tics, tremor
Suppressible	Tics, other movements to limited degrees
Nonsuppressible	Most other movement disorders
Positional	Some tremors, myoclonus, tics, and dystonia
Nonpositional	Most other movement disorders
Synchronous	Some myoclonias, tremor
Asynchronous	Some myoclonias, most other movement disorders

are fast and of brief duration, but *slow and sustained* movements can betray dystonia and some forms of tics. *Repetitive* movements may represent dystonia, myoclonus, tics, akathisia, HFS and, of course, tremor, but *nonrepetitive* movements are typical of chorea. *Large amplitude* violent movements signal ballismus, severe akathisia, and less commonly dystonia, tics, and severe chorea, whereas *small amplitude* movements are more typical of chorea, dystonia, myoclonus, tremor, and HFS. *Proximal* joint excursions usually indicate ballismus and sometimes dystonia, whereas *distal* movements usually suggest chorea and tremor. *Complex* movements may signal complex tics or dystonia, whereas *simple* movements suggest chorea, myoclonus, simple tics, and tremor. *Suppressible* movements are generally tics, but other movements may be minimally suppressible, especially in the context of "trick" maneuvers that patients with dystonia and tremor acquire. Some movements such as tremor, myoclonus, and dystonia may be *positional* and myoclonus can be *synchronous or asynchronous.*

3. Table 10.2 lists the prevalences of the more common hyperkinesias.

4. The *etiologies* of movement disorders are beyond the scope of this manual. Aside from multiple mutations in many of the primary movement disorders, there are multiple etiologies (including genetic) of secondary movement disorders. The genetics of movement disorders are evolving so rapidly that texts are outdated before they are even printed. A search of contemporary journals is the only way to track the panoply of mutations associated with certain movement disorders. Although movement disorders are usually not purely localizable to *lesions* of a single structure, chorea is most often associated with caudate, dystonia with putamen, and ballismus with subthalamic nucleus lesions.

5. Although the pathophysiologies are significantly complex, the rudiments are provided for each disorder in the subsequent text.

TABLE 10.2   Prevalence of Hyperkinetic Movement Disorders

Disorder	Prevalence per 100,000 Population
Huntington disease	4.1−7.5
Primary torsion dystonia	25−33
Blepharospasm	13.3
Myoclonus	8.6
Tourette syndrome	29−2,990
Essential tremor	415
Hemifacial spasm	7.4−14.5
Restless legs syndrome	9,800 (after the age of 65)

In contrast to Parkinson disease, where there is reduced activation of the supplementary motor cortex (SMA), it is believed
that the cortex is overactivated in the hyperkinesias.

6. Hyperkinesias include other less common dyskinesias that are
outside the scope of this manual and are considered elsewhere.[1]

B. Tremor

1. *Tremors* are rhythmically repetitive movements.

2. The pathophysiology of tremors has been linked to the thalamic
nucleus ventralis intermedius as a final common pathway, with
inputs from the globus pallidus and cerebellum.

3. Tremors are *classified* by whether their peak amplitude occurs
when the affected limb is in repose, or during activity (see
Table 10.3). Those most apparent in repose and attenuating with
activity are *resting tremors*, generally involving the hand in a
side-to-side alternating movement of 4 to 6 Hz. *Rabbit tremor* is
a focal perioral rest tremor resembling the rapid sniffing movements of a rabbit. Most tremors, however, reach peak amplitude
with activity and are further classified by the type of activity
that provokes maximal amplitude. Those activating only with
specific limb postures, such as sustention of the arms, are *postural tremors* (also called *positional tremors*). *Orthostatic tremor* is

TABLE 10.3   Diagnostic Characteristics of Tremors

Tremor	Description
Resting tremor	4–6 Hz, peak amplitude at rest, attenuates with movement, typical of Parkinson disease and antipsychotics, often apparent in index fingers, an *alternating* tremor with side-to-side movement of hand; termed *rabbit tremor* when confined to perioral musculature
Action–postural tremor	8–12 Hz (but some variants), peak amplitude on arm sustention and limb movement, typical of most tremors including lithium and other drug-induced tremors, attenuates at rest, a *co-contracting* tremor with up-and-down movement of the hand; *orthostatic tremor* is 12–20 Hz in legs on standing, and *essential tremor* is familial, often involving hands, head, and voice
Terminal kinetic tremor	Tremor evident on finger-to-nose examination when approaching target, attenuates at rest and in midrange of movement, typical of cerebellar systems disease
Rubral tremor	Combined features of resting, action–postural, and terminal-kinetic tremors, typical of midbrain lesions in vicinity of red nucleus (nucleus ruber)
Task-specific tremor	A tremor with properties of dystonia, usually occurring in a specific muscle group only during specific actions, such as in musicians playing only certain notes or chords
Physiologic tremor	A tremor with action–postural properties present in normal individuals apparent only during periods of stress

a postural tremor of the legs and trunk of 12 to 20 Hz evident when the patient is standing. Tremors that activate consistently throughout the range of a movement, such as the finger-to-nose examination, are *action tremors*, often presenting as an up-and-down movement of the distal fingers of 8 to 12 Hz when the arms are extended and further intensifying with action. *Essential tremor* is an autosomal dominant action–postural tremor. Tremors reaching peak amplitude only at the end of the movement, such as when nearing the target finger or nose, constitute *terminal kinetic tremor* (also called *intention tremor* or *cerebellar intention tremor*). Tremors occurring only during selective tasks, such as when playing only certain notes on a musical instrument represent focal *task-specific tremor*. *Physiologic tremor* is an action–postural tremor evident in normal individuals and is brought out by conditions of stress, anxiety, or caffeine. *Rubral tremor* usually combines the features of resting, postural, action, and terminal kinetic tremors. On rare occasions, rhythmic myoclonus and polyminimyoclonus involving distal fingers occur and can be mistaken for tremor.

4. There are many etiologies of various tremors.[1] *Resting* and *rabbit tremors* are seen in Parkinson disease (see Chapter 10) and in drug-induced parkinsonism related to dopamine D_2 receptor antagonist drugs. Most tremors are *action–postural tremors* and there are many causes of these (e.g., essential tremor, toxins, lithium, valproate, β agonists, stimulants, antihistamines, hypoglycemia, thyrotoxicosis, pheochromocytoma, steroids, cyclosporin, interferon, other movement disorders, amyotrophic lateral sclerosis [ALS], and peripheral injury). *Essential tremor* is familial and has been linked to ETM and FET1 mutations. *Terminal kinetic (intention) tremor* generally occurs with cerebellar systems disease. *Task-specific tremor* may represent a form of dystonia. *Physiologic tremor* in normal individuals is made apparent by stress, anxiety, or caffeine. *Rubral* tremor is seen with midbrain lesions in the vicinity of the red nucleus, accounting for the term *rubral*. Prognosis of each tremor generally depends on the underlying cause.

5. The treatment of tremor first involves addressing the underlying cause. After that, treatment is symptomatic. *Resting tremor* is ameliorated with anticholinergics or dopamine agonists (levodopa or direct acting agonists), *action–postural* and *orthostatic tremors* with β-blockers, clonazepam, or gabapentin, *rubral tremor* by treating resting and action components, and *task-specific tremor* with botulinum toxin. For *essential tremor*, propranolol and primidone are effective for limb tremor and second-line treatments include alprazolam, atenolol, gabapentin, sotalol, and topiramate; propranolol is useful for head tremor and botulinum toxin A has been used for hand tremor and vocal tremor in *essential tremor*.[2] No satisfying treatments have been found for *terminal kinetic tremors*. Botulinum toxin, deep brain stimulation (DBS) of the Vim thalamus, internal pallidum, or

subthalamic nucleus and thalamotomy are sometimes useful for some intractable tremors.

6. The *neuropsychiatric features* of tremor are presently ill defined and are otherwise those of the underlying etiology and its treatment.

C. **Choreoathetosis**

1. *Choreoathetosis* ranges from fast dance-like *chorea* to slower writhing movements termed *athetosis*. Choreatic movements generally flow freely from limb to limb, are arrhythmic, and are difficult to suppress.

2. The pathophysiology of chorea generally reflects striatal disease leading to disinhibition of the external globus pallidus, producing a direct γ-aminobutyric acid (GABA)-mediated over-inhibition and indirect (through the subthalamic nucleus) glutamatergic understimulation of the internal globus pallidus. This in turn disinhibits glutamatergic thalamocortical stimulatory activity projecting to the SMA and other loci.

3. Chorea can be diagnosed by certain features. It can be *activated* or *facilitated* by having the patient walk or perform other maneuvers, such as the finger-to-nose examination or finger tapping. The Abnormal Involuntary Movement Scale (AIMS) examination used to diagnose tardive dyskinesia (TD) (TD usually involves choreiform movements) is an appropriate procedure for evaluating chorea: Observe the patient at rest with wrists supported by the knees and hands hanging down, then provoke movements with facilitatory maneuvers, then observe the patient when standing, followed by walking. Observe for activation with facilitation and on walking. So-called *piano-playing* movements may be apparent in the fingers. *Facial* and *orolingual* movements may be apparent, as may *limb* chorea, *truncal* movements, and a choreic *gait*. Patients may attempt to make the movements look as though they were intended by incorporating a choreic excursion into some other sequence of movement, termed a *parakinesia*, such as voluntarily running their hand through their hair. Chorea is associated with *motor impersistence*, manifest in fixation instability, tongue protrusion, and milkmaid's grip. In *fixation instability*, the patient is generally unable to fixate their gaze on a target for more than 30 seconds without breaking off the target, called a *saccadic intrusion*. These can also be apparent on testing extraocular movements, where the eyes suddenly break off the target because of a saccadic intrusion. Motor impersistence is also manifest in the patient's inability to maintain *tongue protrusion* for more than a 30-second interval. *Milkmaid's grip* refers to involuntary relaxations and sudden compensatory contractions when asked to grip the examiner's fingers, with the patient producing a grip similar to milking a cow. *Paroxysmal kinesigenic* and *nonkinesigenic choreas* are paroxysmal choreic events that occur either with or without exercise.[1]

4. The etiologies of chorea are legion (see Table 10.4). The chorea of Huntington disease (HD) and Sydenham chorea represent two of the best-known choreic disorders (see section **IC4a** and **IC4b**). Choreic primary etiologies include *hereditary* (including HD, benign familial chorea and a diversity of neurologic or systemic diseases), *drug induced* (e.g., dopaminergic agents, stimulants, anticonvulsants, steroids, opiates, antihistamines, and digoxin), *metabolic* (e.g., sodium, hypocalcemia, hypomagnesemia, glucose, hepatic, renal, propionic acidemia, glutaric aciduria, GM1 gangliosidosis, and kernicterus), endocrinologic (e.g, hyperthyroidism, parathyroid, pseudohypoparathyroidism, hypocortisolemia, and pregnancy), *nutritional* (e.g., niacin, thiamine, Vitamin B_{12}, and D deficiencies), *infectious/immunologic* (e.g., human immunodeficiency virus (HIV), Sydenham chorea, bacterial, tubercular, viral), *cerebrovascular* (e.g., infarct, transient ischemic attack [TIA], migraine, arteriovenous malformation [AVM], polycythemia vera, and lupus), *traumatic, neurodegenerative* (e.g., Pick disease, thalamic centrum medianum nucleus degeneration), and *physiologic* (e.g., senile essential chorea, and physiologic chorea of infancy). There are a number of *genetic mutations* associated with non-HD choreas (e.g., HDL1, HDL2, CHAC, a 4p.15.3 autosomal recessive gene, a 14q autosomal dominant gene, etc.). In TD, usually developing after at least 3 months of antipsychotic administration, the movements are most commonly oral-buccal-lingual in distribution, but involvement of the extremities and trunk is also seen in more severe cases.

   a. **Huntington disease.** HD is a dominantly inherited CAG trinucleotide repeat disease affecting the *IT15* gene at 4p16.3.[3] An expanded repeat sequence of 37 or more CAG repeats is 100% specific and 98.8% sensitive for HD. Longer repeats correlate with early onset and death. Genetic anticipation (progressively earlier onset in each successive generation) is associated with paternal transmission. HD generally presents between the ages of 35 and 50. The course averages 15 years, with some patients surviving up to 40 years. In addition to chorea, myoclonus, dystonia, or parkinsonism may occur. Childhood-onset HD is associated with parkinsonian rigidity, cerebellar signs, rapid cognitive decline and seizures. As HD progresses, patients become demented, mute, achoreic, and often parkinsonian. On magnetic resonance imaging (MRI), there is striatal degeneration with striking dilatation of the frontal horns of the lateral ventricles, with milder secondary cortical atrophy. The intercaudate to outer-table distance ratio measured at the frontal horns has traditionally formed the basis for the radiologic diagnosis of HD. Laboratory testing involves southern blotting to determine the CAG repeat expansion. Presymptomatic genetic testing is available, but genetic counseling is an essential element of this procedure.

TABLE 10.4 Heredodegenerative Disorders Associated with Movement Disorders

	D	P	C	M
X-linked dominant				
Rett syndrome	D			
X-linked recessive				
Lubag (DYT3 X-linked dystonia-parkinsonism)	D	P		
Deafness-dystonia syndrome (Mohr-Tranebjaerg syndrome)	D			
Pelizaeus-Merzbacher disease	D		C	
Autosomal dominant				
Juvenile parkinsonism	D	P		
Huntington disease	D	P	C	M
Dystonia	D	P		M
Neuroferritinopathy (adult-onset basal ganglia disease)	D			
Machado-Joseph disease (SCA3)	D	P	C	
Dentatorubro-pallidoluysian atrophy	D		C	M
Other spinocerebellar degenerations	D	P	C	M
Familial Fahr syndrome (basal ganglia calcification)	D	P	C	
Benign familial chorea			C	
Tuberous sclerosis			C	
Paroxysmal nonkinesigenic choreoathetosis			C	
Porphyria			C	
Autosomal recessive				
Wilson disease	D	P	C	M
Niemann-Pick type C (dystonic lipidosis, sea-blue histiocytosis)	D			
Juvenile neuronal ceroid lipofuscinosis (Batten disease)	D	P	C	M
GM1 gangliosidosis	D		C	M
GM2 gangliosidosis	D		C	M
Metachromatic leukodystophy	D		C	
Lesch-Nyhan syndrome	D		C	
Homocystinuria	D		C	
Glutaric academia	D		C	
Triosephosphate isomerase deficiency	D			
Methylmalonic aciduria	D			
Hartnup disease	D		C	
Ataxia telangiectasia	D		C	M
Hallervorden-Spatz disease (pantothenate kinase associated neurodegeneration)	D	P	C	M
Neuroacanthocytosis	D	P	C	
Neuronal intranuclear hyaline inclusion disease	D			
Hereditary spastic paraplegia with dystonia (onset 10–12 y)	D			
Sjogren-Larsson syndrome (ichthyosis, spasticity, retardation)	D			
Progressive pallidal degeneration	D			
Olivopontocerebellar atrophies	D	P	C	M
Cystinuria			C	
PKU			C	

TABLE 10.4   (*Continued*)

Argininosuccinic acidemia		C		
Mucolipidoses		C		
Galactosemia		C		
Sphingolipidoses (Krabbe disease)		C	M	
Globoid cell leukodystrophy		C		
Gaucher disease		C		
Hemoglobin SC disease		C		
Xeroderma pigmentosum		C		
Sulfite-oxidase deficiency		C		
Lafora body disease			M	
Sialidosis ("cherry red spot")			M	
Unverricht-Lundborg disease			M	
Citrullinemia				T
Mitochondrial				
Leigh disease	D	C		
Leber disease	D	P		
Deafness, dystonia, retardation, blindness syndrome	D			
Other mitochondrial encephalopathies	D	P	C	M
Other				
Fragile X permutation (CGG repeat—X-linked)	P		M	T
Pyruvate dehydrogenase deficiency (X-linked, X-inactivation dependent)		C		
Trisomy 21 (Down) (nondisjunction)				T
Kleinfelter syndrome (nondisjunction)				T
XYY (nondisjunction)				T
Triple X and 9p mosaicism (nondisjunction)				T
9p monosomy (nondisjunction)				T
Sturge-Weber syndrome		C		
Ataxia-Myoclonus syndrome		C	M	
Coeliac disease (multifactorial)			M	
Partial trisomy 16 (breakage and nondisjunction or chromosomal breakage and translocation)				T
Beckwith-Wiedemann syndrome (imprinting and microdeletion; autosomal dominant with variable expressivity; contiguous gene duplication)				T
Mucopolysaccharidoses (autosomal recessive, except Hunter X-linked)		C		
Familial striatal necrosis (autosomal recessive or mitochondrial)		C		
Paroxysmal kinesigenic choreoathetosis (autosomal dominant with variable penetrance suggested)		C		
Paroxysmal dystonic choreoathetosis (Mount-Reback)	D	C		

P, parkinsonism; D, dystonia; C, chorea; M, myoclonus; T, tics; PKU, phenylketonuria.
Appreciation is expressed to Dr Linda R. Adkison, Ph.D. for her help in the correct genetic classification of these disorders and to Gail Sheffield for assistance in preparing this table.

The differential diagnosis of HD includes spinocerebellar atrophies (e.g., SCA2 and SCA3), HD-like autosomal dominant HDL2, HD-like autosomal recessive HDL3, dentato-rubro-pallido-Luysian atrophy (presenting with varying constellations of movement disorders, seizures, cognitive impairment, and cerebellar signs, with primary pathology in the structures identified in its name), and neuronal intranuclear inclusion disease.

b.   Sydenham chorea is poststreptococcal (group A β-hemolytic), with antibodies directed against the striatum. Chorea is typical during the acute infection, and tics, dystonia, and a tendency to re-eventuate chorea have each been observed in the postinfection phase.

5.   The treatment of chorea involves identifying and treating underlying etiologies. Beyond this principle, its treatment[3] can be inferred from the treatment of HD (see section IC5a). Sydenham chorea is discussed later (see section IC5b). *Paroxysmal kinesigenic choreoathetosis* responds to anticonvulsants (including small doses of phenytoin, phenobarbital, carbamazepine, oxcarbazepine, topiramate, and other agents). The treatment of TD involves discontinuation of the offending agent, or when psychosis precludes this, switching to clozapine. If a switch to clozapine is not possible, switching to an atypical antipsychotic carries essentially half the risk of producing or exacerbating TD than classical neuroleptic agents. It can generally be said of TD that approximately 33% will resolve after drug discontinuation, 33% will gradually improve, and 33% will continue unabated after 2 years.

a.   The treatment of HD involves treating the movements (explained here) as well as the neuropsychiatric features of the disease (see section IC6a). Movements can be followed using the Unified Huntington Disease Rating Scale. Haloperidol in doses of 1.5 to 10 mg per day has been demonstrated to reduce the *chorea*. Apomorphine has reduced chorea and motor impersistence.

b.   The treatment of *Sydenham chorea*[4] is divided into treating the acute and convalescent phases of the illness (explained here) as well as the neuropsychiatric features of the disease (see section IC6b). In the *acute phase*, steroids, haloperidol, and valproate have been used to ameliorate acute phase symptoms. Following the acute phase, long-term treatment with penicillin is needed to prevent future attacks and to prevent rheumatic heart disease. Immune therapies have been applied, including intravenous immunoglobulin (IVIG) and plasma exchange. In treating late sequelae such as *psychosis*, atypical antipsychotics should be used cautiously, monitoring for antipsychotic intolerance reactions (e.g., parkinsonism, neuroleptic malignant syndrome).

6. *Neuropsychiatric features* and treatment of hyperkinesias remain
    to be defined; however, there are some data in HD (see section
    IC6a) and Sydenham chorea (see section **IC6b**).

    a. **Huntington disease**

        (1) Neuropsychiatric features are common in HD.[3] *Person-*
             ality changes have been reported in 70% and include
             irritability (severe in one third of HD patients) and
             aggressiveness (in one third of institutionalized HD
             patients), sometimes conforming to the diagnosis of *in-*
             termittent explosive disorder (found in 31% in one study).
             The patient may deny irritability, and spouses may not
             admit to it unless interviewed separately from the pa-
             tient. *Violence* including assault, arson, and homicide
             attempts have been described in the literature. *Apathy*
             may develop in half of the patients, as can *disinhibi-*
             tion. Hypersexuality was observed in 12% of men and
             7% of women in one study. *Delirium* in HD is usually
             ascribable to alcohol or substance abuse, dehydration,
             medications, subdural hematoma, or infectious etiolo-
             gies. HD is typified by a *subcortical dementia,* often
             without the cortical signs of aphasia and agnosia. Ini-
             tially, there is a reduced speed of cognitive processing
             and set shifting, with *dysattention* and *dysexecution.* The
             reverse serial seven task of the Mini-Mental State Ex-
             amination (MMSE) is usually the first item of this test to
             be affected. *Memory* is characterized by *retrieval deficit*
             errors, wherein lack of spontaneous recall of items can
             be improved by cueing the memory with helpful hints.
             Memory, *visuospatial abilities,* and *judgment* are each
             affected as the illness progresses. *Alexithymia* may de-
             velop. *Schizophrenia* has been documented in 9% of
             patients with HD, and *psychotic symptoms* in 25%. Pa-
             tients with *hallucinations* and *delusions* usually have
             depression. Psychotic symptoms are more common in
             early onset HD. *Mood disorders* occur in 40%, and the
             prevalence of *bipolar disorder* is 10% (elevated 10-fold
             over normative populations). Depression is often pro-
             dromal to the onset of the movement disorder. *Major*
             depressive symptoms appear to be similar to the pattern
             seen in primary major depression; however, completed
             suicide rates have been reported to be as high as 13%.
             The *suicide risk* is of special concern in older patients
             and those with *witzelsucht. Adjustment disorders* can also
             occur. Certain families may carry a proclivity toward
             obsessive-compulsive disorder (*OCD*) in HD, but preva-
             lences of OCD, *generalized anxiety disorder* (*GAD*), and
             panic disorder have not been established. *Anxiety* has
             been reported in 12% of patients with HD, was found
             to be the most common prodromal symptom, and

has been correlated with longer survival. *Mixed anxiety depression* has been associated with akinetic-rigid HD (usually early, childhood-onset HD). *Hypersexuality* and *paraphilias* have been reported, and male patients may become aggressive toward their partners, although patients usually lose interest in sex as the disease progresses, and become *impotent. Hypoactive sexual disorder* was found in 82% in one series.

(2) Anecdotal data support the use of sertraline for *irritability,* and sertraline, buspirone, and propranolol for *aggression.* Whereas clozapine reduced chorea in one study, functional capacity deteriorated. Other data support the efficacy of clozapine for *psychotic features,* and *delusions* may respond better than *hallucinations* to neuroleptics. Anticonvulsants have been preferred to lithium for *mood stabilization* to avoid lithium toxicity. Selective serotonin reuptake inhibitors (SSRIs) and nortriptyline have been recommended as first-line treatments for depression, with monoamine oxidase inhibitors (MAOIs) as a second line, but there is essentially no experience with newer generation antidepressants. *Delusional depression* has responded well to electroconvulsive therapy (ECT). *Anticipatory anxiety* can be managed by delaying the informing of the patient about an event until immediately before it happens. SSRIs and clomipramine have been used to effectively treat *OCD* in HD. Medroxyprogesterone or leuprolide have been useful in reducing *sexual disinhibition.*

b. **Sydenham chorea**
(1) In the *acute syndrome,* features include chorea, tics, *irritability, obsessions, compulsions,* and *psychotic symptoms.* Transient *intellectual impairment* has been reported on occasion. The rate of psychiatric symptoms in general, and *schizophrenia* in particular, has been found to be significantly higher following this disease than in matched controls. Impairment on the Bender-Gestalt test and abnormal electroencephalograms (EEGs) have been observed in the convalescent phase. *OCD* features and spectrum disorders including *body dysmorphic disorder* have been found to be elevated following Sydenham chorea, in contrast with controls who had rheumatic fever without chorea. These poststreptococcal, postchoreic phenomena have been related to the pediatric autoimmune neuropsychiatric disorders associated with streptococcal throat infections (PANDAS) syndrome.
(2) Experience in treating the neuropsychiatric features of Sydenham chorea is limited and controlled data are needed. Given obvious central nervous system (CNS)

neuropathology, cautious conservative initial dose and escalation strategies would seem prudent.

D. Dystonia

1. *Dystonia* involves forceful, twisting, torsional, repetitive movements, and muscle spasms that often manifest sustained postures but may be more brief and sudden, resembling chorea.

2. The pathophysiology of dystonia is thought to relate to excessive striatal activity that leads to GABAergic overinhibition of the globus pallidus, especially the internal pallidum, reducing GABAergic inhibition on glutamatergic stimulatory thalamocorticals projecting to the SMA and other loci. However, there are functional imaging data suggesting that some areas of cortex are activated, whereas others show reduced activation, suggesting a blending of choreic and parkinsonian pathophysiologies.

3. Dystonia is diagnosed by the form of the movement (see section ID1) and its many manifestations.[5] It can manifest in *lordotic* or other postures and is associated with *scoliosis*. *Hypertrophy* of involved muscles is an important sign. Dystonia can be brought out by repetitive movements such as running in place and opening and closing the hands (*facilitating* or *activating* procedures). *Dystonic tremor* may be present. *Action specificity* is generally seen early in the course of dystonia, so that leg dystonia may only be apparent when a patient walks forward, but not sideways or backwards. Another peculiar feature of dystonia is *geste antagoniste*, or the ability to adopt certain compensatory postures or actions that alleviate the dystonia. The inconsistent manifestation of dystonia because of action specificity and geste antagoniste frequently lead to misdiagnosis as a conversion disorder or other psychogenic dystonia. Adding to the confusion, *psychogenic movements* can sometimes develop in the presence of an already extant movement disorder.

    a. *Primary dystonias* are of various genetic types, whereas *secondary dystonias* occur in other diseases. *Hemidystonia* is unilateral secondary dystonia. Some secondary dystonias present as *dystonia-plus* syndromes, involving additional neurologic features.

    b. *Generalized dystonia* has its onset in childhood and usually begins in a leg, then progresses rostrally, eventually involving both sides and all parts of the body. Limbs are often contorted, *torticollis* may be apparent in the neck, *orofacial* features may include *risus sardonicus* (a dystonic sardonic grin) and eyebrow raises, the *gait* may be affected, feet and fingers may be involved, and *fast dystonic jerks* may be evident. These features may be worse with facilitation or other activities, and a tremor, often worse when the patient tries to oppose the muscle contractions, may be apparent.

    c. *Segmental dystonias* involve two or more contiguous body parts and tend to have their onset in the fourth and fifth decades of life, often involving the neck, upper extremities, chest, and head. *Meige* or *Brueghel syndrome* is a segmental *oromandibular* dystonia (with dystonic jaw closure, opening, or lateral deviation) usually accompanied by *blepharospasm* (dystonic closure of the eyelids) and is often accompanied by lingual dystonic movements (often fast dystonic movements) or torticollis.

d. *Focal dystonia* is confined to a single body part, such as isolated blepharospasm.

e. *Dystonic tremors* tend to be of the action–postural type.

f. *Spasmodic dysphonia* refers to dystonic vocal cord contractions, leading to vocal hoarseness (adductor dysphonia) or a whispering, breathy quality to the voice (abductor dysphonia).

g. *Peripheral dystonia* usually occurs in a distal extremity. Paroxysmal *dystonic choreoathetosis* is a rare condition that is manifest only paroxysmally and is associated with choreoathetosis.

h. *Oculogyric crisis* is a form of dystonia wherein the eyes roll up superiorly in the orbits.

i. *Task-specific dystonias* are seen with repetitive use of limbs or fingers, and may be action specific, such that the fingers become involved in a dystonic contraction only when they are used a certain way, called *action specificity*.

j. *Acute drug-induced dystonias* often involve the tongue, jaw, neck, trunk, or upper extremities. *Tardive dystonias* generally involve the back, trunk, and neck, frequently with retrocollis.

4. The etiologies of dystonia are diverse (Table 10.4), and certain features guide diagnosis.

a. *Primary dystonias* are of genetic origin (DYT1-15, etc.). *Secondary dystonias* warrant a workup (see section **ID4b**) and occur in the context of other diseases (e.g., putamenal stroke, inborn errors of metabolism, other genetic syndromes [Table 10.4], etc.). *Hemidystonia* usually indicates a structural lesion etiology. *Dystonia-plus* syndromes generally signify *heredodegenerative disorders* (Table 10.4). Dystonia is occasionally encountered in the parkinsonisms, especially corticobasal degeneration (CBD) (see Chapter 9). *Generalized dystonia* is often associated with inborn errors of metabolism and other pediatric illnesses. *Peripheral dystonia* usually signifies a preexisting sensory or other traumatic injury.

b. The *workup of primary dystonia* is generally confined to identifying the genetic type. The *workup of secondary dystonia* involves MRI when the neurologic examination suggests findings in addition to dystonia or the presentation is atypical. When dystonia presents in childhood (typified by *generalized dystonia*), the workup is more aggressive, including MRI, 24-hour urine for copper, serum ceruloplasmin level, serology, CBC/DIFF, erythrocyte sedimentation rate, antinuclear antibody (ANA), uric acid, routine chemistry profiles, and toxicology, to exclude etiologies of secondary dystonia (Wilson disease, Lesch-Nyhan syndrome, postanoxic state, infection, allergic reactions, toxins, hemolytic uremic syndrome, sickle-cell anemia, acidosis, striatal necrosis, Fahr syndrome, HD, etc.), If the cause remains cryptic, additional investigations can be carried out looking for Hallervorden-Spatz disease, Leigh syndrome, ceroid lipofuscinosis, gangliosidoses, metachromatic leukodystrophy, ataxia telangiectasia, neuroacanthocytosis, dystonic lipidoses, mitochondrial cytopathies, endocrinopathies, chromosomal aberrancies, and so on (Table 10.4).

   c. *Drug-induced acute dystonias* occur predominantly with dopamine D_2 receptor antagonists (antipsychotics, metoclopramide) and with SSRIs. *Tardive dystonias* are encountered after long-term exposure to D_2 antagonists.

   d. *Psychogenic dystonia* can be signaled by incongruities in dystonic features and by the presence of a coexisting psychiatric disorder, but extreme caution is needed in making this diagnosis because many dystonia patients have been misdiagnosed as conversional, factitious, or malingering disorders. Moreover, dystonia is associated with a diversity of psychiatric disorders (see section **ID6**). An electromyographic feature consistent with dystonia is the abnormality of *loss of reciprocal inhibition* such that both agonist and antagonist muscles simultaneously *co-contract* in dystonia, in contrast with normal physiology, and absence of this finding may indicate psychogenic dystonia.

5. The treatment of dystonia involves addressing the underlying disorder in the case of secondary dystonias,[1,5] and providing symptomatic treatment for the dystonia itself.

   a. *Focal, segmental,* and *task-specific dystonias* are treated with local injections of botulinum toxins (e.g., Botox, Dysport). Antibody resistance occurs in 10%, at which point patients can be switched to a different serotype (e.g., from A to F or B). Side effects include transient dysphagia (or if severe, systemic botulism in rare events).

   b. Some dystonias are levodopa/carbidopa responsive (e.g., *dopa-responsive dystonia* which is sometimes attended by diurnal variation in the dystonia and may respond to doses of <300 mg per day) and levodopa/carbidopa should be tried up to 25/250 mg q.i.d. over several months before trying other agents. Most dystonias will require additional treatments, but a levodopa trial is recommended as an initial treatment trial.

   c. Oral agents can be used and these include anticholinergics, benzodiazepines, dopamine agonists, baclofen (ranked from most effective to least effective), and sometimes neuroleptics, lithium, carbamazepine, valproate, and clozapine. The former two agents may require quite high doses, and so it is necessary to start with small doses and gradually titrate upward, allowing the development of tolerance to side effects and the judging of a response before escalating the dose higher. Some dystonias may require doses of tri-hexyphenidyl as high as 120 mg per day, and diazepam as high as 60 mg per day. Obviously, precautions for side effects must be taken. Dopamine agonists are effective in *cranial dystonias* but less so in torticollis. Neuroleptics have been useful in approximately half of torticollis, segmental, and generalized patients. Benzodiazepines are useful for *paroxysmal dystonic choreoathetosis.* Intrathecal baclofen has been used in severe cases, and both bilateral subthalamic nucleus DBS and pallidotomy have been useful.

d.   *Acute dystonia* because of neuroleptics is generally best treated with 1 to 2 mg of benztropine IM, or 50 mg of diphenhydramine IM, unless otherwise contraindicated.

e.   For *tardive dystonia,* clozapine is sometimes useful, especially in cases of schizophrenia that require an antipsychotic. The first step in tardive syndromes is to reduce the etiologic antipsychotic as much as possible. Thereafter, anticholinergics have been most useful, supplemented with dopamine depleters and botulinum toxin.

f.   *Psychogenic dystonias* remit in approximately 25% of cases, and those with conversion disorders and depressive illnesses have the best prognosis, whereas somatization, factitious disorders, and malingering have a poor prognosis.[5] In order of benefit (from most to least), the use of suggestion, formal psychotherapy, physiotherapy, placebo, antidepressants, and behavior modification proved useful in a series of 21 patients. Abuse issues are common. Hypnotherapy has been reported as beneficial.

6.   A number of distinct *neuropsychiatric syndromes* occur in primary dystonia,[5,6] but no studies regarding their treatment exist.[5] *Intelligence* is preserved in primary dystonias, but may vary in the secondary dystonias. *Psychotic features* are unusual in primary dystonias, but may occur in secondary dystonias. Initial data in primary dystonia indicates a risk for *bipolar disorder,* with at least a 10-fold increased prevalence, as in HD. Rapid cycling has also been observed. *Major depression* has been encountered in 30%, whereas *dysthymia* has been observed in 15%. Occasional cases of *atypical depression* may be seen. There is the suggestion that higher prevalence of depression is associated with more cranial dystonic distributions, in contrast to more peripheral involvement. Some studies have suggested a relationship to disability, whereas others do not find this. Depression in torticollis has been characterized by self-blame, self-accusation, self-punishment, and negative body image. GAD was present in 25%, a four-fold increase over normative rates, whereas *social phobia* was seen in 18% in one study of patients with primary segmental dystonia, consistent with previous psychological findings

of high rates of anxiety in cervicocranial dystonia.[5] *Obsessive compulsive features* and *eating disorders* have been reported in dystonia, but it is unclear if they are truly associated with this movement disorder. OCD has been associated with myoclonic dystonia. *Substance abuse* and *dependence* can complicate dystonia, especially alcohol if alcohol improves dystonic spasms, as in myoclonic dystonia. Personality features include *obsessional, schizoid,* and *sociopathic personality traits. Histrionic features* have been observed in two thirds of female patients in one study. Torticollis patients have been reported to have "neurotic" profiles. *Conversional* or *somatization* symptoms may occur. *Psychogenic dystonia* is associated with sudden onset, precipitating events, rapid progression, fixed postures, pain (which can occur in organic dystonia), leg dystonia despite adult onset, paroxysmal worsening, multiple somatizations, and other conversional neurologic signs.

E. **Ballismus**
1. *Ballismus* is recognized by large amplitude, ballistic, flinging excursions of the limb from proximal joints and is usually unilateral (*hemiballismus*).
2. The pathophysiology of ballismus involves reduced function of the subthalamic nucleus, resulting in reduced glutamatergic stimulation of the internal globus pallidus, thereby reducing GABAergic inhibition on glutamatergic stimulatory thalamocorticals projecting to the SMA and other loci.
3. Ballismus is diagnosed by its characteristic presentation.
4. The *etiology* of ballismus is usually a vascular lesion involving the contralateral subthalamic nucleus, pallidosubthalamic projections, and adjacent internal capsule. Less common etiologies include tumor, abscess, encephalitis, vasculitis, systemic lupus erythematosus (SLE), AVM, trauma, hyperglycemia, basal ganglia calcification, tuberous sclerosis, and multiple sclerosis.
5. The treatment of ballismus generally involves the use of a neuroleptic, such as haloperidol, or atypical antipsychotics, dopamine depleters (e.g., reserpine), and sometimes valproate or clonazepam. The prognosis for spontaneous remission is good. Two thirds of patients experience remission, although half of these may be left with chorea. In intractable cases ventrolateral (VL) thalamotomy might be considered as a last resort.
6. Mania has been reported in association with ballismus and can be treated with the conventional treatments for ballismus.

F. **Myoclonus**
1. *Myoclonus* is recognized by explosive shock-like muscle contractions that sometimes occur in trains, which can be rhythmic or arrhythmic, with multiple jerks synchronized in time or that occur asynchronously.
2. The pathophysiology of myoclonus is quite complex and can be of cortical, subcortical, medullary, spinal, or peripheral origins, and can be related to epileptic and nonepileptic etiologies.

3. Myoclonus is diagnosed by its characteristic presentations and is a complex condition.[1] Myoclonus is distinguished from tics in that it cannot be suppressed. Myoclonus has been classified as *symptomatic myoclonus, familial myoclonic epilepsy,* and *essential myoclonus,* in order of most frequent to least frequent. Clinical types include *stimulus-sensitive myoclonus* (activated by pin prick), *reflex myoclonus* (activated by deep tendon reflexes), *ballistic overflow myoclonus* (activated by fast movements such as asking the patient to touch your rapidly moving finger), *action myoclonus* (activated by activity of a limb), *palatal myoclonus* (rhythmic myoclonus of the palate accompanied by a clicking sound that can be auscultated at the external auditory meatus, often at 1 to 3 Hz), *epileptic myoclonus* (manifest in a number of seizure disorders), *alcohol responsive myoclonus, familial myoclonus, intermittent rhythmic myoclonus* (e.g., described in Picks disease in the context of SSRIs), and many other types. Drug-induced myoclonus can occur most frequently with serotonin agonists (e.g., SSRIs) and in excessive serotonin release, such as in *serotonin syndrome.* Myoclonic types of treatment importance include: *Ballistic overflow myoclonus, palatal myoclonus, cortical myoclonus* (diagnosed by EEG back-averaged cortical prepotentials preceding myoclonic jerks on electromyography (EMG) accompanied by enlarged somatosensory evoked potentials), *brainstem reticular myoclonus* (diagnosed in the absence of cortical prepotentials and in the context of myoclonic jerks transmitted in sequential order from CN XI rostrally, and limb and axial musculature from superior muscles caudally), *propriospinal myoclonus* (diagnosed by jerks initially in the thoracic musculature, spreading both rostrally and caudally from this site), and *segmental spinal myoclonus* (myoclonus is restricted to a particular body segment, usually because of local radiculopathy, plexopathy, or neuropathy). *Psychogenic myoclonus* is diagnosed by variable latencies of stimulus-evoked jerks, latencies longer than voluntary reaction time, and presence of the *Bereitschaftspotential* (a potential preceding voluntary actions characterized by frontal negativity, also referred to as the *readiness potential*) before EMG bursts on jerk-locked back-averaged EEG.
4. Myoclonic etiologies are provided in Table 10.4. Several types of primary myoclonus are associated with genetic mutations, including EPM1, EPM2A, tRNA(Ser[UCN]), FAME, and so on. *Symptomatic myoclonus* etiologies include storage diseases, spinocerebellar degenerations, basal ganglia diseases, dementias (Alzheimer disease [AD], Creutzfeldt-Jakob disease [CJD]), viral encephalopathies, metabolic disorders, toxins, drugs (e.g., SSRIs and serotonin syndrome, levodopa), trauma, hypoxia, stroke, thalamotomy, and tumors.
5. The treatment of myoclonus primarily involves treating the underlying cause. Thereafter, certain drugs are useful for the movement disorder itself, depending upon the type of myoclonus. For *cortical myoclonus,* valproate or clonazepam are first-line

choices, followed by primidone, phenobarbital, piracetam, or 5-hydroxytryptophan (5-HTP) with carbidopa. In *brainstem reticular myoclonus*, valproate or clonazepam are first line, with 5-HTP as second line. For *ballistic overflow myoclonus*, benztropine or trihexyphenidyl are first-line treatments, followed by clonazepam or 5-HTP. In *palatal myoclonus*, first-line agents include phenytoin, carbamazepine, clonazepam, diazepam, trihexyphenidyl, or baclofen. For *propriospinal myoclonus*, clonazepam is the treatment. In *segmental spinal myoclonus*, clonazepam is the first-line agent and diazepam, carbamazepine, or tetrabenazine are second-line treatments. The treatment for drug-induced myoclonus is to remove or reduce the offending agent.

6. The *neuropsychiatric features* of myoclonus remain to be defined and are otherwise those of the underlying etiology and its treatment.

G. **Tics**
1. *Tics* generally occur repetitively, and may be simple, such as eye blinks or throat clearing, or complex actions or vocalizations.[7] They tend to wax and wane over time, and can migrate throughout the body. They can be preceded by a premonitory sensation, in 80% of patients in one study. They are usually distractible and are often suppressible or preceded by an urge to perform the tic. They are frequently associated with obsessions or compulsions.

2. The pathophysiology of tics is not known but is thought to relate to excessive dopaminergic release at the level of the striatum.

3. Tics are diagnosed by their clinical features. Gilles de la Tourette syndrome (GTS) is the prototypic tic disorder. In the Diagnostic and Statistical Manual of Mental Disorders, 4th edition (DSM-IV), GTS is diagnosed by the presence of multiple motor and vocal tics occurring together or separately at some time during the illness. Tics occur in recurrent bouts multiple times during the day at least intermittently over the course of 1 year and are never absent for >3 consecutive months. Tics have their onset before the age of 18, are not attributable to substances or other medical conditions, and produce significant personal, social, occupational, or other functional impairment. Other tic disorders fulfill less than the full complement of GTS criteria. Standard structural imaging (MRI) is unrevealing in primary tic disorders.

4. The etiologies of tics include primary and secondary causes. GTS has been associated with an autosomal dominant mutation at 11q23. Secondary tic etiologies include chromosomal disorders (Table 10.4), stroke, trauma, carbon momoxide (CO), drugs (stimulants, levodopa, carbamazepine, phenytoin, phenobarbital, lamotrigine, dopamine antagonists), infections (neurosyphilis, encephalitis, CJD, Sydenham chorea), tuberous sclerosis, mental retardation, static encephalitis, neurodegenerative diseases (HD, neuroacanthocytosis, Hallervorden-Spatz, and Wilson disease), neurocutaneous syndromes, Duchenne muscular dystrophy, Aspergers syndrome, and psychosis.

5. The treatment of GTS involves both pharmacologic and psychotherapeutic interventions. *Neuroleptics* are effective against motor tics, generally leading to 50% to 80% improvement.[7] *Atypical antipsychotics* including olanzapine, risperidone, and ziprasidone have resulted in 40% to 60% improvement with fewer side effects than neuroleptics. *Behavior therapy* (habit reversal therapy) has also been effective for tics, leading to approximately 70% improvement. Other agents may be employed adjunctively. *Noradrenergic α-2 agonists* such as guanfacine and clonidine have led to approximately 30% improvements, and there have been mixed results for the norepinephrine reuptake inhibitor desipramine. Dopamine agonists (apomorphine, ropinirole, pergolide), presynaptic dopamine depleters (tetrabenazine, α-methyl-*para*-tyrosine), baclofen, and botulinum toxin have also demonstrated benefit.

6. The neuropsychiatric features of GTS and their treatment are becoming clearer.

   a. Patients can display *aggressive* and *disinhibited behavior.* Although IQ is normal, *cognitive impairments* may occur in GTS and include *visuomotor disintegration, impaired fine motor skills, executive dysfunction,* and, in patients with attention deficit-hyperactivity disorder (ADHD) or OCD, a risk for *learning disorders. OCD* or OCD symptoms have been observed in more than half of patients, and *ADHD* in approximately 20%. *Learning disorders* in GTS are associated with OCD and ADHD and impose more functional morbidity than the tics, indicating the need for early evaluation and treatment.

   b. OCD in GTS has been successfully treated with SSRIs; the use of risperidone with or without SSRI has occasioned benefit, too. In GTS patients with ADHD, methylphenidate, clonidine, and desipramine have been used.

H. Akathisia

1. *Akathisia* is an uncomfortable inner sensation of restlessness often localized to the legs or abdomen.[1] The subjective inner restless sensation is usually accompanied by abnormal restless movements that may include shifting postures, pacing, rocking, shifting weight from foot to foot (marching in place), repetitive crossing and uncrossing of legs or arms, and other behaviors.

2. The pathophysiology of akathisia is unknown but is thought to relate to insufficient dopamine stimulation in the basal ganglia.

3. Akathisia is diagnosed by its defining clinical features.

4. Akathisia etiologies can be inferred from conditions associated with it. Akathisia is associated with restless legs syndrome (RLS), Parkinson disease, iron deficiency, dopamine receptor D_2 antagonists, dopamine depleting agents, and SSRIs. *Antipsychotic-induced akathisia* can be difficult to distinguish from psychotic agitation, a true dilemma in terms of whether to lower or increase the antipsychotic; the use of lorazepam, while therapeutic, is noninstructive because this agent will ameliorate either

condition. The diagnosis is best made by the patient's report of the subjective akathisic sensation, not always possible in the acutely psychotic patient. Agitation and RLS are the primary entities to be excluded in the differential diagnosis of akathisia. Although RLS and its associated periodic leg movements can be classified as a movement disorder, they are defined in this manual as a sleep disorder and are therefore included in the Appendices (Appendices A and B).

5. Treatment of akathisia. *Antipsychotic-induced acute akathisia* is best treated by lowering the dose of the drug, as much as possible. The use of β-blocker or benzodiazepine for residual akathisia is generally considered more effective and better tolerated than anticholinergic or antihistaminic agents. Propranolol in doses up to 80 mg per day is usually effective, and there seems to be no real difference in efficacy between β-1 and β-2 antagonists. Clonidine, cyproheptadine, and nicotine have also been reported as helpful. The same measures may be employed when treating *tardive akathisia*, in addition to discontinuing the offending antipsychotic, or switching it to clozapine when a psychosis is present. Propranolol has been useful.

6. The *neuropsychiatric features* of akathisia are unknown except that suicide attempts have been reported. Otherwise, the neuropsychiatric features are those of its associated conditions and its treatment.

I. **Hemifacial spasm**

1. *HFS* is a condition wherein one half of the face is involved in repetitive eyewinking and simultaneous grimacing behavior.[1] These are usually clonic jerks that start around the eye and then spread to the mouth, but on occasion progress in the reverse fashion. They are irregular and unpredictable, and often triggered by facial movement. Mild facial weakness develops. It is more common in women than in men (3:2) and rarely remits.

2. The pathophysiology of HFS in 95% of cases is attributed to vascular pulsatile compression of CN VII by the anterior (AICA) or posterior (PICA) inferior cerebellar or vertebral arteries, whereas 5% have been associated with cerebellopontine angle tumors or AVMs, brainstem multiple sclerosis, or as a sequela of Bell palsy.

3. HFS is diagnosed by its defining clinical characteristics.

4. The etiologies of HFS are inferred from its pathophysiology.

5. The treatment of HFS involves symptomatic treatment and neurosurgical address of the underlying cause. Botulinum toxin has been useful for symptomatic treatment. Haloperidol and carbamazepine have rarely proved useful. Neurosurgical posterior fossa microvascular decompression is the only other effective treatment.

6. The *neuropsychiatric features* of HFS are unknown and are those of its associated conditions and its treatment.

References

1. Watts RL, Koller WC, eds. *Movement disorders: Neurologic principles and practice*, 2nd ed. New York: McGraw-Hill; 2004:1–994.
2. Zesiewicz TA, Elble R, Louis ED, et al. Practice parameter: Therapies for essential tremor: Report of the Quality Standards Subcommittee of the American Academy of Neurology. *Neurology.* 2005;64:2008–2020.
3. Anderson KE. Huntington's disease and related disorders. *Psychiatr Clin North Am.* 2005;28:275–290.
4. Jordan LC, Singer HS. Sydenham chorea in children. *Curr Treat Options Neurol.* 2003;5:283–290.
5. Lauterbach EC. Psychiatric management in dystonia. In: Lauterbach EC, ed. *Psychiatric management in neurological disease.* Washington, DC: American Psychiatric Press Group; 2000:179–218.
6. Lauterbach EC, Freeman A, Vogel RL. Differential DSM-III psychiatric disorder prevalence profiles in dystonia and Parkinson disease. *J Neuropsychiatry Clin Neurosci.* 2004;16:29–36.
7. Sandor P. Pharmacological management of tics in patients with TS. *J Psychosom Res.* 2003;55:41–48.

RESTLESS LEGS SYNDROME

1. RLS generally involves restless movements and shifting positions of the legs in response to akathisia. Akathisia is associated with RLS, which in turn is associated with periodic movements of sleep.[1] RLS develops in middle age or later in two thirds of patients, and may be aggravated by periods of rest.
2. RLS pathophysiology is unknown, but RLS is associated with low cerebrospinal fluid (CSF) ferritin and high CSF transferrin levels.
3. RLS is diagnosed by its defining features and its association with periodic leg movements of sleep (PLMS).
4. The etiologies of RLS are unclear, but it has been linked to a susceptibility locus on 12q13-23. In most cases, RLS is transmitted in autosomal dominant fashion. Other etiologies may include anemia, pregnancy, chronic myelopathy, peripheral neuropathy, gastric surgery, uremia, chronic respiratory disease, and drugs, including antipsychotics, antidepressants (especially SSRIs), lithium, and anticonvulsants.
5. The treatment of RLS involves addressing the underlying cause and symptomatic treatment of the movement disorder. In cases of iron deficiency, iron constitutes a useful treatment. Symptomatic treatments include levodopa, direct acting dopamine agonists (bromocriptine, pergolide, pramipexole, ropinirole), codeine, clonazepam, carbamazepine, baclofen, and clonidine.
6. The *neuropsychiatric features* of RLS are ill-defined and presently are those of the underlying etiology and its treatment.

PERIODIC LEG MOVEMENTS OF SLEEP

1. PLMS usually involve big toe and foot dorsiflexion and/or leg extensions or flexions during sleep. These occur at regular periodic intervals every 20 to 40 seconds, but may migrate throughout the body during the night. PLMS tend to occur during sleep Stages I and II, but have also been seen in drowsiness. The movements generally awaken the bed partner. Their prevalence increases with age, and they are rare before the age of 30, occur in 5% between the ages of 30 and 50, and in 30% over age 50. They may be associated with peripheral neuropathies.
2. The pathophysiology is unclear.
3. PLMS is diagnosed by its defining clinical features.
4. PLMS etiologies are unclear.
5. The treatment of PLMS involves treating an underlying cause (Appendix A) and symptomatic treatments, which include levodopa, ropinirole, pergolide, valproate, gabapentin, and oxycodone have proved to be helpful. Separate beds for the bedmates can also attenuate the partner's nocturnal awakenings.
6. The *neuropsychiatric features* of PLMS are ill defined and are presently those of the underlying etiology and its treatment.

Chapter 11

CHANGES
IN PERSONALITY

John J. Campbell, III

I. BACKGROUND

A. **Definitions**
1. *Personality* refers to the characteristics of a person that are enduring, pervasive, and distinctive. Personality has been defined as "the dynamic organization within the individual of those psychophysical systems that determine his unique adjustments to his environment."
2. Those characteristics are known as *traits*. Traits occur throughout the population in a bell-shaped data distribution. Traits have probabilistic influences on behavior that are known as *tendencies*. These tendencies produce patterns of behavior that are consistent over time.
3. *Temperament* factors are heritable biases in information processing reflected as automatic, preconceptual responses to social stimuli. Four dimensions of temperament include novelty seeking, harm avoidance, reward dependence, and persistence.
4. *Character* refers to behavioral tendencies related to concepts of the *self*. Initially, temperament influences the development of character. Eventually, insights gained through the developing character can modify the temperament. Three dimensions of character are self-directedness, cooperativeness, and self-transcendence.

B. **Classification of changes in personality**
1. Efforts to establish a lexicon for personality change related to neurologic disorders have culminated in the Diagnostic and Statistical Manual of Mental Disorders, 4th edition, text revision (DSM-IV-TR) diagnostic criteria for the diagnosis of personality change because of a general medical condition. These criteria include a persistent personality disturbance that represents a change from the individual's previous characteristic personality pattern with evidence from the history, physical examination, or

laboratory findings that the disturbance is the direct physiologic consequence of a general medical condition. The disturbance must not occur exclusively during the course of delirium and is not better accounted for by another mental disorder. Further, the disturbance must cause clinically significant distress or impairment in social, occupational, or other important areas of functioning.

2. There are five specified types of DSM-IV-TR personality change because of a general medical condition. The *labile type*, is characterized by affective lability, the *disinhibited type*, if the predominant feature is poor impulse control, the *aggressive type*, if aggressive behavior predominates, the *apathetic type*, are characterized by marked apathy and indifference, and the *paranoid type*, if suspiciousness or paranoid thinking are prominent. In addition, there is an *other type*, if a feature not noted above is present, a *combined type* if more than one feature predominates the clinical picture, and an *unspecified type*. This new diagnostic nomenclature can be used to provide a formal DSM-IV diagnosis of acquired changes in personality.

3. The neuropsychiatric perspective presented in the subsequent text relies more strongly on established brain-behavior relationships than upon description of the acquired symptoms in the DSM-IV paradigm, which has not yet been widely applied to research populations.

C. **Epidemiology.** Little is known about the prevalence of changes in personality within neuropsychiatric populations. The few published reports vary in nomenclature and methodology and therefore preclude accurate conclusions. It is clear from these reports, however, that personality change is a common occurrence in most, if not all, neuropsychiatric disorders, particularly in those conditions that involve the prefrontal–subcortical neural networks.

D. **Prognosis.** Only a small literature exists on the course and prognosis of personality changes associated with neuropsychiatric disorders, primarily in the area of traumatic brain injury (TBI). These limited data suggest that personality changes can be chronic and disabling.

II. NEUROBIOLOGY AND PATHOPHYSIOLOGY OF PERSONALITY CHANGE

A. **Normal personality.** The neurobiology of human personality is not fully understood. The basis for all human behavior unequivocally involves the final product of the processing and integration of information by widely distributed neural networks within the human brain. Disorders that affect the physical or neurochemical balance within these networks will alter the otherwise stable expression of personality and therefore provide astute clinical observers with signs of incipient neuropsychiatric conditions.

Numerous case reports and case series with clinicopathologic correlation have implicated the neural networks of the prefrontal cortex as a major contributor to human personality and behavior. Alexander and Crutcher have defined these networks as distinct

cortico-striato-pallido-thalamo-cortical loops or circuits. Three of these circuits, involving the dorsolateral convexity of the frontal lobe, the mesial frontal cortex, and the orbitofrontal cortex, have the capacity to mediate "executive" or metacognitive functions that enable us to achieve success in our social environment.
B. **Dysexecutive syndromes.** Prefrontal cortical gray matter, subcortical gray matter (striatum), and white matter are each vulnerable to particular kinds of pathology. Therefore there are numerous conditions that damage these networks and may ultimately manifest as changes in personality. The term *frontal lobe syndrome* has become synonymous with acquired changes in personality and there is no doubt that focal lesions involving the prefrontal cortex produce predictable changes in executive cognition and behavior. However, sufficient evidence exists demonstrating that lesions distant from the frontal cortical mantle may produce similar clinical findings. Hence the term *dysexecutive syndrome* is a more appropriate descriptor for patients who manifest personality changes with executive cognitive deficits.

This nomenclature is more consistent with current theories that describe large scale distributed neural networks subserving behavior. The nomenclature also provides a more rational template for evaluating patients who acquire changes in personality and the complex behaviors reliant upon executive cognition. Although functional divisions within the prefrontal system have been identified, in clinical practice lesions are seldom confined to any one of these systems. As a result, patients are likely to manifest the clinical features of more than one of the symptom clusters defined in the subsequent text. With this in mind, three distinct dysexecutive syndromes have been identified (see Table 11.1).
1. **Disorganized type.** The high-level cognitive functions mediated by the dorsolateral prefrontal lobe and its connections include cognitive flexibility, temporal ordering of recent events, planning ahead, regulating actions based on environmental stimuli, and learning from experience. Patients exhibiting dysfunction

TABLE 11.1   Primary Clinical Features of the Regional Prefrontal Syndromes

Dorsolateral Convexity Disorganized Type	Orbitofrontal Disinhibited Type	Mesial Frontal Apathetic Type
Personality change: Disconcerted or rigid	Personality change: Crass or volatile	Personality change: Lazy or unconcerned
Poor judgment, planning, organization, and insight	Environmentally driven behavior	Limited spontaneity
		Diminished verbal output
Cognitive impersistence	Loss of social comportment	Prolonged response latency
Neglect of hygiene	Distractible	Emotionally bland
	Emotional lability	

in these cognitive domains are concrete and perseverative and show impairment in reasoning and limited mental flexibility. People who were once punctual and successful come to appear stubborn or "scattered" to acquaintances. In addition, they often will "lose set" and engage in purposeless or disorganized activities. The common denominator for these deficits appears to be metacognitive disorganization. It is therefore reasonable to refer to this cognitive and personality symptom cluster as the "dysexecutive syndrome—disorganized type."

Examples of this behavior may include slowly progressive loss of ability to manage a checking account, having utilities occasionally cut off because of nonpayment of bills, neglecting home maintenance and personal hygiene, or having a qualitatively or quantitatively limited supply of food at home. In the setting of a disorganized dysexecutive syndrome, old habits and simple patterns predominate. Hot tea and toasted bread become the *de facto* diet for many elderly people with executive cognitive impairment.

2.   **Disinhibited type.** The orbitofrontal cortex has discrete connections with paralimbic cortex and limbic structures. The orbitofrontal cortex therefore plays a role in the elaboration and integration of limbic drives. Patients with orbitofrontal pathology exhibit poor impulse control, explosive aggressive outbursts, inappropriate verbal lewdness, jocularity, and a lack of interpersonal sensitivity. Because this syndrome is characterized primarily by impulse dyscontrol it would be appropriate to describe it as the "dysexecutive syndrome—disinhibited type."

Examples of this behavior may include making unwelcome public statements about the appearance of strangers, use of vulgar language, or using inappropriate humor. This syndrome has been described as "pseudopsychopathic," and it causes great distress to caregivers who observe the loss of the premorbid personality and its evolution into crassness and vulgarity.

3.   **Apathetic type.** Mesial frontal pathology often affects the functional balance between the cingulum and the supplementary motor area. In a sense, this system represents the behavioral outflow of the executive cognitive system and these structures appear to participate in an exploratory system involving a link between motivation and action. Disruption of this neural network frequently leads to a dysmotivational picture ranging from apathy to akinetic mutism (see Chapter 1). These patients often appear outwardly depressed, yet they lack the dysphoria, negative cognitions, and neurovegetative signs of a major depression, such as anorexia or insomnia. This syndrome has also been described as "pseudodepressed." Because the predominant characteristic of this syndrome is behavioral inertia it is appropriate to describe it as the "dysexecutive syndrome—apathetic type."

Family members are often frustrated by the inertia of the apathetic patient and mistakenly interpret the patient's apathy as deliberate. The patient's emotional blunting is often erroneously perceived as a lack of caring or concern. The striking lack of spontaneity often contrasts sharply with the premorbid personality.

C. **Gastaut-Geshwind syndrome.** Electrical pathology in the brain, in the form of partial complex seizures originating in the anterior temporal lobe, may also influence personality expression. An "Epileptic Interictal Personality," also known as the Gastaut-Geschwind syndrome, has been described in which a person has a moral or religious preoccupation, diminished libido, propensity to write, verbosity, blandness, and difficulty disengaging from conversations. Attempts to further define this syndrome with the Minnesota Multiphasic Personality Inventory have revealed mixed results, with abnormalities frequently noted on the depression, paranoia, schizophrenia, and psychasthenia scales. However, this instrument does not provide a sensitive index of behavioral parameters for this clinical presentation.

Geschwind et al. hypothesized that these changes reflect an enhanced connection between temporolimbic and cortical heteromodal association areas. This "hyperconnection" could result in a heightened (right hemisphere focus) or diminished (left hemisphere focus) response to the social environment. These hypotheses remain controversial. Still, clinicians who treat patients with temporal lobe epilepsy have little doubt about the existence of interictal disorders of personality. This syndrome is not universal, however, and many patients with temporal lobe epilepsy do not demonstrate these traits.

References
1. American Psychiatric Association. *Diagnostic and statistical manual of mental disorders*, 4th ed. Text Revision. Washington, DC: American Psychiatric Association; 2000.
2. McRae RR, Costa PT. *Personality in adulthood: A five factor theory perspective.* New York, NY: The Guilford Press; 2003.
3. Cloninger CR, Svrakic DM, Przybeck TR. A psychobiological model of temperament and character. *Arch Gen Psychiatry.* 1993;50:975–990.
4. Duffy JD, Campbell JJ. The regional prefrontal syndromes: A clinical and theoretical overview. *J Neuropsychiatry Clin Neurosci.* 1994;6:379–387.
5. Waxman SG, Geschwind N. The interictal behavior syndrome of temporal lobe epilepsy. *Arch Gen Psychiatry.* 1975;32:1580–1586.

III. MANAGEMENT

A. **Principles of management.** In general, the management of personality change in patients with neurologic illness should begin with a clinical interview of the patient and collecting collateral history from an acquaintance or family member. The clinician should then conduct a formal assessment of mental status and cognition, a sensorimotor examination, relevant laboratory and neuroimaging studies, and a biopsychosocial formulation and treatment plan.
   1. **Perform a diagnostic evaluation**
      a. The diagnosis of personality change in patients with neurologic illness is especially challenging. Personality change

secondary to a neurologic illness is a *diagnosis of exclusion* and should be offered only when delirium, and other mood, anxiety, and substance use disorders have been ruled out.

b. The clinical interview should establish as clearly as possible the change in the patient's premorbid personality. While self-report scales have been developed to assess personality, temperament, and character, they are of limited use in this clinical situation. Patients with neurologic illness affecting personality often demonstrate lack of insight and cannot reliably complete these instruments. Further, the personality change precludes objective assessment of premorbid personality, which, in essence, no longer exists. Independent reports of spouses and other collateral informants are required to complete the picture.

c. Validated instruments can provide a useful framework for collecting data. The Five-Factor Model captures five domains of personality—*agreeableness, conscientiousness, openness to experience, extraversion,* and *neuroticism.* Alternatively, the temperament and character inventory, developed by Cloninger et al. measures seven domains of personality. Four temperament dimensions are defined—*novelty seeking, harm avoidance, reward dependence,* and *persistence.* The model defines three dimensions of character—*self-directedness, cooperativeness,* and *self-transcendence.*

d. A general physical and neurologic examination should be performed with special attention to the cognitive (including executive cognition) and motor examinations.

e. *Laboratory tests* are indicated only to confirm the presence of a general medical disorder, suspected neurologic disorder, or substance use disorder as suggested by the history or examination, or to characterize the status of a known disorder.

f. Evaluate the *safety* of the patient or caregiver. Problems with impulsive, risk-taking behavior and aggression are common dimensions of personality change that can imperil safety.

g. Evaluate the emotional status of the caregiver, who are usually under considerable stress and may require individualized interventions.

2. **Implement a biopsychosocial treatment plan**
   a. Determine and continually evaluate the *treatment setting* (inpatient vs. outpatient) based on the patient's clinical status, safety, available support systems, ability to care adequately for self, and willingness and ability to cooperate with treatment plan.
   b. While few evidence-based treatments exist for personality change secondary to neurologic illness, I recommend a biopsychosocial model that is, the combined use of appropriate biological (somatic) treatments (including acute phase and continuation or maintenance phase treatment),

psychological treatments, and social interventions. Develop contingency plans with caregivers for dealing with acute situations such as aggression or violence.

c.   Evaluate and address functional impairments in interpersonal relationships, work and living conditions, and other health-related needs.

d.   Provide education and support to patient, family, and caregivers.

e.   Enhance treatment adherence by simplifying the treatment regimen, minimizing the cost of the treatment, minimizing side effects, and identifying relevant community support services.

f.   *Coordinate the care* with other clinicians. Patients with a neurologic disorder will typically be receiving care from multiple clinicians, including an internist, a neurologist or neurosurgeon, a rehabilitation medicine specialist, a physical therapist, or speech therapist. Coordination of care among these many providers is essential to ensure that the care is safe and effective.

IV. PERSONALITY CHANGE IN PATIENTS WITH NEUROLOGIC ILLNESS

A.   **Alzheimer disease**

1.   **Clinical background**

a.   Personality change in Alzheimer disease (AD) is almost universal and occurs early, often preceding the clinical diagnosis. Personality changes may aid in the early detection of AD, which could facilitate early treatment.

b.   The *occurrence* of personality change in AD appears to be related to premorbid personality features, with a "coarsening" of premorbid personality being reported.

c.   The *phenomenology* of personality change in AD is characterized by increases in neuroticism and decreases in extraversion and conscientiousness on the Five-Factor Model. Apathy and intellectual rigidity are common. Cognitive impairment is not a good predictor of overall personality change.

d.   **Course and prognosis.** The personality changes typically persist until late in the course of the disease, when profound apathy occurs. The changes are usually negative and cause great distress for caregivers. Being a caregiver who is experiencing stress is an independent risk factor for caregiver mortality, and caregivers under duress are less effective at meeting the needs of the patient.

2.   **Pathogenesis of personality change secondary to Alzheimer disease**

a.   The *pathophysiology* of personality change in patients with AD is not known, but may involve damage to executive cognitive neural networks and monoaminergic nuclei caused by neuritic plaques and neurofibrillary tangles. Research suggests that these personality changes may be the result of serotonergic dysfunction in areas of the brain processing emotional information.

3. **Diagnosis**

   a. The diagnosis is clinical and based on the history as provided by the patient and caregivers familiar with the patient.

   b. Clinicians may conclude a patient has personality change secondary to AD after other conditions have been excluded. Patients must be screened carefully for mood disorders such as depression. Medication side effects can affect personality and behavior. For example, dopaminergic therapy for parkinsonian symptoms can cause agitation and agents with anticholinergic properties can cause delirium. The clinician should ensure the personality change is not the result of thyroid disease or other general medical conditions. Chronic pain is associated with dysphoria and demoralization and should be adequately treated before diagnosing a personality change secondary to AD.

4. **Treatment**

   a. Optimize the physical health of the patient and ensure that all underlying general medical and neurologic disorders have been optimally treated. Caregivers should be directed to the local chapter of the Alzheimer's Association (they have a very useful website, www.alz.org).

   b. Caregivers should be instructed in the *behavioral management* of the patient's behavioral problems, including prevention and modification of the adverse behaviors by identifying triggers and developing techniques at redirecting untoward behaviors. Caregivers should be offered a combination of social support and assistance with problem solving on the basis of a systematic review by Cooke et al., which concluded that these psychosocial interventions are the most likely to improve psychological well-being.

   c. *Psychotherapeutic interventions* should be offered to the patient. Patients should be offered reality orientation therapy when they are diagnosed with personality change secondary to AD. A systematic review conducted by Specter et al. found that reality orientation has benefits for both behavior and cognition for patients with dementia of various etiologies, including AD.

   d. Optimize the use of *cholinesterase inhibitors* (see Chapter 5). I recommend initial treatment with *donepezil* on the basis of its safety and efficacy at the initial 5 mg once daily dose. Controlled data suggest that these agents may improve neuropsychiatric symptoms (including negative personality change) and functional status, as well as cognition.

   e. If problems persist after these initial steps, then *somatic therapy* should be initiated.

   f. There are no U.S. Food and Drug Administration (FDA)-approved medications for the treatment of personality disturbance in patients with AD. Choice of medication is guided by side effect profile and data regarding efficacy. Despite numerous controlled trials examining the efficacy of somatic therapy on agitation and aggression secondary to dementia of multiple etiologies, there is very little published empirical evidence for the effectiveness of any somatic therapy as a treatment for personality change in the setting of dementia. I recommend sertraline 25 to 100 mg daily on the basis of its safety profile and the results of two small randomized controlled trials showing its efficacy in treating irritability and agitation in patients with AD. If the primary personality disturbance is apathy (in the absence of depression) then I recommend methylphenidate 2.5 to 15 mg twice daily on the basis of a small series of "N of 1" trials published by Jansen, et al. Patients with a history of cardiac disease, including arrhythmia, should be evaluated by a cardiologist before starting methylphenidate.

References

1. Cooke DD, McNally L, Mulligan KT, et al. Psychosocial interventions for caregivers of people with dementia: A systematic review. *Aging Ment Health*. 2001;5(2):120–135.
2. Finkel SI, Mintzer JE, Dysken M, et al. A randomized, placebo-controlled study of the efficacy and safety of sertraline in the treatment of the behavioral manifestations of Alzheimer's disease in outpatients treated with donepezil. *Int J Ger Psychiatry*. 2004;19:9–18.
3. Jansen IH, Olde Rikkert MG, Hulsbos HA, et al. Towards individualized evidence-based medicine: Five "N of 1" trials of methylphenidate in geriatric patients. *J Am Geriatrics Soc*. 2001;49(4):474–476.
4. Lanctot KL, Herrmann N, van Reekum R, et al. Gender, aggression and serotonergic function are associated with response to sertraline for behavioral disturbances in Alzheimer's disease. *Int J Ger Psychiatry*. 2002;17(6):531–541.
5. Mittleman MS, Ferris SH, Shulman E, et al. A comprehensive support program: Effect on depression in spouse-caregivers of AD patients. *Gerontologist*. 1995;35(6):792–802.
6. Purandare N, Bloom C, Page S, et al. The effect of anticholinesterases on personality changes in Alzheimer's disease. *Aging Ment Health*. 2002;6:350–354.
7. Spector A, Davies S, Woods B, et al. Reality orientation for dementia: A systematic review of the evidence of effectiveness from randomized, controlled trials. *Gerontologist*. 2000;40(2):206–212.

B. **Lenticulostriatal disorders (e.g., Huntington disease, Wilson disease)**
   1. **Clinical background**
      a. Personality changes are common in lenticulostriatal disorders and have significant clinical consequences. The *prevalence* of personality changes in lenticulostriate disorders

can be as high as 100%. Many patients receive a psychiatric evaluation before diagnosis.

b. The *occurrence* of personality change in lenticulostriatal disorders may reflect an acceleration and coarsening of changes otherwise expected to occur much later in life.

c. The *phenomenology* of personality change in lenticulostriatal disorders is typically characterized by increases in apathy, depression, and irritability. Aggressive behaviors are common and troubling with lenticulostriatal disorders such as Huntington disease (HD) or Wilson disease. Although not a primary lenticulostriatal disorder, Parkinson disease has been associated with apathy.

d. **Course and prognosis.** The personality changes typically persist until late in the course of the disease, when extrapyramidal motor symptoms predominate. These changes lead to unsafe and often antisocial behaviors, including assault and homicide, that frequently require hospitalization.

2. **Pathogenesis of personality change secondary to lenticulostriate disorders**

a. The *pathophysiology* of personality change in patients with lenticulostriate disorders may relate to reduced ventrobasal striatal glucose metabolism and orbitofrontal dysregulation in HD. Lesions of the putamen and globus pallidum correlate with personality changes in Wilson disease.

3. **Diagnosis**

a. The diagnosis is clinical and based on the history as provided by the patient and caregivers familiar with the patient. The diagnosis of a lenticulostriatal disorder is often difficult early in the course of the disease until more classical neurologic and somatic signs occur.

b. Clinicians may diagnose personality change secondary to a lenticulostriate disorder after other conditions have been excluded. Depression, a very common complication of lenticulostriate disorders, should be thoroughly evaluated and treated. Other medical conditions that can cause or mimic mood disorders, such as thyroid disease, should be ruled out. The presence of substance abuse confounds the diagnosis of personality change secondary to a lenticulostriatal disorder. Chronic pain, if present, should be adequately treated before diagnosing a personality change secondary to a lenticulostriatal disorder.

c. Personality changes may arise directly from medications used to treat motor aspects of lenticulostriate disorders. Dopaminergic therapies for parkinsonian symptoms can be associated with significant behavioral toxicity in the form of agitation, psychosis, and aggression. Pramipexole has been implicated in the development of pathologic gambling. Antipsychotic medications can produce a dysphoric, apathetic state manifesting as a personality change. Apathy may be worsened in patients with Parkinson disease treated with subthalamic nucleus stimulation.

4. **Treatment**

   a. Optimize the physical health of the patient and ensure that all underlying general medical disorders, including mood disorders and substance abuse, have been optimally treated. Caregivers should be directed to the HD Society of America (www.hdsa.org), the Wilson disease Association (www.wilsonsdisease.org), or the Parkinson Disease Foundation (www.pdf.org).

   b. It is essential to *coordinate the care* with other clinicians. Patients with lenticulostriate disorders should receive care from a neurologist. Somatic therapies for movement disorders often adversely affect personality and behavior. Somatic therapies that improve behavior often cause extrapyramidal symptoms. This can place the neuropsychiatrist at odds with the movement disorders specialist, leaving the patient and caregiver stuck in the middle. To optimize the quality of life for the patient and caregiver, the neuropsychiatrist, neurologist, patient, and caregiver need to agree on the best course of treatment, balancing the often unavoidable need to sacrifice some motor improvement to improve behavior, or vice versa. Other care providers can include rehabilitation medicine specialists, physical therapists, occupational therapists, speech and swallowing specialists, and home health nurses. Input from these providers is necessary to ensure that the treatment of personality change secondary to a lenticulostriatal disorder is optimal.

   c. Caregivers should be instructed in the *behavioral management* of the patient's behavioral problems, including prevention and, when possible, modification of the adverse behaviors. Contingency plans should be developed for violent behavior, including acute psychiatric hospitalization and seeking police assistance if necessary.

   d. *Psychotherapeutic interventions* for patients or caregivers have not been formally studied. However, early in the course of the disease psychotherapy should be useful to aid patients and caregivers in coping with the disease, particularly HD, which is progressive and unrelenting. The literature does not identify any specific type of psychotherapy that can be recommended on the basis of efficacy. Therefore, nonspecific factors, such as convenience and availability for the patient and caregiver, and their satisfaction with the therapy, will be important considerations when deciding to refer a patient for psychotherapy.

   e. Despite the almost universal occurrence of psychiatric symptoms in lenticulostriate disorders, there are few published investigations of the effectiveness of *somatic therapies* for personality change secondary to lenticulostriate disorders and no FDA-approved medications for the treatment of secondary personality disturbance. No definitive conclusions can be drawn. Choice of medication is based primarily on safety, side effect profile, and data regarding efficacy.

f. *Sertraline* at doses of 50 to 100 mg daily is a safe and well-tolerated initial treatment for irritability and agitation in the setting of lenticulostriate disorders. *Sertraline* was an effective treatment in two consecutive cases of severe aggression in HD. I recommend a trial of sertraline for similar symptoms secondary to other lenticulostriate disorders, such as Wilson disease, where no literature exists. In case reports, *propranolol* has been shown to reduce aggression secondary to HD. Long-acting propranolol capsules should be started at 60 mg daily and increased weekly by 60 mg increments, as tolerated, until the target symptoms improve sufficiently or side effects such as symptomatic hypotension occur. Doses up to 800 mg daily have been useful, this titration may occur over several weeks before success is achieved. *Atypical antipsychotics* may be useful, given their effectiveness in treating symptoms of agitation and aggression in the general psychiatric population, ability to diminish choreiform movements, and lower incidence of parkinsonian side effects. Olanzapine, at doses up to 30 mg, has been shown to improve motor symptoms of HD. While no effect on personality change and behavior has been studied, it is reasonable to initiate an olanzapine trial if other somatic treatments have not been successful for a lenticulostriate disorder. Aggression can be a significant complication of lenticulostriate disorders and must be treated to lower the risk of violence. *Antikindling anticonvulsants* such as valproic acid or carbamazepine have been shown to effectively treat aggression in a variety of neuropsychiatric populations although controlled trials for lenticulostriate disorders are lacking. Valproic acid can be started at a dose of 250 mg daily and increased over several days to 250 mg three times daily as side effects of sedation and gastrointestinal disturbance permit. Valproic acid may be further increased every 3 or 4 days by 250 mg increments until the target symptoms are sufficiently improved or intolerable side effects appear. Carbamazepine may be started at 200 mg daily and increased by 200 mg increments every 3 or 4 days up to 800 mg twice daily as tolerated. Chelation therapy for Wilson disease has a mixed psychiatric outcome. Psychiatric sequelae resolve more often in patients without dysarthria, behavior dyscontrol, or hepatic symptoms. Irritability appears particularly refractory to chelation. *Methylphenidate* has been shown to successfully treat apathy in a variety of neuropsychiatric conditions although no controlled trials have been conducted for Parkinson disease. On the basis of a single case report, *methylphenidate*, begun at

5 mg twice daily, can be recommended to treat clinically significant apathy secondary to Parkinson disease. Patients with a history of cardiac disease, including arrhythmia, should be referred to a cardiologist before starting methylphenidate.

References

1. Akil M, Schwartz JA, Dutchak D, et al. The psychiatric presentation of Wilson's disease. *J Neuropsychiatry Clin Neurosci.* 1991;3:377–382.

2. Cummings JL. Behavioral and psychiatric symptoms associated with Huntington's disease. *Adv Neurol.* 1995; 65:179–186.

3. Kuwert T, Lange HW, Langen K-J, et al. Cerebral glucose consumption measured by PET in patients with or without psychiatric symptoms of Huntington's disease. *Psychiatry Res.* 1989;29:361–362.

4. Lindenmayer JP, Kotsaftis A. Use of sodium valproate in violent and aggressive behaviors: A critical review. *J Clin Psychiatry.* 2000;61(2):123–128.

5. Oder W, Prayer L, Grimm G, et al. Wilson's disease: Evidence of subgroups derived from findings and brain lesions. *Neurology.* 1993;43:120–124.

6. Paleacu D, Anca M, Giladi N. Olanzapine in Huntington's disease. *Acta Neurologica Scand.* 2002;105(6): 441–444.

7. Ranen NG, Lipsey JR, Treisman G, et al. Sertraline in the treatment of severe aggressiveness in Huntington's disease. *J Neuropsychiatry Clin Neurosci.* 1996;8:338–340.

8. Stewart JT. Huntington's disease and propranolol. *Am J Psychiatry.* 1993;150:166–167.

C. **Multiple sclerosis**

1. **Clinical background**

a. Personality change in multiple sclerosis (MS) has been reported since 1926, when Cottrell and Wilson examined 100 consecutive outpatients and noted unusual cheerfulness and optimism. However, controversy exists and other studies discern no particular personality change to distinguish MS from other central nervous system disorders.

b. The *occurrence* of personality changes in MS does not appear to be related to premorbid personality characteristics. Controlled trials demonstrate divergent conclusions. Philopousis et al. found only 55% of MS patients had good premorbid social functioning compared with 85% of controls.

c. The *phenomenology* of reported personality changes in MS is characterized by elevations in neuroticism and diminished agreeableness, empathy, and conscientiousness when the five-factor personality inventory is used as an assessment tool for patients and informants. These personality changes were associated with executive cognitive dysfunction.

d. **Course and prognosis.** The course of the personality changes is not known. One hypothesis, as yet unproved, proposes that the emotional stress of these personality changes may precipitate exacerbations of the disease and lead to worse neurologic outcomes.

2. **Pathogenesis of personality change secondary to multiple sclerosis**

   a. The *pathophysiology* of personality change in patients with MS is not well established. The presence of demyelination in emotional and executive cognitive neural networks is strongly suspected to affect personality. This is supported by studies that correlate personality changes to cognitive dysfunction.

3. **Diagnosis**

   a. The diagnosis is clinical and based on the history as provided by the patient and caregivers familiar with the patient. Early in the course of the disease, the diagnosis of MS is often delayed until more classical neurologic signs occur.

   b. Clinicians may diagnose personality change secondary to MS after other conditions have been excluded. Depression is a common complication of MS and is also a side effect of immunomodulators used to treat MS. Depression should be thoroughly evaluated and treated. Other medical conditions that can cause or mimic mood disorders, such as thyroid disease, should be ruled out. The presence of substance abuse confounds the diagnosis of personality change secondary to MS. Chronic pain, if present, should be adequately treated before the diagnosis is made.

4. **Treatment**

   a. Optimize the physical health of the patient and ensure that all underlying general medical disorders have been optimally treated. Carefully review the patient's medications.

   b. It is essential to *coordinate the care* with other clinicians. Patients with MS should be receiving care from a neurologist. Somatic therapies for MS often adversely affect personality and behavior. Interferon-β can cause severe depression with suicide attempts. Glatiramer acetate can cause anxiety. Mitoxantrone can cause fatigue that could be misdiagnosed as apathy or depression. Methylprednisolone can cause depression, euphoria, or psychosis. To optimize the quality of life for the patient and caregiver, the neuropsychiatrist, neurologist, patient, and caregiver need to agree on the best course of treatment, balancing the need to prevent disease progression with the need to minimize neuropsychiatric side effects. Other care providers can include rehabilitation medicine specialists, physical therapists, occupational therapists, speech and swallowing specialists, and home health nurses. Input from these providers is necessary to ensure the treatment of personality change secondary to MS is optimal.

   c. Educate the patient and caregivers about the disease and its effects on nonmotor functions such as cognition, mood, and personality. The National Multiple Sclerosis Society has a very useful website for patients and families at www.nmss.org.

d. Caregivers should be instructed in the *behavioral management* of the patient's behavioral problems, including prevention and modification of the adverse behaviors. For example, reducing noise and stimulation and communicating clearly and calmly can assist a patient who has trouble tolerating frustration and filtering sensory stimuli.

e. *Psychotherapeutic interventions* should always be considered for a patient with MS. I recommend individual cognitive behavioral therapy based on one small ($n = 41$) controlled trial showing lower perceived stress and improved coping in patients given cognitive behavioral therapy.

f. *Somatic therapy* for personality change in MS has not been formally studied. Patients having *unusual cheerfulness and optimism* would not be expected to require somatic therapy. Treatment for *depression* secondary to MS or immunomodulation therapy for MS is reviewed elsewhere in this handbook. *Executive dysfunction* has been associated with elevations in neuroticism and diminished agreeableness, empathy, and conscientiousness. Improvements in executive function were demonstrated in a 12-week open label trial of donepezil. I recommend a trial of donepezil begun at 5 mg daily for 4 weeks, then at 10 mg daily with a reassessment of the patient's symptoms of personality change and executive cognition at 12 weeks. At that point the treatment may be continued if improvements are noted.

References

1. Benedict RH, Carone DA, Bakshi R. Correlating brain atrophy with cognitive dysfunction, mood disturbances, and personality disorder in MS. *J Neuroimaging*. 2004; 14(Suppl 3):36–45.
2. Benedict RH, Priore RL, Miller C, et al. Personality disorder in multiple sclerosis correlates with cognitive impairment. *J Neuropsychiatry Clin Neurosci*. 2001; 13:70–76.
3. Cottrell SS, Wilson SAK. The affective symptomatology of disseminated sclerosis: A study of 100 cases. *J Neurology Psychopathol*. 1926;7:1–30.
4. Foley FW, Bedell JR, LaRocca NG, et al. Efficacy of stress-inoculation training in coping with multiple sclerosis. *J Consult Clin Psychol*. 1987;55:919–922.
5. Greene YM, Tariot PN, Wishart H, et al. A 12-week, open trial of donepezil hydrochloride in patients with multiple sclerosis and associated cognitive impairments. *J Clin Psychopharmacology*. 2000;20(3):350–356.
6. Phillopousis GS, Wittkower ED, Cousineau A. The etiologic significance of emotional factors in onset and exacerbation of multiple sclerosis. *Psychosomatic Med*. 1958;20:458–474.

7. Minden SL. Psychotherapy for people with multiple sclerosis. *J Neuropsychiatry Clin Neurosci.* 1992;4: 198–213.

D. Traumatic brain injury

1. **Clinical background**

    a. Personality change is a common sequela of TBI, occurring in 40% to 80% of patients in published reports.

    b. The *occurrence* of personality change secondary to TBI is more likely with increasing severity of injury.

    c. The *phenomenology* of personality change secondary to TBI is characterized by emotional lability to be the most common change, followed by aggression and disinhibition, apathy, and paranoia.

    d. **Course and prognosis.** The personality changes resolve slowly in a minority of patients over a period of years. Thomsen reported that 65% of adults, identified as having personality change following TBI, remained symptomatic after 10 to 15 years of follow up. These changes can be significant and often prevent affected individuals from returning to work and interfered with positive interpersonal relationships.

2. **Pathogenesis of personality change secondary to traumatic brain injury**

    a. The *pathophysiology* of personality change in patients with TBI is the result of mechanical trauma to emotional and executive cognitive neural networks in the prefrontal–subcortical system.

3. **Diagnosis**

    a. The diagnosis is clinical and based on the history as provided by the patient and caregivers familiar with the patient.

    b. Clinicians may conclude that a patient has personality change secondary to TBI after other conditions have been excluded. Patients must be screened carefully for mood disorders such as depression. Insomnia is a common sequela of TBI that should be treated before diagnosing a personality change. Posttraumatic epilepsy should also be thoroughly evaluated and treated. Medication side effects commonly affect the personality and behavior of patients with TBI. Antiepileptic medications and agents with anticholinergic properties can cause delirium. The clinician should ensure that the personality change is not the result of substance abuse, thyroid disease, or other general medical conditions. Chronic pain, often secondary to headache, is associated with dysphoria and demoralization and should be adequately treated before diagnosing a personality change secondary to TBI.

4. **Treatment**

    a. Optimize the physical health of the patient and ensure that all underlying general medical and underlying neurologic

disorders, such as posttraumatic epilepsy have been optimally treated.

b. It is essential to *coordinate the care* with other clinicians. Patients with posttraumatic seizures should be receiving care
from a neurologist. Somatic therapies for seizure disorders
often adversely affect personality and behavior. This complication can place the neuropsychiatrist at odds with the
epilepsy specialist, leaving the patient and caregiver stuck
in the middle. To optimize the quality of life for the patient
and caregiver, the neuropsychiatrist, neurologist, patient,
and caregiver need to agree on the best course of treatment, balancing the need to prevent seizures with the need
to optimize behavior. Other care providers can include
rehabilitation medicine specialists, physical therapists, occupational therapists, and home health nurses. Input from
these providers is necessary to ensure that the treatment of
personality change secondary to a TBI is optimal.

c. Caregivers should be instructed in the *behavioral management*
of the patient's behavioral problems, including prevention
and modification of adverse behaviors. For example, as with
other neuropsychiatric conditions, reducing noise and stimulation, and communicating clearly and calmly can assist
a patient who has trouble tolerating frustration and filtering sensory stimuli. Contingency plans should always be
developed for violent behavior, including acute psychiatric
hospitalization and seeking police assistance if necessary.

d. *Psychotherapeutic interventions* should also be offered to
the patient. Psychotherapy is often impeded by cognitive
impairments and difficulty tolerating strong emotions. Behavioral interventions may be helpful in this population in
modifying untoward behaviors. Patients having problems
with anger management should be offered a cognitive behavioral intervention, based on a controlled trial by Medd
and Tate demonstrating its efficacy.

e. Optimize the use of *cholinesterase inhibitors* (see Chapter 5).
I recommend initial treatment with *donepezil* on the basis of
its safety and efficacy at the initial 5 mg once daily dose.
Controlled data suggest that these agents may improve neuropsychiatric symptoms (including fatigue and diminished
initiation) and functional status, as well as cognition.

f. If problems persist after these behaviors, then *somatic therapy*
should be initiated. There are no FDA-approved medications for the treatment of personality disturbance in patients
with TBI. Patients with TBI are often sensitive to the side
effects of medications. Therefore, beginning with lower
doses and slowly titrating the dosage upward is the optimal approach. Randomized, placebo-controlled trials for
neuropsychiatric sequela of TBI are rare in general and
nonexistent for aspects of personality change.

g. I recommend a trial of amantadine titrated to 100 mg three times daily if *apathy or abulia* are present, based on its safety profile and a single "N of 1" double blind, placebo-controlled study showing benefits across four independent raters. Anticonvulsants have been shown to be helpful in reducing *aggressive behavior* in TBI. Carbamazepine is recommended on the basis of two reports, an open label case series of 7 patients with acute TBI who showed a good response (Chatham–Showalter), and an open label trial showing subjective improvement in 12 of 14 patients with chronic TBI receiving carbamazepine (Persinger). Effective doses ranged from 200 mg PO b.i.d. to 300 mg PO t.i.d. Valproic acid is a generally well-tolerated alternative for patients who do not respond adequately to a trial of carbamazepine. Valproic acid is recommended on the basis of an open label case series showing striking efficacy in reducing aggression in five patients with TBI (Wroblewski et al.). Finally, buspirone has been shown to be helpful in reducing agitation and aggression in neuropsychiatric populations including TBI. Ratey et al. have shown effectiveness at doses as high as 60 mg. Patients occasionally develop transient worsening of symptoms when starting this drug.

References

1. Chatham-Showalter PE. Carbamazepine for combativeness in acute traumatic brain injury. *J Neuropsychiatry Clin Neurosci.* 1996;8(1):96–99.
2. Franzen MD, Lovell MR. Cognitive rehabilitation and behavior therapy for patients with neuropsychiatric disorders. In: Yudofsky SC, Hales RE, eds. *Textbook of neuropsychiatry and clinical neurosciences*, 4th ed. Washington, DC: American Psychiatric Press; 2002:1237–1253.
3. Katz IR, Jeste DV, Mintzer JE, et al. Comparison of risperidone and placebo for psychosis and behavioral disturbances associated with dementia: A randomized, double-blind trial. *J Clin Psychiatry.* 1999;60:107–115.
4. Max JE, Robertson BA, Lansing AE. The phenomenology of personality change due to traumatic brain injury in children and adolescents. *J Neuropsychiatry Clin Neurosci.* 2001;13:161–170.
5. Medd J, Tate RL. Evaluation of an anger management programme following acquired brain injury: A preliminary study. *Neuropsychol Rehab.* 2000;10(2):185–201.
6. Persinger MA. Subjective improvement following treatment with carbamazepine (Tegretol) for a subpopulation of patients with traumatic brain injuries. *Percept Motor Skills.* 2000;90(1):37–40.
7. Ratey JJ, Leveroni CL, Miller AC, et al. Low dose buspirone to treat agitation and maladaptive behavior in brain-injured patients: Two case reports. *J Clin Psychopharm.* 1992;12(5):362–364.

8. Tenovuo O. Central anticholinesterase inhibitors in the treatment of chronic traumatic brain injury—clinical experience in 111 patients. *Prog in Neuropsychopharm Biol Psychiatry.* 2005;29(1):61–67.

9. Thomsen IV. Late outcome of very severe blunt head trauma: A 10–15 year second follow up. *J Neurol Neurosurg Neuropsychiatry.* 1984;47:260–268.

10. Van Reekum R, Bayler M, Garner S, et al. N of 1 study: Amantadine for the amotivational syndrome in a patient with a traumatic brain injury. *Brain Inj.* 1995;9(1):49–53.

11. Wroblewski BA, Joseph AB, Kupfer J, et al. Effectiveness of valproic acid on destructive and aggressive behaviours in patients with acquired brain injury. *Brain Inj.* 1997;11(1):37–47.

Chapter 1.

PAIN

Kevin J. Black

I. BACKGROUND

A. Pain as a neuropsychiatric phenomenon

1. Pain is defined as "an unpleasant sensory and emotional experience associated with actual or potential tissue damage, or described in terms of such damage." Pain "is always a psychological state" and "is always subjective".[1]

2. As this definition notes, pain is much more than a pure sensory phenomenon. Rather, pain is a very complex phenomenon that involves every level of the nervous system from primary sense organs through association and limbic cortex. In fact, it has been observed that the great irony of pain is that it is primarily mediated by an organ that has no nociceptors (the brain).

3. **Components of pain.** Consider the pain felt when a finger comes too close to a hot stove. Listed in the subsequent text are some of the components that contribute to the perception of pain in this situation.

   a. **Detection.** Sufficient heat activates small diameter nerve fibers in the skin that send signals through the spinal cord and thalamus to primary sensory cortex.

   b. **Tissue responses.** A burn that produces tissue damage may provoke inflammation or other responses that themselves produce ongoing activation of sensory, including pain, fibers.

   c. **Gating.** Some pain signals are blocked, for instance, at the spinal cord, before ever reaching the brain.

   d. **Attention.** Common experience shows that distraction can prevent our noticing an injury in some situations, whereas staring at the burned finger and thinking about it can worsen the perception of pain.

   e. **Sensory illusions.** Analogous to optical illusions, somatic sensory illusions demonstrate how the brain (mis) interprets the actual physical environment. For instance, an alternating grid of cool and warm metal contacts appropriately spaced can produce the sensation of pain although the cool contacts themselves are not painfully cold and the warm contacts alone are not painfully hot.

f. **Cognition.** Someone who has burned his finger many times may benefit from the knowledge that a burn of a certain severity is not likely to cause permanent damage and that the pain is transient. By contrast, an individual with a severe burn in the past may erroneously predict a higher severity of pain or consequent disability than actually occurs, thereby affecting the degree of attention to the sensation and the affective response.

g. **Emotion.** Fear, worry, anxiety, and sadness intensify the perceived severity of pain.

h. **Societal responses.** Adults who observe someone incurring a first-degree burn from the stove tend to respond very differently depending on whether the unfortunate party is a 5-year-old or a 35-year-old. After acute painful injury, others' sympathies are engaged and they may provide help, such as fetching things from across the room. Physicians also respond in various ways, such as provision of medications or certification of disability. Whether these societal responses can be helpful or not depends on the situation.

4. Importantly, these components of pain allow useful treatment interventions at several levels, from local anesthesia to physical therapy to family therapy.

5. We rely on patient report for assessment and measurement of pain. Many excellent questionnaires and rating scales are available to facilitate description of pain and monitoring of therapy.

6. **Types of pain.** There are numerous types of pain that probably represent distinct mechanisms both at the peripheral (nociceptors) and central (brain) levels. For instance, visceral pain (e.g., duodenal ulcer) differs substantially from acute skin pain (e.g., paper cut). Various other distinctions can be made where different pain syndromes differ qualitatively as well as in spatial and temporal distribution (e.g., migraine, pharyngitis, angina, pleurisy, dysuria, childbirth, and various types of superficial lesions, such as accompany burn, stab, crush, or freeze injuries).

B. **Pain as an adaptive response**

1. **Pain can be useful.** Pain leads us, *now*, to withdraw a hand that gets too near a hot stove and, *later*, to stay a little farther from the stove next time we cook. A sunburn may prompt us to move into the shade as it develops and may encourage more liberal use of sunscreen the next time we visit the beach. Pain can keep us from putting too much weight on a sprained ankle. In fact, patients with impaired pain perception risk severe injury.

2. **Pain is not always useful.** The examples in the preceding text are of acute pain with a clear, modifiable, external cause. In other situations, pain is less useful. After diagnosis, pain in a cancer patient is not often helpful to the patient. Similarly, pain that lingers for years after an acute back injury usually does not benefit the patient.

3. Both patients and doctors often develop maladaptive responses to pain. These responses do not necessarily reflect evil intent on either part; in fact they are often benevolent but misguided responses.

C. Pain is a major public health problem
1. Back pain alone is one of the five most common reasons for visits to a physician.
2. Neck pain is estimated to disable over 4% of all adults in Saskatchewan.
3. Indirect costs such as disability payments and lost work account for about half of the estimated costs of chronic pain.
4. The annual cost of low back pain in the United States was estimated at $100 billion.
5. Back pain has been estimated to consume 2% of the entire gross national product of the Netherlands.
6. Medical and disability costs of just 95 Irish patients attending a multidisciplinary pain clinic totaled £1.9 million, with £1.5 million attributed to 22 younger, unemployed patients.

II. PREVALENCE

A. Exact prevalence of many pain syndromes is hard to determine confidently because of variable definitions and methods.
B. Acute pain is ubiquitous.
C. Subacute pain is also very common. Low back pain "on most days for at least 2 weeks" occurs at some point in at least one seventh of the population.
D. Chronic benign pain (no identifiable dangerous substrate) has been estimated to occur in up to 40% of the population.
E. Approximately 15% to 20% of women of childbearing age have chronic pelvic pain.
F. Occurrence of pain appears to be relatively similar in different cultures (with some important differences). However, medical care seeking and disability vary substantially across cultures.

III. ETIOLOGY AND PATHOPHYSIOLOGY

A. **Nociception.** Pain related to identifiable stimuli begins with stimulation of nociceptors in skin, viscera, and other organs. Small-diameter neurons activated by these nociceptors synapse in the dorsal horn of the spinal cord, where local interneurons can modulate signal transmission to the brain. Pain signals from the dorsal horn proceed to the thalamus through the contralateral spinothalamic tract but also to the medulla, brainstem, and hypothalamus.
B. **Central pain anatomy.**[2] Sensory thalamic nuclei pass pain signals to primary and secondary somatosensory (S2) cortex. However, neuroimaging studies have revealed that other brain regions such as anterior cingulate cortex and insula are at least equally involved in the perception of pain. The anterior cingulate, insula, S2 and thalamus are most commonly involved. The posterior insula is needed to represent basic features of pain including intensity,

whereas the anterior insula has a demonstrable role in emotional and learned effects on pain perception. Many investigators have discussed a lateral and a medial pain pathway, the lateral representing more sensory and discriminative processes and the medial pathway subserving affective and cognitive influences. Both pathways can be activated in the absence of nociceptive stimuli, for example by empathy for pain in others.

C. **Descending influences.** Specific brainstem nuclei reciprocally innervate the dorsal horn and send descending influences that enhance or suppress pain. Abnormal function of these descending pathways has been demonstrated in animal models of sensitization to pain and more recently in a human functional magnetic resonance imaging (fMRI) study of secondary hyperalgesia. Descending modulatory influences of higher centers are harder to study, but recent studies have suggested that thalamus, hypothalamus, amygdala, and limbic and prefrontal cortical areas can all modulate the perception of painful stimuli.

D. **Neurotransmitters.** Opioid analgesics exert their effects at μ-subtype opioid receptors in the dorsal horn and at other central nervous system (CNS) sites. Cyclo-oxegenase (COX) enzymes are inhibited by nonselective COX inhibitors (such as aspirin) and by selective COX-2 inhibitors. These agents can decrease tissue inflammation in addition to direct central effects. Other neurotransmitters with a significant role in pain perception or treatment include norepinephrine (centrally acting drugs can reduce pain), glutamate (through N-methyl-D-asparate [NMDA] receptors), dopamine (involved in central pain processing), and γ-aminobutyric acid (GABA) (agonists act at GABA receptors in the dorsal horn).

E. **Changes in pain pathways in chronic pain.** Pain can actually modify the body system that perceives it, sometimes leading to changes that sustain a long-term painful response to an initially transient injury. Chronic pain affects the nervous system at all levels. Patients with chronic pain show increased sensitivity to various visceral and peripheral painful stimuli, and activate pain-related brain nuclei in a different manner than do healthy controls. One fascinating recent study of patients with chronic back pain found a 5% to 11% decrease in brain gray matter volume, most obvious in dorsolateral prefrontal cortex and thalamus, and correlating significantly with duration of chronic pain.

F. Psychological and social contributors to chronic pain
1. Patient and physician beliefs and expectations about pain are often incorrect and have been shown to affect recovery.
2. Compensation (on average) prolongs disability. In one study of patients with back pain, the average time off work was 14.9 months for strain injuries incurred at work, versus only 3.6 months for strain injuries incurred away from work.

IV. DIAGNOSIS AND DIFFERENTIAL DIAGNOSIS

A. **Diagnostic evaluation**
1. **Medical history**

    a. Typical medical historical elements include the following:
- (1) Onset, location, quality, severity
- (2) Timing of pain, associated features, activities that aggravate or relieve the pain
- (3) Psychiatric history
- (4) Substance use history
- (5) Past medical and surgical history, family history, review of systems

    b. Additional useful information includes the following:
- (1) Patient's fears
- (2) Patient's expectations from the doctor for diagnostic workup and treatment
- (3) Social history including work history (in children, school attendance), presence of current litigation or disability applications, social supports
- (4) Quantification of pain severity
  - (a) A simple bedside question is "please rate the severity of your pain from zero (no pain) to ten".
  - (b) More comprehensive pain measures are available as described in reference 3.

2. **Physical examination.** This will be guided by the specific pain complaints (e.g., pelvic pain vs. headache) and includes routine mental status examination. For select patients one can include additional steps, such as quantification of function or observation without patient's awareness (e.g., in the waiting room).

3. **Diagnostic laboratory, neurophysiologic and imaging studies.** Whether or which laboratory studies are performed depends on the specific pain complaints. Generally such procedures should be limited to assessing for specific hypothesized diagnoses that fit the history and examination, especially dangerous or highly treatable disorders.

4. **Placebo challenge.** Placebo response is generally *not* a helpful diagnostic tool because healthy individuals have robust and physiologically mediated responses to placebos, for example in studies of tooth extraction or appendectomy pain. Therefore the positive predictive value of placebo response is low (American Pain Society Position Statement).[4]

B. **Differential diagnosis.** Pain in cancer patients is common and a major determinant of quality of life, and is often discussed separately from other pain syndromes. A useful distinction for diagnosis and treatment of other pain syndromes is acute versus chronic pain. Because neuropsychiatrists are less often involved in the management of acute pain or cancer pain, after a brief summary the remainder of this chapter will focus on chronic pain.

V. CANCER PAIN AND ACUTE PAIN

A. In cancer and terminal illness, the goal of pain management is usually relief of suffering and there is less concern for long-term side effects.

B. A large part of medical education and training is devoted to diagnosis and management of acute illness.

C. In both these settings, several risks of opioid medication are minimized, and these are often the most appropriate treatment. Despite substantial educational efforts, studies continue to find that pain is often undertreated in both cancer care and acute medical care settings.

D. The American Pain Society recently published guidelines for management of acute pain and cancer pain.[5]

VI. CHRONIC PAIN

A. **General principles**

1. Change of emphasis—As pain becomes chronic, the approach to patient management must change from what is useful in the acute pain setting.

   a. Curative to rehabilitative—The following quote admirably describes this shift in emphasis: "An analogy to other chronic diseases must be drawn. A diabetic has an incurable condition but patients with diabetes can minimize the effects of the disease by making the right choices—eating properly, foot care, etc. Conversely, they can jeopardize their health and increase chances for diabetic complications by making poor choices. Similarly, those with chronic pain can make choices to magnify their painful experience or mitigate it. To use a phrase from a family practitioner friend of mine: The pain is there—misery and suffering are optional. ... We (medical professionals) must act as guides to help each patient live a good life despite experiencing chronic pain as opposed to living in misery with it."[6] Patients taught that it is okay to return to work before pain completely remits are more likely to have successful treatment outcomes.

   b. Sensory to functional—The focus must shift more to what the patient is able to do than exclusively on the presence and severity of pain.

   c. Diagnostic to surveillance—After initial diagnostic workup indicated by the history and physical examination, the risk–benefit ratio increases quickly for repeated or invasive diagnostic studies, but continued observation is appropriate for new symptoms or signs that may clarify management.

   d. Subspecialty to collaborative—Care must be coordinated by a single physician to avoid mixed messages and unintentional drug interactions, yet collaboration with psychology, physical therapy, psychiatry, anesthesiology, and neurosurgery can be extremely helpful.

2. Collaboration with the patient—One of the most important aspects of managing chronic pain is establishing reasonable treatment goals on which the patient and physician can agree. Identifying and specifically addressing patients' expectations and fears are important.

3. Chronic use of opioid analgesics raises the risk–benefit ratio because of the development of physiologic tolerance.

4. Treat comorbid illness including anxiety and mood disorders.
5. The choice of specific strategies is debated. Generally, if pain and disability are mild, treatment begins with simpler, better proven, safer, and less expensive modalities. Combination therapies or invasive treatments are used for pain associated with greater impairment or lack of treatment response.[7]
6. Multispecialty specialized pain clinics can be invaluable.
7. Treatment of children with chronic pain is discussed elsewhere.[8]

B. **Specific syndromes that should be considered in differential diagnosis**
1. The discussion that follows assumes that treatable nociceptive stimuli have been identified and appropriately addressed.
2. Neuropathic pain—Unfortunately, neuropathic pain is used to mean both "pain due to a lesion of the nervous system" and "pain with qualities that suggest nerve injury," such as burning, tingling, shocking, crawling, or other unusual and hard-to-ignore sensations, often with sensory deficit or hypersensitivity phenomena. This section focuses on neuropathic pain with a defined nervous system lesion. Examples are followed by a general treatment strategy.
    a. Trigeminal neuralgia—Episodic severe pain follows distribution of the trigeminal nerve on one side of the face; responds well to oxcarbazepine or carbamazepine.
    b. Off-period pain in Parkinson disease—Pain, often neuropathic (burning, tingling, electrical or rasping in quality, or with hypersensitivity phenomena) but occasionally cramping or stiff, linked temporally to lower blood levels of antiparkinsonian medication or "off" periods with lower mobility; occurs in approximately 33% of all Parkinson disease (PD) patients, often comorbid with anxiety or depression; first step in treatment is smoothing out diurnal fluctuations in antiparkinsonian medications for example by sustained release levodopa with selegiline or catechol-O-methyltransferase (COMT) inhibitors, or dopamine agonists.
    c. Thalamic strokes—Pain following a neuroanatomically appropriate distribution (contralateral hemibody) developing subacutely after the stroke.
    d. Phantom limb pain—Pain (or other somatic sensations) felt as if occurring in a limb that has been severed or denervated.
    e. Pain with other known nervous system lesions (e.g., diabetic neuropathy; postherpetic neuralgia; spinal injuries).
    f. **Treatment.** Most chronic neuropathic pain responds poorly to opioids, and response to specific treatments is variable. Therefore treatment consists of successive empirical trials of agents reported to produce some benefit. An initial approach is outlined here. See also references 9 and 10.
        (1) In all patients, attend to "General principles" for pain management (see section **VIA** in preceding text). For trigeminal neuralgia or off-period pain in PD see sections **VIB2a** or **VIB2b** in the preceding text.

(2) For pain with hypersensitivity to pressure or heat consider topical treatments (see Table 12.1).

(3) For patients with hypersensitivity to cold, pinprick or light brushing of the skin consider NMDA receptor antagonists (Table 12.1).

(4) For pain distal to a normal segment of spinal cord or nerve consider referral for transdermal electrical nerve stimulation (TENS) treatment (see section **VII**, in subsequent text).

(5) In patients with swelling or change in temperature or color of a painful extremity consider systemic

TABLE 12.1   Pharmacologic Treatments for Chronic Pain

Class	Drug	Comments; Usual Final Dose
Topical	Capsaicin ointment	Available over the counter
	Lidocaine cream	Solution, jelly, ointment, or patch formulations
α_1-Antagonists	Prazosin	1 mg PO b.i.d.—5 mg t.i.d.
	Tamsulosin	0.4–0.8 mg PO q.d
Central α_2-agonist	Clonidine	0.1–0.3 mg PO b.i.d.
	Guanfacine	1–2 mg PO b.i.d.-t.i.d.
Monoamine reuptake inhibitors (norepinephrine)	Desipramine	Contraindicated in patients with cardiac conduction delay; 150–200 mg total daily dose or by blood levels
	Atomoxetine	80–100 mg p.o q.d
Monoamine reuptake inhibitors (serotonin)	Clomipramine	Contraindicated in patients with cardiac conduction delay; 100–250 mg po qhs
	Fluoxetine	20–60 mg PO q.d
	Citalopram	20–60 mg PO q.d
	Fluvoxamine	50–150 mg PO b.i.d.
	Sertraline	50–200 mg PO q.d
	Escitalopram	10–20 mg PO q.d
Monoamine reuptake inhibitors (serotonin-norepinephrine)	Nortriptyline	Contraindicated in patients with cardiac conduction delay; 50–150 mg PO q.d or by blood levels
	Venlafaxine	75–375 mg total daily dose
	Duloxetine	40–120 mg PO total daily dose
N-methyl-D-asparate receptor antagonists	Dextromethorphan	30 mg PO q6h
	Amantadine	100 mg PO b.i.d.-t.i.d.
Other	Gabapentin	300–1200 mg PO t.i.d
	Baclofen	10 mg PO t.i.d.-20 mg PO q.i.d.
μ-Opioid agonists	Oxycodone SR	5–160 mg PO q12h
	Fentanyl transdermal	25–100 mcg/h patch q3d

α_2-agonists or α_1-antagonists (Table 12.1) or referral for a phentolamine infusion.

(6) In the remaining patients with chronic neuropathic pain consider trials of monoamine reuptake inhibitors, gabapentin, or the treatments mentioned in the preceding text.

(7) Patients failing in the strategies mentioned in the preceding text should usually be referred to a specialty pain management treatment center.

3. **Malingering** (see Chapter 14). It is important to note that most patients presenting with a pain complaint do *not* show any suggestion of malingering. Furthermore, patients with otherwise typical, medically explained pain can exaggerate symptom reports, especially when they perceive doctors as unresponsive. However, given its subjective nature, pain can be simulated intentionally and this can be difficult to detect. Generally this diagnosis can be made only in a few fairly uncommon situations: A patient who admits a conscious intent to deceive, a patient whose symptoms resolve immediately when obvious secondary gain is achieved, or perhaps a patient who consistently shows no evidence of pain when he is unaware of observation.

4. Somatization disorder (see Chapter 14). Somatization disorder, or Briquet syndrome, is a common pain disorder. It affects approximately 2% of all women in unreferred clinical samples and is characterized by numerous attempts to seek medical care, beginning before age 30, for a variety of symptoms in several different organ systems. Current (Diagnostic and Statistical Manual of Mental Disorders, 4th edition [DSM-IV]) diagnostic criteria require the presence at some point in life of pain in several unrelated body parts in addition to other features such as pseudoneurologic (i.e., classical conversion) symptoms. Somatization disorder is diagnosed only when, after adequate investigation, the criterion symptoms have no known pathophysiologic explanation. Somatization disorder is discussed in Chapter 14 of this volume but some aspects are discussed here given its importance and probable underrecognition in patients seen for pain.

a. This diagnosis is important to consider, because it provides valuable prognostic information. In one follow-up study 7 years after initial diagnosis, the physical symptoms in 94% of patients with somatization disorder were still best attributed to this diagnosis. Family studies and other clinical evidence further support the validity of this diagnosis.[11]

b. Two prospective studies have diagnosed somatization disorder in approximately 1 in 10 women in specialty pain clinics, but this may be an underestimate.[12]

c. Requiring accepted criteria for diagnosis is important. Patients with a single conversion symptom, or a single unexplained pain symptom, are much more likely to eventually be diagnosed with a specific, accepted, medical cause than are patients who meet full criteria for somatization disorder.

    d.   Treatment for somatization disorder is discussed in Smith, 2001.[13] The most important aspect of management is to avoid unnecessary invasive procedures for diagnosis or treatment ("first, do no harm"). The most important reason for recognizing somatization disorder is that these patients already have a valid explanation for their pain. This explanation substantially reduces the prior probability that extensive, invasive testing is needed to find another cause. Generally by the time the diagnosis is made, patients have been subjected to a number of invasive procedures that, in retrospect, could best have been avoided.

    5.   Pain related to general medical illness.

C. Residual pain syndromes

    1.   After appropriate evaluation, pain in many patients cannot be appropriately characterized with a specific, physiologically explainable cause. Obviously, in such patients it is more advisable to seek consultation if needed, or to maintain vigilance in the expectation that a specific disease will declare itself. Nevertheless, often reasonable diagnostic measures have been taken and there is no evidence of dangerous illness.

    2.   A number of diagnoses have been invented to describe such patients in the hope of allowing further research, including treatment studies. Somatization disorder (discussed in preceding text) has long-term diagnostic stability and predictive value. By contrast, there is little evidence for diagnostic validity for many of the diagnoses in the subsequent text, whether they arise from psychiatric consensus or consensus in other clinical fields.

    a.   DSM-IV-TR describes three varieties of pain disorder, of which only the first two are classified as mental disorders. This classification may be seen as helpful because it does not require a nonexistent duality (i.e., the false idea that pain must be entirely "real" or entirely "in your head"). Nevertheless, the classification still assumes that the doctor can reliably detect "psychological factors," a problematic assumption. The following DSM-IV-TR pain disorders are defined as their names suggest:

        (1) Pain disorder associated with psychological factors

        (2) Pain disorder associated with both psychological factors and a general medical condition

        (3) Pain disorder associated with a general medical condition

    b.   A final DSM-IV-TR category for certain pain presentations is factitious disorder with predominantly physical signs and symptoms (or, with combined psychological and physical signs and symptoms). Factitious disorder is defined by intentional production of signs of illness (e.g., creating infections or self-poisoning), or intentional feigning of symptoms (e.g., pain). It differs from malingering in that malingerers are rewarded with money, release from jail, or other obvious benefits, whereas in factitious disorder there is no apparent external motivation for the behavior. The apparent goal is only to assume the sick role. This disorder is uncommon, resistant to treatment, and—because the definition relies on the person's intent—can be hard to separate from other disorders both conceptually and operationally.

c. Other patients with pain not referable to specific organ lesions have been classified on the basis of physical symptoms.[14] The main difficulty with these classifications is in knowing whether these diagnoses are different from, or add useful information to, better-validated diagnoses. Diagnostic reliability is also an issue; one well-designed multicenter study showed a positive predictive value for complex regional pain syndrome of only approximately 40%. Probably in many cases the motivation for using these diagnoses is to avoid psychiatric stigma or the recognition of diagnostic uncertainty. Nevertheless many of these syndromes have developed their own burgeoning clinical literature, and some useful treatment studies are available (e.g., refer the American Academy of Pain Management's text).[15] A thorough review is outside the scope of this chapter. Many such diagnostic entities have been championed, and will be described in the subsequent text divided by whether the pain is neuropathic in quality or not.

3. Chronic neuropathic pain of unknown cause—Here "neuropathic" describes the quality of the pain rather than a demonstrable cause which includes the following examples:

a. Complex regional pain syndromes (including the former "reflex sympathetic dystrophy"). This is a controversial diagnosis[16] but specific treatments have been proposed as noted in section **VIBf5** in the preceding text.

b. Some chronic low back pain is neuropathic in quality.

4. Chronic non-neuropathic pain of unknown cause—Includes chronic pain referable to other organs. Examples include the following:

a. Low back pain[17,18]
b. Chronic pelvic pain[19]
c. Chronic daily headache
d. Fibromyalgia
e. Prostatodynia
f. Irritable bowel syndrome

5. Treatment for all the residual chronic pain syndromes is generally similar, although expert recommendations specific to common presentations are discussed in the American Academy of Pain Management's text.[15] The "General Principles" in section **VIA** in the preceding text are crucial in all these patients. In addition, empiric trials of the nonspecific treatments in the subsequent text may be helpful (Table 12.1).

VII. NONSPECIFIC TREATMENTS

A. **Overview.** As noted in the preceding text, pain can occur in the absence of peripheral stimuli. Therefore it may be no surprise that interfering with the mechanisms of peripheral pain transduction may not cure pain, especially in chronic pain. One usually needs a comprehensive approach that includes attention to pain mechanisms in the brain, including psychological factors.

B. **Pharmacologic**

1. Local anesthetics can prevent transmission of nociceptive stimuli from peripheral nerves. When a specific anatomic source of pain can be identified these drugs can be injected locally. They can also be given in the epidural space, usually done for a limited period of time.

2. Acetaminophen reduces pain centrally, but patients have usually tried it before consulting a physician.

3. COX inhibitors reduce prostaglandin synthesis. Therefore, they reduce inflammation peripherally, consequently decreasing activation of nociceptors, and in the CNS reduce fever and some forms of secondary hyperalgesia. Examples are aspirin, ibuprofen, and celecoxib. Glucocorticoids can have similar effects.

4. Baclofen is a GABA-B receptor agonist that inhibits excitatory neurotransmission in the dorsal horn and is given either orally or intrathecally.

5. Most marketed antidepressant drugs are monoamine transporter inhibitors. In addition to their specific use in the treatment of comorbid mood and anxiety disorders, several studies have shown efficacy in different pain syndromes, sometimes at sub-antidepressant doses.

6. Noradrenergic drugs such as clonidine can limit sympathetic activity, reduce pain when given intrathecally, and can produce beneficial central effects including sedation when given orally.

7. Opioid agonists such as morphine are the most efficacious pharmacologic treatments for pain. They can be administered by various routes. At times opioid agonists are appropriate in chronic pain management.[20] Drug abuse by DSM-IV criteria is not common in those without prior abuse of other substances, although physiologic dependence (i.e., withdrawal on cessation) is common. However, prior substance abuse is present in a substantial minority of patients with chronic pain. There are additional drawbacks to chronic opioid treatment including peripheral side effects and frequent development of tolerance to the antinociceptive effects. Mixed agonist/antagonist drugs may reduce the risk of certain side effects including respiratory depression and psychological dependence. European chapters of the International Association for the Study of Pain have published guidelines for the use of opioids in chronic noncancer pain, and suggest that they generally should not be seen as a lifelong treatment.[21]

8. Many other medications have been applied in chronic pain, including benzodiazepines, other antiepileptic agents, antiarrhythmic agents such as mexiletine, and those discussed as treatments for neuropathic pain (see section **VIB2f** under Chronic Pain, in preceding text).

C. **Mechanical**

1. Exercise, mobilization, and manipulation of joints, as well as massage of soft tissues, all show benefit in reducing various pain complaints in many patients. A brief evidence-oriented review is available in reference 22.

2. Locally applied heat and cold have commonly appreciated uses especially in acute pain management. Both can be generated by a variety of methods.

D. **Neurophysiologic stimulation**

1. **Peripheral and spinal stimulation.** Mechanical, thermal, chemical or electrical stimuli that excite peripheral nerves can reduce the perception of pain even if applied distant from the pain site. One such method is TENS, where 1 to 120 Hz electrical stimuli are applied to the skin at an intensity below the noxious threshold. This procedure has found widespread application despite important questions about to what extent the benefit exceeds that of a placebo treatment of similar magnitude. Spinal cord stimulation for example with implanted epidural electrodes is also used.

2. Repetitive transcranial magnetic stimulation (rTMS) of the motor cortex appears to have at least short-lived effects on nociception. Clinical applications are still being defined.

3. Increased familiarity with implanted deep brain stimulation (DBS) has led to renewed interest in DBS of various cortical or subcortical targets. In highly selected patients success rates of 40% to 87% have been reported.

E. **Surgical**

1. **Specific lesion-oriented.** Lesions of nerves or spinal cord tracts have been employed for treatment of focal pain, often in patients with neuropathic or cancer pain. These procedures include facet denervation and dorsal root entry zone (DREZ) sections, and moderate success has been reported in some patients, although complications and diminished effect over time are relatively common.

2. **Central.** A variety of ablative lesions to the cerebrum and brainstem have been applied to various types of pain. Stereotactic neurosurgical techniques have made these safer. Still, there are thought to be very few current indications for such surgery.

3. **Problems with surgery.** Unfortunately, many patients are dissatisfied with results of surgery, including surgery for pain. Surgical complications are felt to be a primary or contributing factor in about a fifth of patients with chronic pain.

F. **Psychological**

1. **Educational.** A major part of pain management is in providing correct information about pain to patients. Studies have shown

that many patients present with specific incorrect beliefs about pain or pain management. Examples are "if it hurts there must be tissue damage" or "if it hurts and I exercise I will damage it further." The physician's main concerns in a new patient evaluation (e.g., is there a specific, medically serious cause) may differ substantially from the patient's (e.g., do I need to stop my daily walk). Therefore physicians are often unaware of the patient's beliefs and concerns or do not address them directly. Questionnaires for assessment and handouts for education are available; in one study, simply providing an informational booklet about pain improved patient outcome. Some patients may benefit from more involved training (e.g., "back school").

2. **Relaxation training is used as one component of many treatment programs.** Biofeedback and hypnosis have been widely used.

3. Behavioral and cognitive-behavioral therapies for chronic pain have been studied intensively. There is high face validity for these procedures because specific maladaptive behaviors and beliefs are common in patients with chronic pain.[23] Different reviews and meta-analyses differ on the strength of the evidence for efficacy of these treatments.

4. **Group therapy.** Comprehensive, multidisciplinary group therapy has been shown to reduce doctor visits and use of pain medications. One university clinic has published a very complete treatment outline.[6]

G. Collaboration with other professionals is built into many successful multidisciplinary pain treatment programs. For treatment-resistant or complex cases, consider referral to psychology, anesthesiology, neurosurgery, or specialized pain management centers.

References

1. International Association for the Study of Pain. Pain terms: A list with definitions and notes on usage recommended by the IASP Subcommittee on Taxonomy. *Pain*. 1979;6:249–252.

2. Tracey I. Nociceptive processing in the human brain. *Curr Opin Neurobiol*. 2005;15(4):478–487.

3. Turk DC, Okifuji A. Assessment of patients' reporting of pain: An integrated perspective. *Lancet*. 1999;353:1784–1788.

4. Sullivan M, Terman GW, Peck B, et al. American Pain Society Ethics Committee: APS position statement on the use of placebos in pain management. *J Pain*. 2005;6(4):215–217.

5. Gordon DB, Dahl JL, Miaskowski C, et al. American Pain Society recommendations for improving the quality of acute and cancer pain management: American Pain Society Quality of Care Task Force. *Arch Intern Med*. 2005;165(14):1574–1580.

6. Brill C, Post SJ, Ferguson T, et al. "Columbia Medical Plan Pain Management Group manual." In: Weiner RS. *Pain management: A practical guide for clinicians*, 6th ed. Chap. 7. Boca Raton, IL: CRC Press; 2001:55–73.

7. Nistler C. Care of the patient with chronic pain. In: David AK, Johnson TA, Jr, Phillips DM, et al. eds. *Family medicine: Principles and practice*, 6th ed. Chap. 61. New York: Springer-Verlag; 2003; Available at http://online.statref.com/document.aspx?fxid=32&docid=300 (accessed 8/22/2005).

8. Suresh S. Chronic pain management in children. In: Benzon HT, ed. *Essentials of pain medicine and regional anesthesia.* Chap. 55. New York: Churchill Livingstone; 1999:433–443.

9. Fields HL. Evaluation and treatment of neuropathic pain. In: Schiffer RB, Rao SM, Fogel BS, eds. *Neuropsychiatry,* 2nd ed. Chap. 16. Philadelphia, PA: Lippincott Williams & Wilkins; 2003:395–404.

10. Woolf CJ, Mannion RJ. Neuropathic pain: Aetiology, symptoms, mechanisms, and management. *Lancet.* 1999;353:1959–1964.

11. Goodwin DW, Guze SB. Hysteria. *Psychiatric diagnosis,* 5th ed. Chap. 4. New York: Oxford University Press; 1996:105–126.

12. Reich J, Tupin JP, Abramowitz SI. Psychiatric diagnosis of chronic pain patients. *Am J Psychiatry.* 1983;140:1495–1498.

13. Smith GR Jr. Somatization disorder and undifferentiated somatoform disorder. In: Gabbard GO, ed. *Treatments of psychiatric disorders,* 3rd ed., Chap. 58 Washington, DC: American Psychiatric Press; 2001; Available at http://online.statref.com/document.aspx?fxid=7&docid=283 (accessed 8/22/2005).

14. Melzack R, Wall PD. *Handbook of pain management.* St. Louis: Churchill Livingstone; 2003.

15. Weiner RS, ed. American Academy of Pain Management. *Pain management: A practical guide for clinicians,* 6th ed. Boca Raton, IL: CRC Press; 2001.

16. Landau WM. Reflex sympathetic dystrophy. *Mayo Clin Proc.* 1996;71(5):524–525.

17. Carragee EJ. Clinical practice: Persistent low back pain. *N Engl J Med.* 2005;352:1891–1898.

18. U.S. Preventive Services Task Force. Primary care interventions to prevent low back pain in adults: Recommendation statement. *Am Fam Physician.* 2005;71(12):2337–2338.

19. ACOG Committee on Practice Bulletins—Gynecology. ACOG practice bulletin no. 51. Chronic pelvic pain. *Obstet Gynecol.* 2004;103:589–605.

20. American Academy of Pain Medicine; American Pain Society; American Society of Addiction Medicine. Public policy statement on the rights and responsibilities of health care professionals in the use of opioids for the treatment of pain: A consensus document from the American Academy of Pain Medicine, The American Pain Society, and The American Society of Addiction Medicine. *Pain Med.* 2004;5:301–302.

21. Kalso E, Allan L, Dellemijn PL, et al. 2002 European Federation of Chapters of the International Association for the Study of Pain. Recommendations for using opioids in chronic non-cancer pain. *Eur J Pain.* 2003;7:381–386.

22. Hooper PD, Haldeman S. Mobilization, manipulation, massage and exercise for the relief of musculoskeletal pain. In: Melzack R, Wall PD, eds. *Handbook of pain management.* Chap. 32. St. Louis: Churchill Livingstone; 2003:485–501.

23. Asmundson GJG, Vlaeyen J, Crombez G, eds. *Understanding and treating fear of pain.* New York: Oxford University Press; 2004.

Chapter 13

SLEEP DISORDERS

Sheldon Benjamin

I. BACKGROUND

Sleep, the collection of brain mechanisms that leads to feeling rested and refreshed in the normal state, becomes a source of complaint in patients with primary sleep disorders and sleep disorders secondary to a number of medical, neurologic, and psychiatric conditions. Clinicians who treat patients with neuropsychiatric conditions should become facile at diagnosis and treatment of sleep disorders.

II. CLASSIFICATION

The most frequently used classification systems for sleep disorders in the United States are the International Classification of Sleep Disorders, 2nd edition (ICSD-2),[1] and the Diagnostic and Statistical Manual of Mental Disorders, 4th edition, text revision (DSM-IV-TR). The ICSD-2 classifies sleep disorders as insomnias, sleep-related breathing disorders, hypersomnias, circadian rhythm disorders, parasomnias, sleep-related movement disorders, and other sleep disorders (see Table 13.1). The DSM-IV-TR classifies sleep disorders as primary and secondary (caused by other psychiatric or medical condition, or substance use) types and lists fewer specific subtypes than does the ICSD-2. This chapter will follow the DSM-IV-TR classification (see Table 13.2).[2]

A. **Definitions**

1. **Dyssomnias** are characterized by insomnia, hypersomnia, or abnormal sleep–wake cycles. The dyssomnias are subdivided into intrinsic, extrinsic, and circadian rhythm–related disorders.

2. **Parasomnias** are abnormal sleep behaviors or physiologic events associated with full or partial arousal that may occur in rapid eye movement (REM) sleep, non-REM sleep, or in transition to or from sleep.

3. **Fatigue** must be distinguished from sleepiness. Fatigue is an imprecise term that may include anergia, easy fatigability, muscle tiredness, exhaustion, decreased endurance, decreased motivation, or even excessive daytime sleepiness (EDS). Table 13.3 lists

TABLE 13.1   International Classification of Sleep Disorders, 2nd Edition[1]

Insomnias	Adjustment insomnia
	Psychophysiologic insomnia
	Paradoxical insomnia
	Idiopathic insomnia
	Insomnia due to mental disorder
	Inadequate sleep hygiene
	Behavioral insomnia of childhood
	Insomnia due to drug or substance
	Insomnia due to medical condition
	Insomnia not due to substance or known physiologic condition
	Physiologic insomnia, unspecified
Sleep-related breathing disorders	Primary central sleep apnea
	Central sleep apnea due to Cheyne-Stokes breathing pattern
	Central sleep apnea due to high-altitude periodic breathing
	Central sleep apnea due to a medical condition, not Cheyne-Stokes breathing pattern
	Central sleep apnea due to drug or substance
	Primary sleep apnea of infancy
	Obstructive sleep apnea
	Sleep-related nonobstructive alveolar hypoventilation, idiopathic
	Congenital central alveolar hypoventilation syndrome
	Sleep-related hypoventilation/hypoxemia due to lower airways obstruction, neuromuscular, and chest wall disorders, pulmonary parenchymal or vascular pathology
	Sleep apnea/sleep-related breathing disorder, unspecified
Hypersomnias	Narcolepsy with or without cataplexy
	Narcolepsy with or without cataplexy due to medical condition
	Narcolepsy unspecified
	Kleine-Levin syndrome
	Menstrual-related hypersomnia
	Idiopathic hypersomnia with or without long sleep time
	Behaviorally induced insufficient sleep syndrome
	Hypersomnia due to medical condition
	Hypersomnia due to drug or substance
	Hypersomnia not due to substance or known physiologic condition
	Physiologic hypersomnia, unspecified
Circadian rhythm sleep disorders	Delayed sleep phase type
	Advanced sleep phase type
	Irregular sleep–wake cycle
	Nonentrained type (free-running)
	Jet lag type
	Shift work type
	Due to medical condition
	Other
	Due to drug or substance

TABLE 13.1   (*Continued*)

Parasomnias	Confusional arousals
	Sleepwalking
	Sleep terrors
	Rapid eye movement sleep behavior disorder
	Recurrent isolated sleep paralysis
	Nightmare disorder
	Sleep-related dissociative disorders
	Sleep enuresis
	Sleep-related groaning
	Exploding head syndrome
	Sleep-related hallucinations
	Sleep-related eating disorder
	Parasomnia, unspecified
	Parasomnias due to drug or substance
	Parasomnias due to medical condition
Sleep-related movement disorders	Restless legs syndrome
	Periodic limb movement disorder
	Sleep-related leg cramps
	Sleep-related bruxism
	Sleep-related rhythmic movement disorder
	Sleep-related movement disorder, unspecified
	Sleep-related movement disorder due to drug or substance
	Sleep-related movement disorder due to medical condition
Other sleep disorders	Physiologic sleep disorder, unspecified
	Environmental sleep disorder
	Fatal familial insomnia

disorders frequently associated with fatigue. Fatigue may be a complaint in up to 20% of all patients seeking medical care.

4. **Sleepiness** refers to a need for sleep or a tendency to fall asleep.

B. **Sleep architecture**

1. Evaluation of sleep disorders requires awareness of normal sleep architecture. A normal night's sleep typically consists of three to five sleep cycles of approximately 90 minutes length. A normal sleep cycle consists of progression from wakefulness through a few minutes of stage 1 sleep, from which people may be easily aroused, to stage 2, which constitutes approximately half of normal sleep. The normal individual then passes into stages 3 and 4 slow wave sleep, which together account for 20% to 25% of sleep time. After a latency of approximately 90 minutes following sleep onset (the REM latency) the individual passes into REM sleep, during which muscles are paralyzed and individuals report dream activity, if aroused. REM is terminated either by brief arousal or by passage into stage 2 sleep to begin another cycle. The stages of sleep are distinguished by electroencephalogram (EEG) patterns and physiologic changes,

TABLE 13.2   Diagnostic and Statistical Manual of Mental Disorders (text revision) Classification of Sleep Disorders[2]

Primary sleep disorders	Dyssomnias	Primary insomnia
		Primary hypersomnia
		Narcolepsy
		Breathing-related sleep disorder
		Circadian rhythm sleep disorders
		Delayed sleep phase type
		Jet lag type
		Shift work type
		Unspecified type
		Dyssomnia NOS
	Parasomnias	Nightmare disorder
		Sleep terror disorder
		Sleepwalking disorder
		Parasomnia NOS
Sleep disorder related to another mental disorder	Insomnia related to another mental disorder	Related disorders
		Major depression
		Dysthymic disorder
	Hypersomnia related to another mental disorder	Bipolar disorder
		Generalized anxiety disorder
		Panic disorder
		Adjustment disorder
		Schizophrenia
		Somatoform disorder
		Personality disorder
Sleep disorder related to a general medical condition	Insomnia type	
	Hypersomnia type	
	Parasomnia type	
	Mixed type	
Substance-induced sleep disorder (alcohol, amphetamine, caffeine, cocaine, opioid, sedative, hypnotic, anxiolytic, or other substance)	Insomnia type	With onset during intoxication
	Hypersomnia type	With onset during withdrawal
	Parasomnia type	
	Mixed type	

NOS, not otherwise specified.

which are listed in Table 13.4. The amount of time spent in each sleep stage varies through the night such that more time is spent in slow wave sleep in the first part of the night and more time is spent in REM sleep during the last part of the night. Infants spend 50% of sleep time in REM. The sleep pattern of the elderly is typically characterized by fragmentation with decreased slow wave sleep. Total sleep time decreases with age.

2. Neurotransmitter function varies with the sleep cycle.[3] Arousal, maintained by the ascending reticular activating system (ARAS),

TABLE 13.3   Disorders Frequently Associated with Complaints of Fatigue

Anemia	Cancer	Chronic fatigue syndrome
Chronic obstructive pulmonary disease	Depression	Epilepsy
Human immunodeficiency virus/acquired immunodeficiency syndrome	Hypothyroidism	Lyme disease
Multiple sclerosis	Myasthenia gravis	Parkinson disease
Postpolio syndrome	Systemic lupus erythematosus	Neuromuscular disease
		Traumatic brain injury

is an acetylcholine-dependent process. ARAS cholinergic activity decreases to initiate sleep. Slow wave sleep involves increased raphé and basal forebrain activity, with activation of serotonergic and γ-aminobutyric-acid-secreting (GABAergic) neurons, and contributions from opiates, α-melanocyte-stimulating hormone (α-MSH), and somatostatin. Serotonergic, adrenergic, and histaminergic activities are high during wakefulness and suppressed during REM sleep. REM sleep is initiated by cholinergic neurons in the pontine tegmentum. Cholinergic neurons are most active during wakefulness and REM sleep. Serotonin, which tends to help dampen sensory input and facilitate motor activity, would need to be suppressed during REM

TABLE 13.4   Physiologic Findings Associated with Sleep Stages

Sleep Stage	Electroencephalogram Findings	Neurotransmitter Changes
Wakefulness	Alpha background at rest eyes closed	Increased ACh, 5-HT, EPI, histamine
1	Low voltage 5–7 Hz theta slowing	Decreased ACh needed for sleep initiation
2	Theta slowing, sleep spindles, K-complexes	
3	20%–50% higher voltage<2 Hz delta slowing	Increased 5-HT and GABA, increases in opiates, α-MSH, somatostatin
4	50% higher voltage delta slowing	Same as stage 3
Rapid eye movement	Low voltage faster activity, with decreased skeletal muscle movements, and eye movements	Increased ACh, decreased 5-HT, EPI, histamine

Ach, acetylcholine; 5-HT, serotonin; EPI, epinephrine; GABA, γ-aminobutyric acid; α-MSH, α-melanocyte stimulating hormone.

sleep to facilitate muscle atonia and dreaming. Monoaminergic activity terminates REM.

III. EVALUATION OF SLEEP DISORDERS

    A.   **Sleep history.** A thorough sleep history is essential to determine the most likely cause and treatment of sleep disorders. Elements of the sleep history are listed in Table 13.5. In evaluating chronic insomnia or circadian rhythm disturbances, it is helpful for patients to maintain and complete a sleep diary for 2 weeks in which bedtime, time of sleep onset, time and duration of awakenings, final awakening time, and times of daytime naps are recorded. The Epworth Sleepiness Scale may be used to quantify the patient's complaints about sleepiness.[4]

    B.   **Use of the sleep laboratory.** Nocturnal polysomnography (PSG) is used for insomnia only if the diagnosis is not obvious from the sleep history. The PSG is mainly used in the evaluation of EDS and parasomnias. The PSG is used in combination with the multiple sleep latency test (MSLT) for evaluation of possible narcolepsy or idiopathic hypersomnia. A mean sleep latency of <5 minutes and the presence of at least two sleep onset REM periods (SOREMPs) out of five measured on the MSLT are suggestive of narcolepsy but do not rule out apnea. A short mean sleep latency on the MSLT is one

TABLE 13.5   **Elements of the Sleep History**

Sleep Hygiene
Bedtime/awakening time
Arrangement of bedroom (television, clock position, lighting, noise and light barriers, nighttime ritual)
Exercise
Sexual activity
Use of stimulants/substances
Nighttime eating
Napping behavior
Shift work, circadian demands

Related Issues
Medical conditions (including pain, nocturia, dyspnea, seizures, etc.)
Medications
Psychosocial stressors
Mood changes

History from Partner
Snoring
Irregular breathing
Movements in sleep
Estimated sleep length and quality
Mood changes/performance changes

Insomnia History
Duration of complaint
Sleep onset insomnia (time to sleep)
Difficulty maintaining sleep
Early morning awakening (time)
Nonrestorative sleep

Hypersomnia History
Irresistible daytime naps
Daytime drowsiness
Situations in which naps occur (sedentary activity vs. driving, talking, eating, etc.)

Narcolepsy Symptoms
Excessive daytime sleepiness
Cataplexy
Hypnagogic/hypnopompic hallucinations
Sleep paralysis

TABLE 13.6   Summary of Cognitive Findings in Major Sleep Disorders[6]

	Attention Impairment	Memory Impairment	Common Deficits
Insomnia	22.8%	20%	Attention span, immediate recall (verbal), vigilance
Sleep-related breathing disorders	35.9%	17.1%	Attention span, divided attention, sustained attention; driving performance (92.9%)
Narcolepsy	44.2%	15.6%	Sustained attention, vigilance, driving performance

Percentage showing more impairment than controls based on analysis of 56 studies.

way of differentiating EDS from fatigue. Guidelines for the use of the sleep laboratory have been published by the American Academy of Sleep Medicine.[5]

C. **Neuropsychological testing.** Impairment of daytime cognitive function is among the major concerns of individuals with sleep disorders. Neuropsychological evaluation may be used to assess the impact of sleep disorders on arousal, vigilance, attention, concentration, recall, and motor performance in sleep disorders. A subset of testing may be repeated following treatment to determine the degree of cognitive benefit. Table 13.6 describes the common cognitive findings in the three principal sleep disorders on the basis of an analysis of 56 neuropsychological studies.[6]

IV. DYSSOMNIAS

A. **Insomnia**

1. **Phenomenology.** *Insomnia,* according to the ICSD, is characterized by difficulty in initiating or maintaining sleep. A broader definition, according to the National Center on Sleep Disorders Research, is inadequate or poor quality sleep characterized by one or more of the following: Difficulty falling asleep, difficulty maintaining sleep, waking up too early in the morning, or nonrefreshing sleep; and having daytime consequences such as tiredness, lack of energy, difficulty concentrating, or irritability. Insomnia can have many causes, and may be transient (several days), short term, or chronic (more than 3 weeks). *Primary insomnia,* according to the DSM-IV-TR, refers to insomnia of at least 1 month duration that causes distress and social or occupational dysfunction, and is not due to another sleep disorder, medical disorder, or substances of abuse.

2. **Prevalence.** Insomnia tends to increase with age, with approximately one third of people older than 65 reporting nearly continuous insomnia. Chronic insomnia tends to occur in approximately 10% of middle-aged adults, is approximately

1.5 times more frequent in women than men, and is a frequent perimenopausal complaint. Sleep onset insomnia is more common in younger individuals. Middle and terminal insomnia is more common in middle-aged and elderly individuals.

3. **Etiology/pathophysiology.** Secondary insomnia may be caused by a number of primary sleep disorders, or psychiatric, neurologic, and medical conditions, with the pathophysiology varying according to cause.

4. **Differential diagnosis.** A thorough sleep history will typically resolve the differential diagnosis. Transient/intermittent insomnia is most often stress or excitement related but can be caused by exposure to high altitudes, shifting time zones or work shift changes, and acute medical illness. Short-term insomnia is also typically stress induced and is also common in bereavement.

   Primary insomnia has a broad differential diagnosis (see Table 13.7). The most common causes of insomnia seen at sleep centers are psychiatric disorders, psychophysiologic insomnia, substance dependence, restless leg syndrome (RLS)/periodic limb movement disorder (PLMD) (see subsequent text), sleep state misperception, and breathing-related sleep disorders. Certain medications, such as corticosteroids, calcium channel blockers, antidepressants, psychostimulants, bronchodilators, and

TABLE 13.7   Differential Diagnosis of Primary Insomnia

Medical Disorders	Psychiatric Disorders
GERD	Substance dependence
COPD, asthma	Mood disorders
Fibromyalgia, rheumatologic diseases	Anxiety disorders
	Psychotic disorders
	Adjustment disorders
Primary Sleep Disorders	**Neurologic Disorders**
Idiopathic insomnia	Dementia
Breathing-related sleep disorders	Stroke
Restless leg syndrome and periodic limb movements of sleep	Parkinson and other extrapyramidal diseases
Parasomnias	Epilepsy
Sleep state misperception	Headache and other pain syndromes
	Myotonic dystrophy
	Fatal familial insomnia
Circadian Rhythm Disturbances	**Behavioral Disorders**
Irregular sleep pattern	Inadequate sleep hygiene
Time zone shift	Psychophysiologic insomnia
Delayed or advanced sleep phase	Adjustment sleep disorder
Shift work	
Environmental disturbances	

GERD, gastroesophageal reflux disease; COPD, chronic obstructive pulmonary disease.

decongestants, have a propensity to cause insomnia. Having ruled out medical, psychiatric, and substance-related insomnia; circadian rhythm disorders (see subsequent text); PLMD (see subsequent text); and central apnea (see subsequent text), most of the remaining patients will have sleep state misperception, complaining of insomnia but shown by PSG not to be insomniac; learned or psychophysiologic insomnia; and primary (idiopathic) insomnia.

5. **Treatment**

a. The treatment of insomnia always begins with instructions on sleep hygiene. Encourage patients to establish a regular sleep–wake schedule on weekdays as well as weekends; ensure a cool, dark, quiet sleep environment; avoid any activities and remove any stimuli from the bedroom not associated with sleep or sexual activity; institute a 30-minute wind down time before sleep; if the patient spends >30 minutes in bed worrying, they should be encouraged to move elsewhere for other quiet activity until sleepiness sets in; limit caffeine to the morning; avoid using alcohol as a sedative; avoid excessive alcohol or cigarette smoking in the evening; try a high tryptophan-containing snack at night (e.g., milk, banana); institute a regular exercise program but try to avoid exercising within 3 hours of bedtime.

b. Psychotherapy may be of use to reduce anxiety and reinforcement of insomnia, and develop alternative sleep strategies. Cognitive behavioral therapy (CBT) and relaxation training are useful for this purpose, with CBT shown to be effective in randomized clinical trials. CBT is considered more useful than medication in the treatment of chronic primary insomnia. In individuals older than 60 years with marginal cognitive function or balance issues, behavioral treatment of insomnia is especially preferred because sedative hypnotic agents tend to increase the risk of cognitive dysfunction and falling.[7]

c. The treatment of secondary insomnias due to other sleep disorders, medical or psychiatric conditions, or substance abuse should be directed to the primary disorder, and should also include instructions for proper sleep hygiene. Sedative hypnotic treatment is generally reserved for transient insomnia, such as that seen in jet lag, stress reactions, or transient medical conditions; for secondary insomnia unresponsive to treatment of the primary disorder; or for chronic primary insomnia that has not responded to sleep hygiene and CBT approaches.

Benzodiazepine hypnotic agents are not indicated for the long-term treatment of chronic insomnia because of the risks of tolerance, dependency, daytime attention and concentration compromise, incoordination, and rebound insomnia. They should be avoided in the elderly, in pregnant or breast-feeding women, in substance abusers, and in patients with suicidal or parasuicidal behaviors. Owing to the risk of respiratory depression benzodiazepines should be avoided in patients with untreated obstructive apnea and chronic pulmonary disease.

When benzodiazepine hypnotics are used, their use should be limited to two to three times per week to avoid the above mentioned risks. Transient insomnia related to anxiety may be treated with benzodiazepine hypnotics (see Table 13.8). Insomnia due to medical or psychiatric conditions may be treated with nonbenzodiazepine short half-life hypnotic agents if treatment of the underlying cause is unsuccessful in improving sleep (Table 13.8). These agents produce less tolerance and rebound insomnia on discontinuation than benzodiazepine hypnotics. For prolonged use in chronic insomnia daily dosage of eszopiclone 1 to 3 mg has been studied over a 6-month period without evidence of tolerance or rebound insomnia on discontinuation. Ramelteon, the first agent released in the new class of selective melatonin agonists, is effective in sleep onset insomnia and does not appear to produce tolerance, withdrawal, or rebound insomnia. It may be safer than benzodiazepine agonists in the elderly or in individuals vulnerable to confusion but does not prolong total sleep time. In selecting an agent for treatment of insomnia, half-life should be taken into account. Short half-life agents are used for sleep onset insomnia. Only zaleplon may be safely taken in the middle of the night without prolonged morning side effects. Intermediate half-life agents (temazepam, zolpidem, eszopiclone) or prolonged release agents (zolpidem ER) are used for sleep onset and sleep maintenance insomnia, and should be taken 8 hours or more before alertness is required the next morning. Mirtazapine 15 to 60 mg may be chosen for treatment of depression when insomnia is a prominent symptom. Serotonergic tricyclic antidepressants, such as amitriptyline and doxepin, may be used for depression when insomnia is a prominent complaint if suicide risk is minimal. Their use should be avoided in PLMD, however, because of a tendency to exacerbate this disorder. Trazodone, another serotonergic antidepressant, has been shown to be effective in combination with selective serotonin reupltake inhibitor (SSRI) agents in depressed individuals if the SSRI alone is not effective for insomnia[8] but it has not been shown to be effective for long-term use in primary insomnia. Serotonergic antidepressants are not U.S. Food and Drug Administration (FDA) approved for treatment of primary insomnia and increase the risk of serotonin syndrome if used in combination with SSRI agents. Sedating neuroleptics (e.g., quetiapine) should not be used to treat primary insomnia in the absence of psychotic symptoms. Diphenhydramine has no proven efficacy in primary

TABLE 13.8   Pharmacologic Treatment of Insomnia

Medication Class	Drug	Dose	Half-life	Active Metabolites
Benzodiazepine hypnotics	Intermediate acting			
	Temazepam	7.5–30 mg	8–12 h	No
	Oxazepam	10–30 mg	5–15 h	No (renal excretion)
	Long acting	0.25–1 mg	12–20 h	Yes
	Alprazolam	0.5–2 mg	10–22 h	No
	Lorazepam	0.5–2 mg	22–38 h	No
	Clonazepam	2.5–10 mg	20–50 h	Yes
	Diazepam	0.5–2 mg	22–38 h	No
		2.5–10 mg	20–50 h	Yes
Nonbenzodiazepine benzodiazepine	Zaleplon	5–20 mg	1–1.5 h	Yes
receptor agonists	Zolpidem	2.5–10 mg	1.5–4 h	No
	Zolpidem ER	1–3 mg	5–7 h	No
	Eszopiclone	1–3 mg	5–7 h	Yes
Melatonin receptor agonist	Ramelteon	8 mg	1–2.6 h	Yes
Serotonergic antidepressants	Trazodone	25–200 mg	3–9 h	Yes
	Doxepin	25–150 mg	6–8 h	Yes
	Amitriptyline	25–150 mg	10–50 h	Yes
	Mirtazapine	15–60 mg	20–40 h	Yes
γ-Hydroxy butyrate	Sodium oxybate	4.5–9 mg	40 min	No

insomnia and may contribute to cognitive dysfunction and gait instability in vulnerable individuals. There is no data to support the use of melatonin or valerian in primary insomnia.

B.   Excessive daytime sleepiness (idiopathic hypersomnia, narcolepsy, breathing-related sleep disorders)

1.   Idiopathic central nervous system hypersomnia (primary hypersomnia)

a.   **Phenomenology.** The diagnosis of idiopathic central nervous system (CNS) hypersomnia is reserved for those individuals with EDS who do not have any other components of the narcolepsy syndrome, or for those whose EDS is not secondary to other disorders. The EDS is characterized by long periods of daytime drowsiness with impaired performance, a tendency to take long daytime naps, complaints of unrefreshing sleep, difficult morning awakenings, and sometimes with sleep drunkenness on being awakened from naps. Patients report automatic behavior during drowsiness with frequent microsleeps, especially when resisting the urge to nap. Onset is typically from ages 15 to 30 and symptoms persist indefinitely.

b.   **Prevalence.** The prevalence of idiopathic CNS hypersomnia is unknown, in part due to the difficulty in establishing the diagnosis with certainty and in isolation from other etiologies of sleep dysfunction.

c.   **Etiology/pathophysiology.** Cerebrospinal fluid (CSF) studies point to the possibility of a dysfunctional norepinephrine system in idiopathic CNS hypersomnia in contrast to the dopaminergic dysfunction suspected in narcolepsy. A small familial subgroup has been shown to have associated headaches, orthostasis, Raynaud phenomenon, fainting, and a shared HLA type. Another subgroup develops idiopathic hypersomnia after Landry-Guillain-Barré syndrome or a viral infection such as mononucleosis.

d.   **Differential diagnosis.** Differential diagnosis of EDS is listed in Table 13.9. Idiopathic hypersomnia is essentially a diagnosis of exclusion. The sleep history and sleep diary should first be reviewed. Medications known to affect the sleep cycle should be withdrawn if possible and patients should be placed on a sleep regimen of at least 7 to 7.5 hours sleep per night for 1 to 2 weeks before obtaining a PSG to rule out breathing-related sleep disorders. An MSLT is done to rule out sleep onset REM and verify short mean sleep latency. Narcolepsy without cataplexy is differentiated from idiopathic hypersomnia by the presence of REM-related features and by the finding of two or more SOREMPS on the MSLT. If appropriate, a urine toxicology screen may also be done to rule out substance-induced hypersomnia.

e.   **Treatment.** Treatment must begin with good sleep hygiene and at least 8 hours of sleep per night; avoidance of CNS

TABLE 13.9   Causes of Excessive Daytime Sleepiness

Breathing-related sleep disorders	Idiopathic hypersomnia
Narcolepsy (with and without cataplexy)	Insufficient sleep
Periodic limb movement disorder	Sleep–wake cycle disorder
Substance use	Periodic hypersomnias (e.g., Kleine-Levin syndrome)
Posttraumatic hypersomnia	Mood disorders
Nocturnal hypoxemia due to COPD or other nonapneic respiratory disorders	Communicating hydrocephalus
Thalamic stroke	

COPD, chronic obstructive disease.

depressants, sleep deprivation, or shift work; and trying to keep naps down to one per day of 45 minutes or less (naps are not refreshing in this syndrome). Begin pharmacologic treatment with modafinil 100 mg per day, increasing as needed to 400 mg per day. Despite a half-life of 8 to 14 hours there is evidence that split dosage (morning and afternoon) produces more uniform symptomatic relief. If unsuccessful, an intermediate half-life stimulant such as methylphenidate SR 20 mg qam or b.i.d. with second dose at noon; or a long half-life stimulant, such as methylphenidate ER 18 to 54 mg qam, may be used. If not effective, dextroamphetamine 15 mg may be used up to three times during the morning and afternoon.idiopathic

2. **Narcolepsy**

    a. **Phenomenology.** *Narcolepsy* is a familial hypersomnia characterized by a tetrad of EDS, cataplexy, hypnagogic hallucinations, and sleep paralysis. The full tetrad occurs in a minority of patients, estimated at 10% to 15%. *Cataplexy* refers to episodic loss of muscle tone in response to emotional stimuli (e.g., laughing at a joke or getting angry) and occurs in 70% of patients. Cataplexy need not involve the entire body but may be limited to just the head or jaw. Deep tendon reflexes are absent during the events, which typically last <30 seconds. *Hypnagogic hallucinations,* found in 30% of patients and more frequently in patients with cataplexy, are vivid dream-like auditory, visual, or somesthetic hallucinations occurring during transition to sleep. Hypnagogic hallucinations are not specific to narcolepsy and may occur in up to 25% of normal individuals. *Sleep paralysis,* found in 25% of patients with narcolepsy, refers to skeletal muscle paralysis (respiratory and ocular movements are preserved) with maintained alertness during transition to or from sleep. Sleep paralysis ceases with noise or with falling asleep. Other sleep disorders such as REM behavior disorder (RBD) and confusional arousals may also occur (see arousal disorders in subsequent text). Patients with narcolepsy have disturbed nocturnal sleep as well, with sleep fragmentation and interruption being common. The narcolepsy complex occurs without cataplexy in 20% to 30% of patients.

b.   **Prevalence.** Narcolepsy occurs in approximately 0.05% of the population with one third of patients having a positive family history and most cases presenting in young adulthood. First-degree relatives of patients have a 60 times greater risk of developing the disorder. Narcolepsy is associated with an increased incidence of other sleep disorders including obstructive sleep apnea, RLS, and REM sleep behavior disorder.

c.   **Etiology/pathophysiology.** Most patients with narcolepsy are positive for HLA type DQB1*0602/DQA1*0102. Despite this finding there is no clear evidence of familial transmission. A defect of the hypocretin (orexin) system has also been demonstrated. Thalamic neurons containing the neuropeptide, hypocretin, project widely to CNS areas associated with sleep–wake cycles. Decreased hypocretin causes symptoms of daytime sleepiness and is associated with intrusion of partial manifestations of REM sleep (e.g., muscle paralysis) during wakefulness. Increased basal ganglia D_1, D_2, and α_2 receptors have also been demonstrated in patients with narcolepsy and dopaminergic dysfunction is suspected.

d.   **Differential diagnosis.** Differential diagnosis of EDS is listed in Table 13.9. A PSG to rule out other treatable sleep disorders with an MSLT the following day is the standard diagnostic procedure. Effective treatment of other diagnosed sleep disorders (e.g., obstructive sleep apnea–hypopnea syndrome [OSAHS]) should be documented before initiating treatment of narcolepsy. An individual with the narcolepsy tetrad, or at least with EDS and cataplexy and positive MSLT may be considered to have narcolepsy. Positive family history and positive HLA test result do not add significantly to the diagnosis. Isolated cataplexy is rarely due to other neurologic causes, with occasional reports in brainstem lesions and Niemann-Pick type C disease.

e.   **Treatment.** Begin with instruction on proper sleep hygiene (see section **IVA5**). Planned 15- to 30-minute daytime naps are an effective adjuvant therapy for narcolepsy-induced EDS and should be recommended. Patient, family, and employer, if appropriate, should be educated about the disorder and the patient's need for naps and medication. An exercise program to minimize weight gain can help prevent the added sleep effects of obesity. Patients with inadequately controlled EDS should be warned not to drive or operate heavy equipment.

Pharmacologic approaches to narcolepsy are aimed primarily at EDS and cataplexy (see Table 13.10). Caffeine has

TABLE 13.10 Pharmacologic Treatments of Narcolepsy

Agent	Half-life	Dose	Symptoms Treated
Sympathomimetic psychostimulants			EDS
Methamphetamine	4–5 h	5–60 mg/d	
D-amphetamine	10–12 h	5–60 mg/d	
Combined amphetamine salts (D-amphetamine sulfate,	10–13 h	5–60 mg/d	
D-amphetamine saccharate, amphetamine sulfate,	3–4 h	10–60 mg/d	
amphetamine aspartate) (Adderall)			
Methylphenidate			
Methylphenidate extended release preparations			
Modafinil	9–14 h	100–400 mg/d	EDS
Selegiline	2–10 h	5–40 mg/d	All narcolepsy components; higher doses necessitate low-tyramine diet

(continued)

TABLE 13.10 *(Continued)*

Agent	Half-life	Dose	Symptoms Treated
Antidepressants			Cataplexy, sleep paralysis, hypnagogic hallucinations
Venlafaxine (SR)	5–11 h	75–225 mg/d	
Atomoxetine	5–21 h	10–80 mg/d	
Duloxetine	8–17 h	40–60 mg/d	
Fluoxetine	4–16 d	20–60 mg/d	
Protriptyline	74 h	5–60 mg/d	
Imipramine	19 h	10–100 mg/d	
Desipramine	19–125 h	25–100 mg/d	
Clomipramine	19–37 h	10–150 mg/d	
Sodium oxybate	40 min	4.5–9 g/night	Insomnia, EDS, cataplexy
Caffeine	3–7 h	1–6 cups (equivalent to 75–450 mg)/d	EDS

EDS, excessive daytime sleepiness; SR, sustained release.

been shown to be effective in mild EDS and most patients with EDS discover caffeine regimens on their own. The absence of dependence, ease of use, general tolerability, and the fact that it appears to activate hypocretin neurons make modafinil 100 to 400 mg per day the drug of first choice for EDS.[9] In the elderly, dosage should begin with 50 mg. Modafinil may not be as effective in severe EDS. Headache, dizziness, nausea, anxiety, or nervousness may limit treatment in some patients. The sympathomimetic psychostimulants are used alone or in combination with modafinil for more severe EDS. Shorter half-life stimulants (e.g., methylphenidate HCl) may be used for immediate effect in combination with a program of napping or longer-acting stimulants. Methylphenidate 5 to 20 mg per dose up to 100 mg per day is experienced as less stimulating than dextroamphetamine but is better tolerated with less anorexia, tachycardia, and hypertension. After titrating methylphenidate to the most effective dose with least side effects, many patients appreciate being switched to a long-acting, once-daily methylphenidate formulation such as Ritalin-LA, Concerta, or Metadate. If methylphenidate is insufficiently alerting, dextroamphetamine 5 to 15 mg per dose up to 100 mg per day may be used. Pemoline is no longer used due to the risk of hepatotoxicity. Stimulants should be given either in the long-acting form as a single morning dose or in the regular form as divided doses with the last dose before dinner so as to wear off before the hour of sleep. Sympathomimetic stimulants should be avoided in patients with hypertension, symptomatic cardiovascular disease, glaucoma, hyperthyroidism, or substance abuse, and should not be used in combination with monoamine oxidase (MAO) inhibitors. These agents can increase abnormal involuntary movements, so their use is discouraged in these patients. Chronic high-dose exposure has been associated with the development of compulsive behavior. Cardiovascular status should be regularly monitored and dose reduction or discontinuation should be considered if cardiovascular status changes. Decreased treatment intensity may also be appropriate if the patient's social or occupational demands are reduced. If EDS increases, the patient should undergo repeat PSG testing to determine whether an additional sleep disorder has developed.

Treatment of sleep onset or sleep maintenance insomnia in patients on psychostimulants should be approached by moving stimulant dosages earlier in the day and refraining from the use of sedative hypnotics when possible. Sodium oxybate (see subsequent text) has several advantages in treating the nocturnal sleep disorder of narcolepsy. If these options are ineffective or contraindicated, a nonbenzodiazepine hypnotic that promotes sleep onset and maintenance, such as eszopiclone may be effective.

Pharmacologic treatment of cataplexy is accomplished using either antidepressants or sodium oxybate, with the former still being used as initial treatment pending further efficacy studies.[9] Treatment should be initiated with a combined serotonin/norepinephrine reuptake inhibitor (venlafaxine, atomoxetine, duloxetine), which are more effective REM suppressants than SSRIs, and safer and better tolerated than tricyclic antidepressants. Although venlafaxine is most frequently used, the specific agent may be selected on the basis of side effect profile, cost, or other patient-specific issues. If ineffective, SSRIs and tricyclics are second choice agents, with clomipramine being the most efficacious of the tricyclics. If antidepressants are inadequately effective or if cataplexy is severe, sodium oxybate should be prescribed. Sodium oxybate (γ-hydroxybutyrate) is effective in both cataplexy and EDS and may ultimately become the drug of first choice for narcolepsy with cataplexy, reducing the need for polypharmacy approaches. Because of its history of inappropriate usage, sodium oxybate is available only through a restricted program from the manufacturer. Prescribing information may be found on the following website: http://xyrem.info/successphys.htm. Treatment is initiated with a dosage of 4.5 g per night in 2 equal doses of 2.25 g taken at bedtime and 4 hours later. The maximum dosage is 9 g per night but increased side effects occur at this dosage. The MAO inhibitor, selegiline, has been shown to be effective in both EDS and cataplexy, but may require doses as high as 40 mg per day and therefore requires a low-tyramine diet.

3. **Breathing-related sleep disorders.** *Breathing-related sleep disorders* include obstructive apnea (most common), central apnea, central alveolar hypoventilation, and upper airway resistance syndrome. Most patients with central apnea also have some obstructive symptoms. Breathing-related sleep disorders are most commonly associated with hypersomnia but the patient may complain of sleep maintenance insomnia as well. Neuromuscular diseases, especially myotonic dystrophy, are often associated with hypoventilation and apnea in addition to daytime fatigue.

    a. **Phenomenology**

        (1) The *OSAHS* is caused by intermittent pharyngeal obstruction during sleep, resulting in daytime sleepiness. Apnea is defined as cessation of airflow for at least 10 seconds and is typically associated with sleep fragmentation and 2% to 4% decreased oxygen saturation. Hypopnea is defined as 30% to 50% reduction in airflow for 10 seconds or more but the definition by some centers requires oxygen desaturation

and arousal to occur as well. OSAHS is characterized by EDS plus an apnea–hypopnea index of at least 5 apneas/hypopneas per hour of sleep. Obesity, increased neck circumference, male gender, hypertension, and family history are associated with increased risk of OSAHS. Symptoms of OSAHS during sleep may include snoring, observed apnea, choking, night sweats, nocturia, restlessness, drooling, and esophageal reflux. Daytime symptoms include fatigue, sleepiness, morning headache, impaired concentration, decreased libido, depression, irritability, clumsiness, and personality change. Alcohol exacerbates OSAHS symptoms. The *upper airway resistance syndrome* may also cause daytime sleepiness. This syndrome includes increased breathing effort due to airway resistance in sleep not resulting in apnea or hypopnea.

(2) *Central sleep apnea* describes repeated apneic episodes (of at least 10 seconds duration) during sleep, resulting from a temporary loss of ventilatory effort that may occur with or without Cheyne-Stokes breathing. Patients with central alveolar hypoventilation (waking hypercapnia) may present with cor pulmonale, peripheral edema, and polycythemia, in addition to daytime sleepiness and snoring. The remainder of patients with central apnea may more often complain of insomnia and restless sleep than daytime sleepiness.

b. **Prevalence.** Obstructive apnea is most frequent among people 40 to 65 years of age with a prevalence in that group of approximately 4% in men and 2% in women, with higher prevalence among obese and hypertensive individuals. Central apnea constitutes 4% to 10% of apnea studied in sleep laboratories.

c. **Etiology/pathophysiology.** Obstructive apnea is caused by intermittent oropharyngeal obstruction due to a combination of normal sleep-related muscle hypotonia and either a congenitally small oropharyngeal opening or factors tending to narrow the opening, such as hypertrophy of tonsils/adenoids, nasal obstruction, enlarged uvula, macroglossia, micrognathia, or retrognathia. Central apnea is not a single entity but may be caused by a variety of disorders of central respiratory control. It may be caused by an underlying cardiac or neurologic disease, or by an increased respiratory drive, resulting in hypocapnia on arterial blood gas analysis. It may also occur as hypoventilation related to obesity and decreased respiratory drive, resulting in hypercapnia on arterial blood gas analysis. A severe congenital form of central alveolar hypoventilation (Ondine curse) also exists. Apnea induces oxygen desaturation, systemic hypertension, pulmonary hypertension, and cardiac dysrhythmia, with bradycardia during the apneic event and tachycardia during recovery of airflow. Sleep apnea is a risk factor for hypertension and is a likely risk factor for cardiac disease and stroke.

d. **Differential diagnosis.** Causes of *hypersomnia* or *EDS* are listed in Table 13.9. Sleep apnea is the most frequent cause with narcolepsy and idiopathic hypersomnia also frequent among patients evaluated in sleep laboratories, and delayed sleep phase (DSP) disorder is sometimes seen. However, insufficient sleep is a common cause of daytime sleepiness that may be suggested by marked differences in sleep on work days and days off.

e. **Treatment**

(1) Treatment of sleep apnea, like insomnia, involves a multimodal approach. Treatment of obesity with weight loss programs and nutritional consultation should be undertaken if appropriate. If the sleep study indicates positional apnea, patients must be trained to sleep on their side, an effort that can be aided by the attachment of a ping pong or tennis ball to the back of the pajama top. Use of alcohol or sedative medications in the evening should be discouraged. Cigarette smoking, which tends to cause airway irritation and can increase the tendency toward obstruction, should be reduced and discontinued at least in the evenings. If EDS impairs driving safety, the patient must be counseled to avoid driving until EDS is reduced. Sleep deprivation, which worsens apnea, should also be avoided.

(2) Continuous positive airway pressure (CPAP) treatment is the mainstay of therapy for obstructive apnea. The CPAP machine delivers sufficient pressure through a nasal or face mask to keep the airway open during sleep. The mask can be uncomfortable and compliance is variable. Heated humidification, patient education, and close medical follow-up have been shown to improve compliance. Bilevel positive airway pressure (BIPAP) devices allow different pressure settings for inspiration and expiration and may increase compliance in some patients although they have not been shown to be superior to CPAP in efficacy. Modafinil has been demonstrated to be an effective adjuvant to CPAP in treating residual sleepiness in sleep apnea, once CPAP compliance and effect have been documented.

(3) Oral appliances for mandible and tongue repositioning may be used to maintain airway patency but the effect should be checked in a follow-up PSG.

(4) Surgical interventions such as uvulopalatopharyngoplasty are available if CPAP is ineffective. They are reported to be approximately 50% effective, but the effect may vary depending on the specific anatomic

obstruction in a particular patient. In severe cases in which all treatment alternatives have been exhausted, tracheostomy may be required.

(5) Patients with central sleep apnea should be treated in consultation with a sleep center or pulmonary specialist.

C. **Circadian rhythm disorders**

1. **Phenomenology.** Circadian rhythm sleep disorders involve a mismatch between the sleep schedule required by the environment and the sleep–wake schedule of the patient. Forms of this disorder include DSP disorder, in which there is a persistent pattern of delayed sleep onset and late awakening time with daytime grogginess and evening alertness ("night people"); the less common advanced sleep phase (ASP) disorder in which there is a persistent pattern of falling asleep early in the evening and awakening very early in the morning ("morning people"); jet lag; shift work sleep disorder; and non-24 hour sleep–wake cycle (nonentrained or free-running circadian disorder), more common in blind or developmentally disabled individuals and some dementias. Difficulty waking up and sleep drunkenness may occur in DSP disorder. Early evening sleepiness is common in ASP disorder. DSP and ASP disorders may not be a source of distress in individuals able to structure their lives in concert with their sleep patterns.

2. **Prevalence.** The prevalence of circadian disorders in the general population is not known. DSP disorder occurs in 7% to 16% of adolescents and young adults and accounts for 10% of sleep lab evaluations for chronic insomnia. ASP disorder occurs in 1% of middle-aged and older adults and increases with age, making it a common cause of terminal insomnia in the elderly. Jet lag is more prevalent and requires longer recovery time in older adults.

3. **Etiology/pathophysiology.** A positive family history is found in 40% of DSP disorder cases. Polymorphisms in the circadian clock gene *hPer3* and other loci are associated with the disorder. Although the exact mechanism is unknown, mismatch of the circadian rhythm and the external environment are implicated as well as altered circadian cycles (with varying light exposures in the early morning and late evening) and sleep recovery after sleep loss. ASP disorder can run in families with autosomal dominant inheritance and in which a mutation in at least one circadian clock gene has been reported. Jet lag is precipitated by a loss of synchrony between circadian rhythm and local time combined with sleep loss. Non–24-hour sleep cycle may result from lack of light input to entrain the circadian pacemaker.

4. **Diagnosis.** These disorders are diagnosed by history and review of the sleep diary and typically do not require sleep laboratory investigation.

5. **Treatment.** Circadian disorders are treated by promoting good sleep hygiene with regular sleep and wake times 7 days per

week. Although additional controlled trials are needed, patients with DSP disorder may benefit from bright light therapy from a 10,000-lux source for 20 to 30 minutes after waking up in the morning, or for 20 to 30 minutes in the evening in case of ASP disorder. Older people accustomed to walking outdoors in the early morning can wear dark glasses to avoid inadvertently advancing their sleep phase further. Although not yet studied for this indication, remelteon has been tried for a few days to attempt to advance the sleep cycle in patients with DSP disorder.

Chronotherapy, in which the patient is placed on a 27-hour day, and the sleep cycle is advanced in 3-hour increments until reaching the appropriate sleep time, may be used for treatment of DSP disorder in patients able to tolerate this schedule. Individuals with non–24-hour sleep cycles may be treated with bright light therapy and melatonin agonists might be of use as in DSP disorders. Patients refractory to these interventions may be referred to a sleep disorders center. Short half-life benzodiazepine hypnotics given at the hour of sleep for the first 3 days has been shown to facilitate adaptation in jet lag. Melatonin therapy has also been helpful.

D.   **Restless leg syndrome and periodic limb movement disorder (dyssomnia not otherwise specified)**

   1.   **Phenomenology**

      a.   *RLS* consists of an irresistible urge to move one's legs while at rest or in the first part of the night, which in most people coincides with transition to sleep (therefore it is a circadian rather than a sleep-limited disorder). Patients frequently report a crawling sensation relieved by moving the legs or walking. The International Restless Leg Syndrome Study Group has defined a set of minimal criteria necessary for diagnosis: Desire to move the limbs associated with paresthesias or dysesthesias; motor restlessness with motor strategies to relieve discomfort; symptoms worse at rest and at least partially relieved by activity; and symptoms worse in evening or at night.

      b.   *PLMD* involves brief (<5 second), periodic (at 20 to 40 second intervals) leg movements that may result in arousal from non-REM sleep. The movements typically involve the great toe as well as the leg. The patient's bed partner may complain of kicking movements during sleep and patients may awaken with the bedclothes in disarray. PLMD often co-occurs with RLS and may be found in patients with narcolepsy, sleep apnea, and RBD.

   2.   **Prevalence.** Although RLS had initially been estimated to affect 5% of the population, bedtime leg restlessness has since been shown to occur in 10% to 15% of population-based survey responders. RLS appears to be responsible for approximately 10% of chronic insomnia evaluated in sleep laboratories, and occurs equally in men and women. Although mean age of onset is 27 to 41, up to 45% of patients with RLS in one large survey had

symptom onset before age 20. The prevalence of PLMD increases with age from 5% of 30- to 50-year olds to 44% of those older than 65. PLMD also increases with anemia, folate deficiency, kidney disease, and use of antidepressants. RLS and PLMD are increased in patients with iron deficiency or on dialysis.

3. **Etiology/pathophysiology.** Sixty-three percent of patients with RLS have at least one affected first-degree relative with suspected autosomal dominant inheritance. Although the underlying pathophysiology remains unknown, the frequency of RLS in patients with peripheral neuropathy suggests a peripheral nerve contribution; the observation of leg movements in spinal cord lesions and spinal anesthesia suggests a spinal contribution, and functional magnetic resonance imaging (fMRI) studies show activation of pontine and red nuclei in waking periodic leg movements and thalamo-cerebellar activation in leg-related sensory symptoms. A CNS pacemaker for periodic leg movements is suspected due to the similarity of movement periodicity to other periodic brain functions. A dopaminergic mechanism is strongly suggested by the efficacy of dopaminergic agents in treating these conditions as well as the tendency of dopamine blockade to cause akathisia. Endogenous opioid system involvement is suggested by the efficacy of opioids in treating these conditions and the ability of naloxone to provoke symptom recurrence in opioid-treated patients. Relatively greater CNS iron deficiency in late life has been found in early onset compared to late-onset RLS, an interesting finding given the capacity of systemic iron deficiency to induce an akathisia-like condition.

4. **Differential diagnosis.** Resolution of the differential diagnosis is based on a thorough sleep history. RLS and PLMD should be distinguished from akathisia due to neuroleptics; hypnic jerks (sudden jerks at sleep onset that occur normally, also called *sleep starts*); nocturnal leg cramps (typically calf cramps); movement due to neuropathic leg pain; and the relatively rare painful legs and moving toes syndrome, which includes severe foot pain, burning, and near continual toe movement but is not necessarily worse at night or relieved by activity. Determination of serum iron and ferritin levels is recommended.

5. **Treatment.** Medicines that increase RLS, including dopamine blockers, tricyclic antidepressants, and SSRIs, should first be discontinued if possible. Avoidance of caffeine, alcohol, and nicotine may also help reduce symptoms. Serum iron deficiency should be corrected so that ferritin level has normalized before starting other treatments. Dopamine agonist and dopamine precursor treatments are the mainstay of treatment with benzodiazepine or anticonvulsant agents used as alternatives.[10,11] The nonergot dopamine agonists Pramipexole (0.125 mg 2 hours before symptom onset, increasing by 0.125 mg q3d until symptoms are relieved or a maximum of 2 mg per day is reached) and ropinirole (0.25 mg 2 hours before symptom onset, increasing by 0.25 mg q3d until symptoms are relieved or maximum of 4 mg

per day is reached) are often better tolerated than the commonly used ergot dopamine agonist, pergolide (0.1 to 0.5 mg h.s.), which has also been shown as effective.[10] Ropinirole is the only FDA-approved medication for RLS. Levodopa/carbidopa combinations of 100/25 to 200/50 h.s. in the regular or extended release form are also used but they may cause daytime augmentation of the RLS symptoms in as high as 80% of patients treated long term, and early morning rebound of symptoms in up to 30%, a problem much less frequently encountered with dopamine agonists. Other common adverse effects of dopaminergic treatment include nausea and daytime sleepiness, with occasional exacerbation of psychotic symptoms. Patients may take a dose of levodopa/carbidopa in the evening while waiting for their dopamine agonist to take effect. If dopaminergic treatment is not tolerated, clonazepam 0.5 to 2 mg h.s., gabapentin 100 to 400 mg h.s. to a maximum of 800 mg t.i.d. (if RLS is associated with neuropathic pain or in hepatic insufficiency), carbamazepine 200 to 400 mg h.s., or opiates (codeine, oxycodone, or propoxyphene) may be effective. Clonazepam may also be added if dopamine agonist treatment alone is not completely effective in severe cases. Owing to the risk of dependence, opiates are not the first choice and should be avoided in the presence of substance abuse history.

V. PARASOMNIAS

Parasomnias are abnormal, complex sensory or motor experiences arising from sleep. The most common parasomnias arising from REM sleep include nightmares, RBD, sleep paralysis, and hypnagogic/hypnopompic hallucinations. Nightmares are anxiety-provoking dreams in which the anxiety persists briefly after becoming alert. *Sleep paralysis* and *hypnagogic hallucinations* have already been described. *Hypnopompic hallucinations* occur during transition to wakefulness. The most common predominantly non-REM arousal parasomnias include confusional awakenings, night terrors (*pavor nocturnus*), and sleepwalking (*somnambulism*).

A.   **Arousal disorders: Sleep terrors, confusional arousals, and sleepwalking**

1.   **Phenomenology.** *Arousal disorders* occur during the first 3 hours of the night when the bulk of stage 3 and 4 sleep occurs. *Sleep terrors* typically begin with a loud cry, followed by the appearance of panic associated with tachypnea, tachycardia, midriasis, and sweating, and usually last approximately 6 minutes. In contrast to nightmares, which occur during REM sleep and are recalled, patients do not recall sleep terrors. Children younger than 5 years may develop similar episodes called *confusional arousals* that can be quite disconcerting to parents. *Sleep drunkenness*, a form of confusional arousal that persists in adulthood, may be associated with serious injury to self or others. Patients with sleep drunkenness may remain confused for up to 30 to 60 minutes following morning awakening. *Sleepwalking*

(*somnambulism*) consists of nocturnal ambulation, movement, or other bizarre behavior that appears to occur without awakening and which are not recalled by the patient in the morning. Like sleep terrors and confusional arousals it occurs more frequently in childhood. Sleepwalkers may walk with eyes open and avoid bumping into objects. However, they may also just sit up in bed and make repetitive movements. Talking, if it occurs at all, is minimal. Sleepwalkers seldom respond to others speaking to them. Arousal by another person may precipitate prolonged confusion or aggressive behavior. Patients seldom have any recall of events during non-REM parasomnias.

2. **Prevalence.** Sleep terrors are estimated to occur in up to 6.5% of children and 2.5% of adults, with the prevalence falling to 1% in adults older than 65. Confusional arousals occur in approximately 17% of children and in 3% to 4% of young adults. Up to 17% of children also sleepwalk with a peak incidence at age 12, and with history of confusional arousals in early childhood a common antecedent. Sleepwalking occurs in 4% of adults and is not necessarily preceded by sleepwalking in childhood. The arousal disorders in general tend to run in families. The risk of sleepwalking is doubled with one affected parent and tripled, to 60%, if both parents are affected.

3. **Etiology/pathophysiology.** In addition to genetic factors, rotating shift work, sleep deprivation, forced awakening, substance abuse, CNS depressants, stress, anxiety, mood disorders, or other sleep disorders—especially DSP disorder and narcolepsy—may predispose patients to arousal disorders. Confusional arousals have occasionally been reported in brainstem and diencephalic lesions but neurologic etiologies are quite rare. Sleepwalking and sleep terrors are thought to involve instability of slow wave sleep with disordered arousals. Sleepwalking in childhood is not necessarily pathologic but may become more problematic if it persists beyond adolescence. Hyperthyroidism, psychotropic medications, migraine, stroke, traumatic brain injury (TBI), and other neurologic disorders may precipitate sleepwalking.

4. **Differential diagnosis.** Because nocturnal seizures can precipitate arousal and transient confusion, a prolonged sleep EEG may be needed. Violent or aggressive behavior occurring during sleep should be evaluated by PSG to determine whether the problem is confusional arousal in slow wave or RBD in REM sleep. Sleepwalking with agitation may be difficult to distinguish from sleep terrors without PSG, because both can begin with a scream and involve bolting from the bed and becoming aggressive. If the behavior occurs during the sleep study without evidence of any of the above, the possibility of malingering should be considered.

5. **Treatment.** Parents should be educated about not trying to arouse the child from confusional arousal episodes and be reassured

that the child will grow out of them. Attempts to awaken an individual during a sleep terror may result in prolonged confusion; so waiting for the episode to end on its own is the best approach. Gently guiding the sleepwalker back to bed is the best management approach for this disorder. If sleepwalking is associated with dangerous behaviors, a secure sleeping environment should be established. Discontinuation of psychotropic agents if clinically appropriate may also decrease sleepwalking. Care should be taken when prescribing sedative hypnotics because many of these agents have been reported to cause sleepwalking.

B. **Rapid eye movement behavior disorder (parasomnia not otherwise specified)**

1. **Phenomenology.** *RBD* is a movement disorder consisting of complex, at times violent, movements occurring during REM sleep and causing risk of physical injury to bed partners or others nearby. Patients may complain of sleep injury or changes in dreaming but not usually of sleep disruption. They may have a dream-like patchy recall of parasomnic behavior.

2. **Prevalence.** Violent behaviors during sleep have been estimated by survey to occur in 2% of adults, with approximately one fourth due to RBD for an estimated prevalence of 0.5%. RBD occurs most frequently in men older than 50 years.

3. **Etiology/pathophysiology.** RBD appears to represent acting out of dreams due to failure of muscle atonia during REM sleep. A dopamine insufficiency mechanism has been postulated.

4. **Differential diagnosis.** RBD has occurred in association with narcolepsy, dementia, stroke, multiple sclerosis (MS), brainstem tumor, brainstem atrophy, serotonergic antidepressants, and alcohol withdrawal. The strongest neurologic association, however, appears to be Parkinson disease and Parkinson-related syndromes, such as Lewy body dementia, occurring before the development of parkinsonian symptoms in some patients. Electromyogram (EMG) activity may be detected by PSG during REM sleep. RBD should be distinguished from other parasomnias as well as nocturnal seizures, nocturnal panic disorder, posttraumatic stress disorder (PTSD), dissociative identity disorder, conversion disorder, and malingering. RBD occurs after the patient has been asleep for at least 2 hours in contrast to the non-REM arousal disorders that occur during the first few hours of sleep. Nocturnal PSG, often for more than one night and with audiovisual observation, is useful in diagnosis.

5. **Treatment.** A safe sleep environment should be established; dangerous objects should be removed from around the bed, pillows should be placed around the bed, and consideration should be given to placing the mattress on the floor. Clonazepam 0.5 to 1 mg h.s. is highly effective in suppressing symptoms of RBD. If clonazepam is ineffective, or causes cognitive side effects, or results in worsening of apnea symptoms, patients should be treated with a melatonin agonist,[12] or as a third choice, with pramipexole.[13]

VI. SLEEP DISORDERS DUE TO PSYCHIATRIC AND NEUROLOGIC CONDITIONS

A. **Sleep disorders due to psychiatric conditions**

1. **Phenomenology.** Most Axis I psychiatric disorders include sleep symptoms. Major depression and dysthymic disorder are associated with sleep onset, maintenance and terminal insomnia, hypersomnia, and nightmares. Mania is associated with decreased need for sleep and decreased total sleep time but the patient is unlikely to complain of insomnia. An association of slow wave sleep arousal disorders with mood and anxiety disorders has been reported. Sleep onset insomnia, sleep interruptions, and nightmares are common in anxiety disorders. Panic disorders carry the additional risk of abrupt awakening in a panic attack, and reexperiencing the trauma through dreams, nightmares, and flashbacks, is part of the core criteria for PTSD. Insomnia, sleep schedule disorganization, and complaints of neuroleptic-induced sedation are common in schizophrenia. Comorbid substance abuse should always be considered in the differential diagnosis of sleep complaints in psychiatric disorders.

2. **Diagnosis.** As in all sleep disorders, diagnosis begins with a thorough sleep history and maintenance and completion of a sleep diary if necessary. Sleep laboratory investigations are only needed when the sleep complaints fail to get better with improvement of the primary psychiatric disorder, when there is evidence of a concomitant primary sleep disorder, or when the sleep symptom may have a separate treatable etiology (e.g., nocturnal seizures). Table 13.11 lists PSG findings in major Axis I disorders.

3. **Treatment.** As in all sleep disorders, patients with psychiatric disorders should be instructed in sleep hygiene. Encouraging a regular sleep cycle may additionally enhance mood stabilization in bipolar disorders. Treatment of the primary psychiatric disorder should be maximized. Many dyssomnia complaints may be resolved simply by moving sedating psychotropic medications to the evening for complaints of hypersomnia, or alerting agents to the morning for complaints of insomnia. Avoidance of caffeine should be part of the treatment of anxiety disorders and bipolar mania. Before adding additional hypnotic or alerting agents consideration should be given to changing from the primary psychotropic agent to one with a more favorable side effect profile for the given sleep complaint. CBT approaches to insomnia may be helpful in this population and relaxation therapy may be particularly useful in anxiety disorders.

   Benzodiazepines (e.g., lorazepam 1 to 2 mg q4h as needed) are often added for sedation and anxiety reduction in the acute stages of mania. Clonazepam 0.5 to 2 mg h.s. may be used for nocturnal anxiety reduction in panic disorder and PTSD if SSRI

TABLE 13.11   Polysomnography Findings in Psychiatric Disorders

Axis I Diagnosis	Polysomnography Findings
Depression	Prolonged sleep latency Decreased slow wave sleep Shortened REM latency Altered REM/slow wave sleep distribution *Polysomnography findings in dysthymic disorder are of a similar pattern but milder*
Mania	Prolonged sleep latency Decreased slow wave sleep Shortened REM latency *Polysomnography is not indicated during manic episodes*
Generalized anxiety disorder	Prolonged sleep latency Frequent awakening Decreased slow wave sleep Decreased REM sleep
Panic disorder	Prolonged sleep latency Increased muscle movement in sleep Abrupt awakenings from early slow wave sleep with tachypnea, tachycardia, and panic symptoms
Post-traumatic stress disorder	Prolonged sleep latency Increased awakenings from both REM and slow wave sleep Increases and decreases in REM sleep and REM latency have been reported
Schizophrenia	Prolonged sleep latency Decreased total sleep time Decreased slow wave sleep Shortened REM latency Decreased REM sleep during psychotic exacerbations

REM, rapid eye movement.

treatment alone is insufficient. Otherwise, the treatment guidelines listed under insomnia, earlier in this chapter, should be implemented if insomnia treatment is needed after the forgoing interventions.

B. Sleep disorders due to neurologic conditions

  1. **Phenomenology**

   a. **Chronic fatigue syndrome and fibromyalgia.** Patients with chronic fatigue syndrome (CFS) and fibromyalgia (FM) complain of nonrestorative sleep, myalgia, arthralgias, and chronic fatigue. Those with FM also have characteristic point-tenderness in areas such as the iliac crests, trapezius, lateral epicondyle, and medial knee fat pads (American College of Rheumatology diagnostic criteria require 11 of 18 known tender points), and a search for these should be part of the physical examination. Some controversy exists as to the nature of these disorders and it is common to see them in patients with other psychiatric, medical, and psychosocial conditions that could by themselves cause sleep symptoms. It is not known whether the sleep symptoms in these syndromes are primary or secondary and whether the two conditions are indeed separate disorders. FM and CFS are more common in women and their etiology remains unknown. Sleep-disordered breathing and PLMD are frequent comorbid conditions.

b. **Parkinson disease.** Sleep complaints, which occur in up to 60% of patients with Parkinson disease, commonly include sleep fragmentation, insomnia, nightmares/sleep terrors, sleep talking, hallucinations, and EDS.[14] Sleep onset insomnia and sleep interruption are the most frequent complaints. EDS affects up to 50% of patients. Sleep disturbances increase with disease progression, on–off phenomenon, and hallucinations. Arousals may occur due to akinesia restricting nocturnal movement. Comorbid sleep disorders include insomnia, sleep apnea, RLS, PLMD, narcolepsy without cataplexy, sleep terrors, circadian rhythm disorders, sleep-related hallucinations, and RBD. RBD may even precede development of parkinsonism in Parkinson disease and Lewy body dementia. Depression and dementia, both very common in this group, also contribute to sleep symptoms. In addition, somnolence is a common side effect of dopaminergic therapy and selegiline, if taken too late in the day, causes sleep onset insomnia. Dopaminergic agents are also REM suppressants and are associated with vivid dreams, nightmares, and sleep terrors in many patients.

c. **Epilepsy.** Epilepsy and sleep are related in a number of ways.[15] Sleep affects the distribution and frequency of seizure discharges while seizure discharges may affect sleep regulation and interrupt sleep. Sleep deprivation lowers the seizure threshold. Transition to sleep is utilized during EEG testing to activate epileptiform discharges. People with epilepsy often complain of EDS or insomnia and sleep apnea is a common comorbid condition. Epileptic seizures are in the differential diagnosis of many parasomnias as well. Seizures occur mostly or exclusively during sleep in 15% to 20% of people with epilepsy. Nocturnal seizures may cause myoclonic jerks resembling hypnic jerks; hypnagogic hallucinations; nightmares; sleep interruption; and EDS. EDS may also reflect recurrent daytime seizures. Some of the components of narcolepsy, such as cataplexy, sleep paralysis, hypnagogic hallucinations, and automatic behavior, may seem to resemble seizures. Kleine-Levin syndrome may resemble the periodic hypersomnia caused by bouts of seizures. Occasionally it is the nocturnal seizures, triggered by oxygen desaturation, which cause sleep apnea to be diagnosed. Enuresis may be the sole clue to nocturnal seizures.

Automatic ambulation occurring during nocturnal partial complex seizures may appear similar to somnambulism. Anticonvulsants may cause either sleepiness or insomnia. Vagal nerve stimulation has been reported to both improve EDS and exacerbate sleep apnea. There appears to be a relationship between epilepsy and breathing-related sleep disorders. Finally, mood disorders associated with epilepsy may by themselves produce sleep symptoms.

d. **Multiple sclerosis.** Sleep disorders occur frequently in multiple sclerosis, with the most common sleep findings being middle insomnia, nocturnal movement disorders, sleep-disordered breathing, narcolepsy with or without cataplexy, and RBD.[16] Sleep symptoms may be affected by pain, nocturia, mood disorder, and disease severity. Sleep disruption may result in increased daytime sleepiness. Fatigue is a complaint in most patients with MS and does not appear to correlate with disease manifestations or severity. A number of medications with sedating side effects may exacerbate the complaint. The etiology is unknown. However, the fact that interferons worsen fatigue may suggest an immune system contribution.

e. **Dementia.** Sleep disruption, with increased percentage of stage 1 sleep, decreased sleep efficiency, and increased arousals, is greater in dementia than in age-matched controls. Given its prevalence in the healthy elderly, it is likely that sleep apnea is more common in dementia than may be appreciated. *Sundowning* is the term generally used to refer to agitation in the early evening hours commonly seen in patients with dementia. Its etiology has been variously posited as due to circadian mechanisms or an artifact of the evening environment. Nocturnal agitation, which may be related to sleep interruption or REM dyscontrol, is another common phenomenon. Forced awakening due to being checked on worsens nocturnal agitation. Some studies suggest greater disruption of sleep–wake cycles in vascular dementia with primarily white matter damage than in Alzheimer disease, presumably due to disruption of connections to the hypothalamic suprachiasmatic nucleus. Breathing-related sleep disorders may also be more common in vascular dementia than in Alzheimer disease. REM dyscontrol in Alzheimer disease may be related to cholinergic deterioration, given the REM initiation role postulated for the cholinergic system. *Fatal familial insomnia* is a rare inherited degenerative disease, thought to be caused by an abnormal prion protein, which causes intractable insomnia, autonomic dysregulation, endocrine dysfunction, and degeneration of thalamic nuclei, culminating in hallucinations, myoclonus, ataxia, and stupor.

f. **Traumatic brain injury.** Disordered sleep has been reported in 36% to 70% of patients following TBI.[17] Problems with sleep initiation are reported more frequently than sleep maintenance. Easy fatigability is part of the postconcussion syndrome, and hypersomnia was found in 47% of patients post-TBI in one study. In addition, sleep-disordered breathing and narcolepsy without cataplexy are associated with TBI. Hypocretin, a deficiency of which occurs in narcolepsy, has been shown to be diminished in the CSF following acute TBI, offering a possible insight into the pathophysiology.

g. **Stroke.** Ischemic stroke occurs most frequently in the morning hours, a phenomenon attributed to circadian rhythms of platelet aggregation, blood pressure, heart rate, catecholamines, and so on. Twenty percent to 40% of ischemic strokes present during the night. Snoring, present in almost half of middle-aged men and in more than one fourth of middle-aged women, may increase the risk of stroke, and may be a sign of OSAHS, which in theory raises blood pressure. Up to 70% of patients with acute stroke have sleep-related breathing disorders. Stroke-related deficits also appear as being able to cause OSAHS by themselves (e.g., brainstem stroke). Cheyne-Stokes respiration, a periodic breathing pattern with apneas and crescendo–decrescendo breathing, is seen in hemispheric infarction, but it may also occur in the elderly, in newborns, and at high altitudes. Because the nature of the strong association between apnea and stroke is not well understood, suspicion of OSAHS may be warranted in all patients with TIA or ischemic stroke.

Hypersomnia occurs after thalamic or midbrain infarction, or following large hemispheric strokes. Insomnia is also quite common, although insomnia as a direct result of CNS damage is less common, and may follow thalamic, midbrain, or pontine strokes. Strokes of the midbrain tegmentum or paramedian thalamus may result in peduncular hallucinosis, a syndrome of complex, dreamlike, often colorful, visual hallucinations occurring in the evening and at sleep onset, and thought to represent waking REM sleep. The *Charcot-Wilbrand syndrome* describes patients with parietooccipital, occipital, or deep frontal strokes, often bilateral, who develop cessation or reduction of dreaming, or in just the visual component of dreaming. These patients may have other deficits such as topographic amnesia or prosopagnosia.

2. **Diagnosis.** The sleep history should be gathered with attention to both the sleep complaints associated with each diagnosis and with other etiologies of sleep disorder or pain, as well as for signs of mood or anxiety disorders. In dementia, a caregiver or spouse must provide the sleep history and complete the sleep diary. In disorders such as MS, Parkinson disease, and TBI that are frequently associated with daytime sleepiness, care should be taken to elicit signs of sleep interruption or breathing-related

sleep disorders that could further increase daytime sleepiness. Particular attention should be directed to the timing of medications that may affect the sleep cycle. Medical conditions may complicate the differentiation of primary sleep disorders from neurologic disorders. For instance, cardiac arrhythmias may cause seizures or masquerade as seizures, whereas seizures may cause arrhythmias. GERD may cause sleep interruption, but nocturnal seizures may cause paroxysmal choking that could be interpreted as a symptom of GERD. Before concluding that a person with epilepsy suffers from a primary sleep disorder, the effect of anticonvulsant level and seizure frequency on the sleep complaint should be determined. Routine issues such as constipation may cause sleep symptoms in dementia or Parkinson disease. A PSG should be done for all patients with neurologic disorders who develop EDS. A sleep EEG is necessary in stereotyped nocturnal episodes to evaluate for nocturnal seizures. Patients with neurologic disorders who develop sleep maintenance insomnia often require PSG evaluation to determine whether arousals are related to their neurologic condition or to a comorbid primary sleep disorder.

3. **Treatment.** Treatment begins with instruction in sleep hygiene, maximization of treatment of neurologic disorder, and altering the dosage time of sedating or alerting medications for other conditions if appropriate. Adhering to a regular sleep schedule and avoiding sleep deprivation may enhance control of neurologic symptoms (e.g., seizures, headaches). Care should be taken to diagnose and treat comorbid mood and anxiety disorders, a frequent cause of sleep complaints in neurologic conditions. CBT is helpful in chronic insomnia. Graded exercise therapy has been shown to improve CFS, and participation in a supervised exercise program (avoiding overheating) can be helpful in MS. Sundowning in dementia should be treated behaviorally with orienting measures (calendar, clock, night light) and attention to proper sleep hygiene. Increased daytime light exposure and reduction of daytime naps may be helpful. For patients with Parkinson disease or dementia who have difficulty getting to the bathroom during the night, a bedside commode may improve sleep symptoms.

    Nonbenzodiazepine benzodiazepine receptor agonists may be used for sleep onset and sleep maintenance insomnia in neurologic disorders. Duloxetine 40 to 60 mg per day should be used for depression associated with pain in FM. If unsuccessful and pain persists, pregabalin 150 to 450 mg per day or gabapentin 100 to 600 mg three times daily should be tried. An extra dose of carbidopa/levodopa (e.g., Sinemet 25/100) at bedtime with repeat if needed in the middle of the night may ease nocturnal akinesia as well as PLMD and reduce sleep interruption in Parkinson disease. If a middle of the night dose becomes necessary, a controlled release formulation is used at bedtime. However, dopaminergic agents may exacerbate psychotic symptoms in Parkinson disease, and may be a cause of sleep onset insomnia or sleep interruption. Melatonergic treatment of insomnia is becoming common in Parkinson disease, dementia, and other neurologic disorders of the elderly where it is desirable to avoid the side effects of benzodiazepine hypnotics. For nocturnal agitation in dementia, mood stabilizers may be used if tolerated. Low dose atypical antipsychotic agents (e.g., risperidone 0.5 to 2 mg h.s.) are often helpful for this problem. However, both typical and atypical antipsychotic agents have been shown to cause a small increase in the risk of cardiovascular death, and risperidone has been associated with an increased stroke risk in the elderly. Antipsychotics should therefore be avoided, if possible, in individuals with prominent cardiovascular risk factors. In Parkinson disease, ramelteon may be effective for both insomnia and RBD, which are otherwise treated as described earlier in this chapter.

Pharmacologic treatment of MS-related fatigue and TBI-related hypoarousal begins with amantadine 50 to 100 mg qam, increasing to a maximum of 300 mg per day if needed. If unsuccessful, modafinil 100 to 400 mg per day may be prescribed. Sympathomimetic psychostimulants are occasionally prescribed as are activating antidepressants such as bupropion.

References
1. American Academy of Sleep Medicine. *International classification of sleep disorders: Diagnostic and coding manual*, 2nd ed. Westchester, IL: American Academy of Sleep Medicine; 2005.
2. American Psychiatric Association. *Diagnostic and statistical manual of mental disorders DSM-IV-TR (text revision)*, 4th ed Washington, DC: American Psychiatric Press, Inc.; 2000.
3. Mignot E, Taheri S, Nishino S. Sleeping with the hypothalamus: Emerging therapeutic targets for sleep disorders. *Nat Neurosci suppl.* 2002;5:1071–1075.
4. Johns M. A new method for measuring daytime sleepiness: The epworth sleepiness scale. *Sleep.* 1991;14:540–545.
5. Kushida C, Littner M, Morgenthaler T, et al. Practice parameters for the indications for polysomnography and related procedures: An update for 2005. *Sleep.* 2005;28(4):499–521.
6. Fulda S, Schulz H. Cognitive dysfunction in sleep disorders. *Sleep Med Rev.* 2001;5:423–445.
7. Glass J, Lanstot K, Herrmann N, et al. Sedative hypnotics in older people with insomnia: Meta-analysis of risks and benefits. *Br Med J.* 2005;331(7526):1169–1173.
8. Saletu-Zyhlarz G, Abu-Bakr M, Anderer P, et al. Insomnia in depression: Differences in objective and subjective sleep and awakening quality to normal controls and acute effects of trazodone. *Prog Neuropsychopharmacol Biol Psychiatry.* 2002;26(2):249–260.
9. Littner M, Johnson S, McCall W, et al. Practice parameters for the treatment of narcolepsy: An update for 2000. *Sleep.* 2001;24(4):451–466.

10. Hening W, Allen R, Earley C, et al. An update on the dopaminergic treatment of restless leg syndrome and periodic limb movement disorder. *Sleep*. 2004;27(3):560–583.
11. Littner M, Kushida C, Anderson W, et al. Practice parameters for the dopaminergic treatment of restless legs syndrome and periodic limb movement disorder. *Sleep*. 2004;27(3):557–559.
12. Boeve B, Silber M, Firman T. Melatonin for treatment of REM sleep behavior disorder in neurologic disorders: Results in 14 patients. *Sleep Med*. 2003;4(4):281–284.
13. Fantini M, Gagnon J, Filipini D, et al. The effects of pramipexole in REM sleep behavior disorder. *Neurology*. 2003;61(10):1418–1420.
14. Kumar S, Bhatia M, Behari M. Sleep disorders in parkinson's disease. *Mov Disord*. 2002;17:775–781.
15. Vaughn B, D'Cruz O. Sleep in epilepsy. *Semin Neurol*. 2004;24:301–313.
16. Fleming W, Pollak CP. Sleep disorders in multiple sclerosis. *Semin Neurol*. 2005;25:64–68.
17. Fichtenberg N, Millis S, Mann N, et al. Factors associated with insomnia among post acute traumatic brain injury survivors. *Brain Inj*. 2000;14:659–667.

Chapter 14

UNEXPLAINED NEUROPSYCHIATRIC SYMPTOMS

Fred Ovsiew, Jonathan M. Silver

I. INTRODUCTION

A. Doctors learn, from the earliest days of medical training, to identify the tissue pathology associated with patients' symptoms to reach a diagnosis. Cases where no such "organic" pathology can be linked to somatic symptoms pose conceptual and practical difficulties for doctors, and of course for patients as well.

B. These "medically unexplained" symptoms have drawn numerous labels. Of these the most famous is "hysteria," a term no longer used in medical circles although widely employed in the humanities and social sciences—"the new hysteria studies," as the historian Mark Micale has called the field. Other appellations for such symptoms include "functional," "psychogenic," and "pseudo-this-or-that." All of these terms have shortcomings. Even the intended neutrality of the term "medically unexplained" could be criticized as inappropriately excluding psychological explanation from the realm of medicine. Some clinicians have investigated which terms patients prefer, but such preferences are likely historically and culturally contingent and, moreover, may be at odds with the doctors' need for clear communication. In this chapter, we will refer to medically unexplained or nonorganic symptoms. Ultimately, diagnostic categorization should derive from understanding the pathogenesis of the conditions; we take up this issue after considering the syndromal presentations of nonorganic symptoms in neuropsychiatric practice.

II. SYNDROMES OF "MEDICALLY UNEXPLAINED" NEUROPSYCHIATRIC SYMPTOMS: PHENOMENOLOGY

For ease of presentation, we will organize these syndromes à la Diagnostic and Statistical Manual of Mental Disorders, 4th edition (DSM-IV). However, little evidence supports considering these psychological and behavioral states as discrete entities or psychiatric "diseases," and time is ripe for reconsideration of the current nosology.

A.   Conversion disorder

   1.   This category refers to motor or sensory symptoms superficially suggestive of nervous system disease although not generated by organic pathology. Rather the symptoms are judged as being due to psychological factors by virtue of the timing of their onset or exacerbation in relation to psychological stressors. The diagnosis excludes symptoms that are deliberately feigned and symptoms limited to pain or sexual dysfunction. Some authors argue, however, that doctors' ability to discern deception and thereby to distinguish conscious from unconscious mechanisms is too limited to form the basis of the nosology. The term *conversion* derives from an early Freudian notion that in this disorder affect, considered as a quantum of energy, is transformed into somatic excitation. No one thoughtfully holds this view or indeed the theory of mental energy where it was embedded, but the term conversion is mummified in the DSM, obscuring our lack of a theoretic consensus about the actual genesis of such symptoms. Alternatively, the International Classification of Diseases (ICD) considers such symptoms under the rubric of dissociation that posits an etiologic theory, although not a well-established one.

   2.   Nonorganic symptoms are common in clinical practice: At least one third of symptoms presented to primary care physicians are medically unexplained.[1] Epidemiologic data for conversion disorder—difficult to obtain because of the requirement that the symptom be medically unexplained, information that may not be accessible by the interview of the sufferer—suggest a relatively low population prevalence, in the vicinity of 1 to 2 per 1,000 in a 12-month prevalence.[2] The frequency in women may exceed that in men. However, among those seeking medical care, and especially in specialty settings, the figures are markedly different. For example, in a consecutive series of 300 outpatients seen in a neurology clinic in Scotland, symptoms were considered "not at all explained" by organic pathology in 11% and only "somewhat explained" by disease in 19%.[3] The point prevalence of conversion disorder among Danish medical inpatients was 1.5%[4] and 2.9% among neurology clinic attenders.[5]

   3.   The outcome of conversion symptoms is not fully known. Studies from tertiary centers may overstate chronicity—a degree of chronicity having been a factor in the patients coming to such a venue—and population-based outcome studies are not available. However, commonly the disorder evolves unfavorably.

Often conversion symptoms do not resolve or, if they do, other somatoform symptoms may develop. If the field of view of outcome is widened, patients are seen to do poorly in regard to other benchmarks, such as mood symptoms, employment, and family functioning.[6] In general, patients with somatoform disorders are as disabled as patients with other major mental disorders.[7]

B. **Somatization disorder and undifferentiated somatoform disorder**

1. Some patients present not an isolated nonorganic symptom but a seeming lifestyle devoted to somatic complaints without explanatory organic disease. These more pervasive disorders are classified as somatization disorder (SD) if they meet arbitrary criteria of severity, or as undifferentiated somatoform disorder (USD). In research settings other categorizations have been proposed; the data appear to show that patients just short of meeting criteria for SD generally resemble their more severely and pervasively affected counterparts. Unsurprisingly, a continuum of severity exists with SD at the most severe end.

2. The formal criteria for SD require the early onset (before age 30 by criterion, but far earlier in most instances) of multiple somatic complaints with consequent medical help-seeking or functional impairment. Specifically, the patient must report four pain symptoms, two gastrointestinal symptoms, one sexual symptom, and one conversion symptom. In each instance, no explanatory disease can be found after appropriate evaluation.

3. The criteria for SD include only somatic symptoms, albeit somatic symptoms without a basis in somatic disease. However, mental symptoms feature prominently in the presentation of patients with somatoform disorders. Briquet—the 19th century French physician who made an inventory of the symptoms of hysteria—knew this well and emphasized the "affective predominance" and lability of the hysteric. Psychogenic amnesia, which cannot be classified as "somatoform" because it is mental, resembles a conversion symptom in all other respects. Rates of mood disorder and other psychiatric syndromes are high in populations with somatoform symptoms (see subsequent text). Less appreciated in textbooks, although well known to clinicians, is the thought disorder, or incapacity to organize coherent narratives (especially of illness), that is highly prevalent in patients with nonorganic somatic symptoms. Such patients provide vague, circumstantial, indirect, and egocentric reports that lead to frustration and puzzlement on the part of the interviewer.[8]

4. As with conversion disorder, the prevalence in medical settings of more pervasive somatization substantially exceeds the population prevalence. In a Dutch general practice survey, 0.5% met the criteria for SD but an additional 17.7% met the broader criteria for USD.[9] In the Scandinavian inpatient study mentioned earlier, the rate of DSM-IV SD was 1.5% and that of USD 10.1%.[4] In a neurology clinic sample, the rates of SD and USD were 1.1% and 17.5% respectively.[5] More than a third met the criteria for

TABLE 14.1   Common Diagnoses
for Multiple Unexplained Somatic Symptoms

Chronic fatigue syndrome
Chronic Lyme disease
Fibromyalgia
Gulf war syndrome
Irritable bowel syndrome
Multiple chemical sensitivities
Sick building syndrome
Systemic candidiasis
Toxic exposure
Toxic mold

one or the other type of the somatoform disorders. The effect of a prevalence of nonorganic disease in medical practice in this range—one patient in six or even one patient in three—is enormous.

5. Patients with somatoform disorders may present with a specific "diagnosis," either provided by a clinician or self-attributed. These putative diseases vary in their evidentiary basis and validity (see Table 14.1). Patients' involvement in Internet groups focused on these diagnoses can complicate assessment and treatment. Further, prognosis may vary inversely with the patient's commitment to a diagnostic label or to a somatic explanation for the symptoms.[10]

Other psychiatric diagnoses are common in patients with somatoform disorders. In the study of patients in a neurology clinic already cited, 60.5% of those with somatoform disorders met criteria for another psychiatric disorder.[5] Anxiety or depressive disorder cooccur in approximately one fourth of the patients,[9] but other conditions, for example eating disorders, should be considered and sought in the psychiatric evaluation.

C. Pain disorder
1. This category comprises patients who report pain, with its associated distress and impairment in function, when psychological factors are judged to be significant in the origin, maintenance, or severity of the pain, and when neither feigning or intentional production of the pain nor an explanatory mood or anxiety disorder is present. A concurrent organic disorder may be present; if so, the psychological factors are nonetheless judged to play a major role in the pain disorder.
2. How is one to judge that the psychological factors are significant? In practice, the nonpsychiatric physician often makes the judgment; the clinician considers that the reports of pain are incompatible with an organic lesion if one is present, or excessive compared with patients with similar disorders whom the physician has treated. Since the psychiatrist's experience is likely to be more limited than, say, the orthopaedic surgeon's

experience of low back pain after surgery, the somewhat odd situation obtains where the nonpsychiatrist offers or clinches the psychiatric diagnosis. Faced with such a patient, the neuropsychiatrist may not find compelling psychological factors by interview. However, as most people have some psychological stressor at any given time, and because the tendency of patients not to acknowledge psychological conflicts must be taken into account, psychiatrists characteristically have a low threshold for attributing causal power to presumed psychological factors. Further consideration of the problem of pain evaluation and management is provided in a separate chapter in this volume.

D. **Factitious disorder and malingering**
1. In these behavioral syndromes, symptoms (whether somatic or mental) are deliberately produced. The production may consist in feigning of symptoms or in creating them by self-injurious behavior, for example, production of fever by self-injection with contaminated material. Factitious disorder is distinguished from malingering by the goal or motivation of the behavior. In the former, the goal is the patient's assumption of the sick role; in the latter some practical incentive, such as financial gain or legal exculpation, is sought.
2. Malingering may be distinctly recognizable and even represent rational problem-solving behavior in certain social settings, such as prisons. Some have argued that external incentives, notably financial ones, drive much pseudosickness behavior, from whiplash through post-traumatic stress disorder. However, the motivations for behavior are rarely easy to discern unambiguously. Although it may seem to some that seeking financial gain is so naturally a preponderant motive that its pursuit demands no further explanation, others believe that the behavior of many patients considered to be malingerers is complexly determined. Outside the prison or similar institutional settings, a life devoted to malingering is sufficiently deviant to raise major psychiatric questions.

III. ETIOLOGY AND PATHOGENESIS OF SOMATIZATION

A. Although patients with nonorganic complaints refer to their current life stresses and may be willing to acknowledge a need for psychological assistance with them, a psychiatric explanation of somatization would be inadequate unless based on an understanding of why the reaction to stress takes the form that it does.
B. Equivocal evidence indicates an effect of current stressors in patients presenting with nonorganic somatic complaints.[11] However, a study performed in a refugee camp showed that even under the most extreme of currently stressful conditions, the propensity to develop medically unexplained symptoms depended on adverse or traumatic experiences in childhood.[12] Most studies find that childhood trauma, notably sexual or physical abuse, plays an important predisposing role in the vulnerability to somatization. Other features of childhood

adversity, including illness in the child or the parents, are also relevant. Of particular interest and importance is the presence of somatization in the mother.[13]

C. These findings, which point to developmental issues that should be explored in the psychiatric evaluation, do not immediately disclose the psychological mechanism by which the vulnerability to somatization is mediated. A process of symptom amplification—an attributional bias to explanation by disease, with a self-confirmatory pattern of excessive attention to somatic signals—has been highlighted, especially in its implications for a cognitive-behavioral treatment approach. How such a preference for a medical narrative of oneself might emerge from childhood experience has been explored in a preliminary way. A deficit in emotional awareness—specifically in the capacity for differentiated identification and elaboration of emotional states—has also been documented to characterize patients with somatoform disorders.[14] The acquisition of mature affect awareness and regulation clearly depends on secure attachment and is disrupted by childhood trauma. Under optimal circumstances, the developing child gains the capacity to recognize, abstract, name, differentiate, and elaborate upon inner states of emotional tension. When this capacity fails to develop normally, the person may be prone to use primitive modes of experience and description, "thinking with the body." From this perspective, the term "somatization" is a misnomer; the problem is rather failure of mentalization.[15]

D. Rief and Barsky summarized the equivocal evidence for biologic abnormalities in patients with somatoform disorders.[16] They and others proposed that symptom amplification amounts to an abnormality of filtering or oversensitivity to somatic signals. Vuilleumier's review of the functional imaging data found insufficient data for firm conclusions but suggested that conversion disorder is marked by intactness of elementary sensory and motor networks along with abnormal activation of limbic regions that are abnormally coupled to higher-order motor representations.[17] Consistent with the idea of abnormal filtering of somatic sensations usually kept out of awareness, this hypothesis, we speculate, amounts to postulating an overactive "somatic marker" system. In contrast with patients with medial frontal-lobe lesions who show decreased response to somatic sensations that should be important in decision making, patients with somatizing show "a kind of primitive protection or avoidance mechanism resulting in a pathologic state of alertness and attention that can modulate their sensory or motor experience and that is reflected in neural activity within specific brain areas such as cingulate cortex and sensorimotor networks."[17] This proposal of a cerebral mechanism for conversion symptoms is not an alternative to a developmental account of their psychology; it addresses the consequences of developmental events for brain organization and the implementation of the psychological mechanisms in brain function.

E. Of particular neuropsychiatric interest is the relationship between conversion disorder and organic brain disease. Many clinicians in the early part of the last century noted that organic disease produced alterations in personality, contributory to hysteria; the English neuropsychiatrist Eliot Slater argued that it was often this personality change in a patient with organic brain disease that led to the abnormal doctor–patient relationship reified as "hysteria." Traumatic brain injury (TBI) has been recognized as a common predisposing factor.[18] Somatoform disorders may be associated with right-hemisphere lesions both in patients with pseudoseizures and in epileptics after lobectomy.[19] Notwithstanding this suggestion, exactly what features of organic brain disease conduce to conversion symptoms and exactly what psychological deficit is entailed remain uncertain.

IV. DIAGNOSTIC APPROACH TO "MEDICALLY UNEXPLAINED" SYMPTOMS

A. From a medical viewpoint, the first and crucial diagnostic issue in patients with "medically unexplained" somatic symptoms is to be sure that a medical explanation is not being missed. Slater asserted that a diagnosis of "hysteria" was fraught with error, not only because it could not be made accurately but also because it indicated little more than poor communication between a doctor and a patient. In that study, 22 of 85 patients (26%) thought to have conversion symptoms proved at long-term follow-up to have organic disease. Slater—writing some four decades ago—famously concluded that the diagnosis of "hysteria" was "a disguise for ignorance, and a fertile source of clinical error. It is in fact not only a delusion but a snare."[20]

Fortunately, contemporary data reassure us that such diagnostic errors occur infrequently. Stone et al. in a recent overview of the literature, showed that studies since 1970 of the accuracy of diagnosis of nonorganic neurologic symptoms find only a 4% error rate.[21] However, concern must continue over the possibility of missing important, even devastating, organic disease because of premature and incorrect closure around a diagnosis of conversion disorder.

B. The inverse risk, also potentially damaging to the patient, is the misattribution of physical symptoms to a false organic diagnosis, that is, missing the psychiatric diagnosis. Somatoform disorders are often unrecognized by nonpsychiatric physicians. In the neurology clinic first-attenders sample mentioned in the preceding text, somatoform disorder correctly identified by the neurologist only in one half of the cases.[5] This outcome is the inverse of the Slater problem: Attachment to a somatic diagnosis not justified by the evidence in lieu of a psychiatric diagnosis that is not unlikely *a priori* (given the prevalence data already reviewed). In our experience, nonpsychiatric physicians often recognize the high likelihood of psychiatric illness in a patient presenting somatically but conduct a comprehensive somatic medical evaluation without pursuing psychiatric evaluation with equal vigor.

C. The following pointers may help in avoiding the pitfalls in the diagnostic process:

1. The diagnosis of somatoform disorders cannot be made without an adequate history. Therefore the presence of obstacles in

history taking should lead to special caution. For example, if the examiner is not fluent in the patient's language, if collateral informants are unavailable, or if medical records cannot be gathered, the diagnosis of a somatoform disorder should be provisional at most.

2. The role of medical records in the diagnostic process deserves emphasis. Patients who somaticize give inaccurate and incomplete histories. In one study of the longitudinal course of nonorganic somatic symptoms, 61% of medically unexplained somatic symptoms reported at the baseline evaluation were not reported at follow-up 12 months later.[22] Medical record review must correct these inaccuracies.

3. The neuropsychiatric evaluation must thoroughly explore potential organic contributors to symptom formation, not only by virtue of direct production of the presenting symptoms but also in respect of personality alteration associated with cerebral disease and conducive to impairment of representational and communicational capacities.

4. A bizarre or unfamiliar appearance of symptoms should not be given undue weight. Familiarity with the counterintuitive appearance of some organic signs is gained only with considerable clinical experience. Dismissing as "bizarre" a patient's inability to walk when the ability to run is unimpaired, for example, would risk missing a characteristic feature of early dystonia.

5. Nonorganic features of the examination represent suggestibility that can be present irrespective of the organic nature of the complaint. Except for signs that directly show nonphysiologic features of the complaint itself, such findings should be given little weight. Therefore, a Hoover sign in a patient with leg weakness counts toward the diagnosis.[23] However, a patient with moderate TBI may be labeled as "exaggerating" because the sensory examination is inconsistent, although the patient never makes complaints referable to the sensory system. In fact, the inconsistent examination may itself be a product of organic disease, not involving sensory systems *per se* but impairing judgment and communication.

6. The mental status examination must be thorough. The substantial excess of other mental disorders in patients with somatoform disorders requires the clinician to seek symptoms and signs of a broad range of psychopathology outside the somatic sphere. Many developmental and current adversities are relevant to the pathogenesis of somatization.

7. However, the discovery of a potential psychological meaning of the symptom is not sufficient for a diagnosis. Clinicians may be biased to look harder to find such factors in these patients; the identification of these factors does not mean that they are explanatory or causative. Psychosocial stressors are common in the general population and their specificity in regard to a diagnosis of conversion disorder is probably low. Similarly, secondary gain may be present with organic disease and cannot

be judged specifically to implicate nonorganic mechanisms in symptom origin. Although psychosocial information is psychiatrically relevant, it is potentially treacherous as a pointer to diagnosis of somatization.

8. Clinicians must be alert to their own biases. Although often useful, the comprehensive biopsychosocial formulation may encourage the clinician to take seriously, or to dismiss, symptoms that seem, or do not seem, to accord with other elements of the patient's life. For example, the patient's history of early sexual abuse may encourage the clinician to prioritize a diagnosis of conversion disorder; the patient's excellent work achievements may lead the clinician to pursue somatic investigations of a complaint of fatigue with exceptional vigor. Although in studies of large numbers of patients such psychosocial factors may be correlated with diagnosis, in the individual case they may not be explanatory and may lead to narrow differential diagnostic thinking. Although the clinician must consider these elements of the case, bias must be avoided.

9. The clinician should avoid the use of unrecognized idiosyncratic diagnoses; standard diagnostic criteria should be used. For example, not everyone who is chronically fatigued has the chronic fatigue syndrome as defined in internationally accepted diagnostic criteria.

10. The possibility of deliberate production of symptoms should be actively considered, especially in cases presenting in a forensic context or with uncooperative patients.

D. Neuropsychiatric referral of patients with somatoform disorders may occur when the clinician supposes that sophisticated testing (in particular, functional brain imaging) will disclose an organic disorder that has evaded diagnosis by other clinicians. In our view, the use of brain imaging to "confirm" the presence of an underlying "biologic" illness in patients with somatoform disorders is not indicated. Although such studies may well reveal abnormalities or at least anomalies of higher-order cerebral function, such findings disclose no "disease" other than the psychiatric diagnosis already known.[17]

V. TREATMENT OF SOMATIZATION

Management of patients with medically unexplained symptoms often proceeds in a manner determined by the prejudices of the evaluator. At its best, this practice is the art of medicine, and all clinicians at times must act without full guidance by directly relevant evidence. In our recommendations, we rely on systematic evidence when available and on our clinical experience when necessary.

A. **Raise psychiatric issues with the patient early in the evaluation.** Many patients with somatoform disorders will not seek or accept psychiatric care. Whether the nonpsychiatric physician's approach to referral is an important determinant of the patient's acceptance is not established by systematic research. In our view, when the physician is undertaking an evaluation of a potentially nonorganic complaint, the issue of psychiatric (or psychological) referral should generally be raised early. Not to do so implies to the patient that the ultimate referral means that the doctor has given up on him or her, for failure to find a "real" disease. The alternative approach is to discuss with the patient early in the evaluation that one possible contributor to the symptom picture is "stress" (or whatever psychological term would be mutually acceptable to doctor and patient). The process of evaluation of this element of the patient's disorder can then be pursued simultaneously with the organic investigations.

B. **Provide, or use, expert advice.** Many patients will not follow up with psychiatrists no matter what the nonpsychiatric physician's view is. Contrary to what the nonpsychiatric physician might wish, primary care physicians or specialists in nonpsychiatric medicine, including neurologists, will conduct the treatment of these patients. Fortunately, controlled trial evidence shows that even a single consultation letter from a psychiatrist can usefully recommend steps that allow such treatment to be more beneficial.[24] Such steps can include seeing the patient regularly, at a scheduled frequency that does not reward the development of new complaints by greater contact with the doctor. Investigations should be limited, preferably to situations where they are indicated by signs rather than symptoms.

C. **Be thorough in the evaluation.** As we have emphasized, patients with somatoform disorders often have other psychiatric disorders and impairments in many aspects of life. Although reducing disability from nonorganic symptoms and reducing inappropriate medical care are worthwhile goals, the treatment approach should keep in mind that the patient may well be suffering in other ways than those most salient medically.

D. **Take a rehabilitative perspective on symptoms.** Management of acute nonorganic symptoms should focus on symptom relief. The treater should not demand acknowledgement by the patient that the symptoms relate to emotional factors; to do so is likely to pose an insuperable obstacle and vitiate the treatment. Rather the patient should be provided with a face-saving way to forego the symptomatic behavior without having to make such an acknowledgement, for example, by participation in physical therapy.

Graded exercise has support as a treatment of fatigue in the chronic fatigue syndrome (and in other conditions).[25] Given the evidence for benefits of exercise in depression and for cardiovascular health, clinicians should have a low threshold for recommending exercise to patients with somatoform disorders.

E. **Consider the person as well as the symptoms.** Many patients will be able to acknowledge "stress" or family difficulties and, in some way, request or accept psychological assistance. Clinicians should remain alert to personality disturbance or frank psychiatric symptoms other than the presenting nonorganic somatic symptom. Even if the latter remits, the former may remain as important obstacles to a successful life course.

F. **Use psychopharmacology judiciously.** Pharmacologic treatment can be of considerable benefit to certain patients for certain symptoms. When a conversion disorder is driven by depression, treatment with an antidepressant may relieve the somatic symptoms. Usually, such patients present with definite depressive symptoms—although at times not mood symptoms and often not spontaneously reported—and their conversion symptoms are of short duration. When somatization is more pervasive and extensive in the patient's history, pharmacotherapy for target symptoms, such as anxiety and depression, may still be worthwhile but expectations for substantial impact on the somatoform disorder should be limited. In some instances, nonorganic somatic symptoms respond to antidepressant treatment, although whether this is because of an effect on anxiety and depression is uncertain.

Approaches to symptoms other than anxiety and depression have less evidence-based support. Many clinicians use amantadine, modafinil, and stimulants for fatigue. Pain complaints often lead to the use of amitriptyline or other tricyclic antidepressants or, more recently, duloxetine. This approach, based on the strong evidence for efficacy of the agents in neuropathic pain, does not have an equally strong basis in the somatoform disorders.

G. **Approach patients' preexisting diagnoses cautiously.** Many patients who present with the diagnostic labels (see Table 14.1) will have undergone, or will request or demand to undergo, treatment with pharmacotherapy deemed specific for the disease. For example, a request for intravenous antibiotics from a patient with claimed chronic Lyme disease will not be surprising. These requests should be handled in accord with the best evidence in general medicine. Patients lacking serologic or other evidence of Lyme disease therefore should not be treated with antibiotics; those with evidence satisfactory to the infectious disease community should.

H. **Use cognitive-behavioral therapy or other psychotherapeutic approaches.** In many instances, physicians believe that patients with somatoform disorders have psychological problems that should be addressed with psychotherapy; it seems fair to state that the patients will be less often convinced or enthusiastic. If patients are willing to acknowledge "stress" or another basis for psychological assistance, referral for therapy should be undertaken. Often, cognitive behavioral therapy (CBT) will be the most acceptable intervention from the patient's point of view, and systematic evidence supports its use in somatoform disorders.[26] The primary goal is to improve function; somatic symptoms reported by patients may or may not improve. Several small controlled trials of psychodynamic psychotherapy for nonorganic symptoms (although not for conversion disorder or SD) showed favorable results;[27] no head-to-head comparisons with CBT are available. Probably, the clinician should use generally applicable principles of treatment choice in differentially referring or treating patients with different forms of psychotherapy. Due regard should be given to the risk of iatrogenic worsening of patients with borderline or primitive personality engaged in poorly chosen psychotherapeutic endeavors.

References

1. Kroenke K. Patients presenting with somatic complaints: Epidemiology, psychiatric comorbidity and management. *Int J Methods Psychiatr Res*. 2003;12(1):34–43.
2. Faravelli C, Abrardi L, Bartolozzi D, et al. The Sesto Fiorentino Study: Point and one-year prevalences of psychiatric disorders in an Italian community sample using clinical interviewers. *Psychother Psychosom*. 2004;73(4):226–234.
3. Carson AJ, Ringbauer B, Stone J, et al. Do medically unexplained symptoms matter? A prospective cohort study of 300 new referrals to neurology outpatient clinics. *J Neurol Neurosurg Psychiatry*. 2000;68(2):207–210.
4. Fink P, Hansen MS, Oxhoj M-L. The prevalence of somatoform disorders among internal medical inpatients. *J Psychosom Res*. 2004;56(4):413–418.
5. Fink P, Steen Hansen M, Sondergaard L. Somatoform disorders among first-time referrals to a neurology service. *Psychosomatics*. 2005;46(6):540–548.
6. Reuber M, Mitchell AJ, Howlett S, et al. Measuring outcome in psychogenic nonepileptic seizures: How relevant is seizure remission? *Epilepsia*. 2005;46(11):1788–1795.
7. Hiller W, Rief W, Fichter MM. How disabled are patients with somatoform disorders? *Gen Hosp Psychiatry*. 1997;19(6):432–438.
8. North CS, Hansen K, Wetzel RD, et al. Nonpsychotic thought disorder: Objective clinical identification of somatization and antisocial personality in language patterns. *Compr Psychiatry*. 1997;38(3):171–178.
9. De Waal MWM, Arnold IA, Eekhof JAH, et al. Somatoform disorders in general practice: Prevalence, functional impairment and comorbidity with anxiety and depressive disorders. *Br J Psychiatry*. 2004;184(6):470–476.
10. Huibers MJH, Wessely S. The act of diagnosis: Pros and cons of labelling chronic fatigue syndrome. *Psychol Med*. 2006; 36:895–900.
11. Roelofs K, Spinhoven P, Sandijck P, et al. The impact of early trauma and recent life-events on symptom severity in patients with conversion disorder. *J Nerv Ment Dis*. 2005;193(8):508–514.
12. Van Ommeren M, Sharma B, Komproe I, et al. Trauma and loss as determinants of medically unexplained epidemic illness in a Bhutanese refugee camp. *Psychol Med*. 2001;31(7):1259–1267.
13. Craig TK, Bialas I, Hodson S, et al. Intergenerational transmission of somatization behaviour: 2. Observations of joint attention and bids for attention. *Psychol Med*. 2004;34(2):199–209.
14. Subic-Wrana C, Bruder S, Thomas W, et al. Emotional awareness deficits in inpatients of a psychosomatic ward: A comparison of two different measures of alexithymia. *Psychosom Med*. 2005;67(3):483–489.
15. Ovsiew F. An overview of the psychiatric approach to conversion disorder. In: Hallett M, Fahn S, Jankovic J, et al. eds. *Psychogenic movement disorders: Neurology and neuropsychiatry*. Philadelphia, PA: Lippincott Williams & Wilkins; 2006:115–121.

16. Rief W, Barsky AJ. Psychobiological perspectives on somato-
     form disorders. *Psychoneuroendocrinology.* 2005;30(10):996–1002.
17. Vuilleumier P. Hysterical conversion and brain function. In:
     Laureys S ed. *Progress in brain research, volume 150: The boundaries
     of consciousness: Neurobiology and neuropathology.* Amsterdam:
     Elsevier; 2005:309–329.
18. Westbrook LE, Devinsky O, Geocadin R. Nonepileptic seizures
     after head injury. *Epilepsia.* 1998;39(9):978–982.
19. Naga AA, Devinsky O, Barr WB. Somatoform disorders after
     temporal lobectomy. *Cogn Behav Neurol.* 2004;17(2):57–61.
20. Slater ET, Glithero E. A follow-up of patients diagnosed as
     suffering from "hysteria". *J Psychosom Res.* 1965;9(1):9–13.
21. Stone J, Smyth R, Carson A, et al. Systematic review of
     misdiagnosis of conversion symptoms and "hysteria". *BMJ.*
     2005;331(7523):989.
22. Simon GE, Gureje O. Stability of somatization disorder and
     somatization symptoms among primary care patients. *Arch Gen
     Psychiatry.* 1999;56(1):90–95.
23. Stone J, Zeman A, Sharpe M. Functional weakness and sensory
     disturbance. *J Neurol Neurosurg Psychiatry.* 2002;73(3):241–245.
24. Dickinson WP, Dickinson LM, deGruy FV, et al. A randomized
     clinical trial of a care recommendation letter intervention for
     somatization in primary care. *Ann Fam Med.* 2003;1(4):228–235.
25. Wallman KE, Morton AR, Goodman C, et al. Exercise prescrip-
     tion for individuals with chronic fatigue syndrome. *Med J Aust.*
     2005;183(3):142–143.
26. Hiller W, Fichter MM, Rief W. A controlled treatment study of
     somatoform disorders including analysis of healthcare utiliza-
     tion and cost-effectiveness. *J Psychosom Res.* 2003;54(4):369–380.
27. Leichsenring F. Are psychodynamic and psychoanalytic ther-
     apies effective?: A review of empirical data. *Int J Psychoanal.*
     2005;86(Pt 3):841–868.

Chapter 1

INTELLECTUAL DISABILITIES OF DEVELOPMENTAL ONSET

Alya Reeve

I. BACKGROUND AND DEFINITION

A. Intellectual disability (ID) is an impairment of cognitive function formerly known by many different names including mental deficiency, mental retardation (MR), developmental disability, cognitive disability, also feeblemindedness, idiocy, and many pejorative labels. It is characterized by limitations in both intellectual functioning and in adaptive function. ID is not something you have, "like blue eyes, or a bad heart" that can be compared across individuals for its own characteristic pathophysiology, nor is it an independent medical disorder (diagnosed, with known etiology). ID is not a clear independent mental disorder, though it is coded on Axis II of the Diagnostic and Statistical Manual of Mental Disorders (DSM) system. Rather, ID reflects the "fit" between the capabilities of individuals and the structure and expectations of their environment (see Table 15.1). Demands of certain settings can minimize or exacerbate the signs and symptoms of ID and affect the degree of limitations in functioning for an individual.

A variety of processes can result in or be associated with ID including:
- Inherited syndromes (e.g., trisomy 21, Fragile X, etc.)
- Metabolic deficiencies (e.g., mitochondrial disorders, vitamin and nutritional deficiencies, etc.)
- Acquired injuries (e.g., anoxia, trauma, hemorrhage, and ischemia)

TABLE 15.1   The American Association on Mental Retardation Definition of Mental Retardation

Mental retardation is a disability characterized by significant limitations both in intellectual functioning and in adaptive behavior as expressed in conceptual, social, and practical adaptive skills. This disability originates before age 18.

Five assumptions essential to the application of the definition

1. Limitations in present functioning must be considered within the context of community environments typical of the individual's age peers and culture.
2. Valid assessment considers cultural and linguistic diversity as well as differences in communication, sensory, motor, and behavioral factors.
3. Within an individual, limitations often coexist with strengths.
4. An important purpose of describing limitations is to develop a profile of needed supports.
5. With appropriate personalized supports over a sustained period, the life functioning of the person with mental retardation generally will improve.

©2002 American Association on Intellectual and Developmental Disabilities. www.aamr.org. Formally changed its name to American Association on Intellectual Disabilities in 2006.

- Exposure to toxins or infection (e.g., lead, or meningitis, measles, etc.)
- Environmental challenge, (e.g., inability to perform to grade-expectations in school)

Emphasis on the intelligence quotient (IQ) ratings for diagnosis has skewed the assessment of ID toward a focus on measures that require education-related skills.

It is important to point out that there is neither a reliable standardized measure (test) of social intelligence (reading person-to-person situations), nor of practical intelligence (functioning in day-to-day activities and problem solving daily living). Many individuals with borderline or low IQ scores have excellent social and practical skills; and do not require assistance to maintain employment or to live independently. In the broadest sense, they function well because the natural supports within society (from family and friends to community and religious affiliations) provide the structure and interests and means to not be limited in their independence. Conversely many individuals with borderline or low normal IQ scores are unable to function independently because of a mismatch between the demands of their environment and significant deficits in social and/or practical intelligence.

B. Defining ID and classifying severity of ID is done in different contexts, with differing meanings and results.
- Clinicians must pay particular attention to whether they are seeking:
  - To answer a question of etiology
  - To assist in access to support services
  - To predict future development or response to treatment intervention

- Identification of syndromes, or etiopathology, may contribute to prevention strategies and improved therapeutic measures.
- Approximately 75% of children classified with ID have no associated medical condition.
- Statistical models define ID based on having IQ two standard deviations below the mean (implies that there is a continuum of cognitive ability in the general population).
- Very frequently, individuals are labeled by the school system (a social systems model) for purposes of classroom expectations, rate of learning, and specialized instruction.

C. The neuropsychiatrist can provide a dynamic clinical model for understanding ID by integrating information from all other models/ definitions of ID.
  - Incorporating neuropsychiatric tools and skills in evaluating the developmental aspects of fluid intelligence include the following:
    ○ Reasoning, problem solving
    ○ Having areas of relative strengths and weaknesses in cognitive abilities
    ○ Explicit and implicit learning techniques
  - Integrating psychiatric functioning, life stresses, normal aging, and activities

D. The bibliography lists several excellent sources for more comprehensive discussion about the issues in integrating multiple sources of clinical and historical information. The focus of this chapter is on the care of patients with ID of developmental onset—much is being learned and the clinician has to *adapt* relevant information into their clinical practice.

II. PREVALENCE

A. Prevalence of ID/MR is estimated at approximately 0.7% to 1.25% of the general population, with some estimates as high as 3%. This rate would estimate that approximately 2 to 3 million individuals in the United States are affected with ID or MR. (The high-end estimate would assume that the death rate for individuals with ID is the same as for the general population; that ID is reliably identified in infancy; that ID does not change with increasing age). Using the 1990 census, 1.5 million people aged 6 to 64 were diagnosed with ID. The rate of ID/MR is underestimated because not all individuals seek assistance. For example, students are often passed on from grade to grade without comprehensive assessment, and if not tracked into special education programs students often drop out of school at their first opportunity. Furthermore, people know they do not want to be labeled as having ID/MR.

There are relatively lower rates for ID reported in western and mountain states in the United States; the highest rates are reported in eastern, southern, and central United States Higher rates of ID are reported in men overall, however, there are no sex-based differences among persons with severe forms of ID.

The life expectancy is increasing for individuals with ID; yet mortality rates are higher than for the general population. Death rates after the first year of life remain elevated for people with ID. In less severe forms of ID the death rate is about twice that of the general population, whereas in severe forms of ID the death rate may be 30-fold greater. There are probably several factors that contribute to this increased death rate including:

- Neurologic disorders and secondary medical complications in those with severe forms of ID
- Aspiration and secondary complications of aspiration related to gastroesophageal reflux disease (GERD), motor dyscontrol, muscle weakness, polypharmacy, excess sedation, seizures, and eating habits

The classification of severity of ID is commonly done based on IQ as follows:

- Mild level of ID corresponds to the range of 55 to 70.
- Moderate level of ID corresponds to the range of 40 to 55.
- Severe level of ID corresponds to the range of 25 to 40.
- Profound level of ID corresponds to <25.

The rationale for this kind of classification scheme was that it could predict life-long performance and capability, and assist in anticipating the medical needs of individuals. Unfortunately these classifications are not as helpful in clinical assessment or educational programming as it was hoped, and the overreliance on simple IQ measures (without taking into account [1] a full neuropsychological assessment, especially an inventory of frontal-executive functions and [2] the environmental supports available), can often result in a mismatch between what functional level is predicted based on IQ score, and the functional level that the person is able to actually demonstrate. Providers often erroneously attribute problematic behaviors to "MR" rather than looking for more specific or relevant diagnoses.

III. ETIOLOGY AND PATHOPHYSIOLOGY—ISSUES FOR PREVENTION

There are approximately 250 to 300 known causes of ID and this number is likely to increase as we learn more about the genetics of cognition. However, in the clinical arena, the cause of ID in most individuals is unknown or considered idiopathic. Some of the major categories of the causes of ID are listed in the subsequent text.

A. **Birth trauma.** The most common problems in birth are blunt trauma or lack of oxygen. The extent of anoxic damage is not predictably detected until several weeks or months have passed. Early motor development may be normal or may evidence signs of cerebral palsy. Often anoxic damage results in only minor motor symptoms and major cognitive delay, such as decreased speed of association, difficulty with new learning, and poor or slowed retention of novel information.

B. **Disorders of development.** Any disorder that affects brain development, myelination, pruning, or preservation of learning, can result in loss of abilities or prevent expected acquisition of knowledge. Onset before the age of 21 qualifies the disorder as a developmental disorder (as opposed to a disorder acquired in adulthood). Note that this is a different age criterion from federal definition of ID/MR. Several of the more common mechanisms are described in the subsequent text.

- *Haemophilus influenzae type b*
  - ○ Cause of bacterial meningitis
    - · Meningitis is 3% to 5% fatal.
    - · Of the survivors, 25% to 35% have permanent brain damage: ID, partial blindness, hearing impairment, speech disorders, hemiparesis, behavioral dyscontrol, seizures.
    - · Preventable by vaccination between age 2 months to 5 years
- Inborn errors of metabolism that require early detection and initiation of intervention during the neonatal period to prevent ID are:
  - ○ Phenylketonuria (PKU)
    - · Autosomal recessive single gene disorder
    - · Untreated, leads to severe ID and cerebral palsy (CP)
    - · Treatment with dietary restriction of phenylalanine permits normal intelligence, but with increased rates of hyperactivity and learning disorders.
  - ○ Galactosemia
    - · Missing enzyme for digestion of dairy products
    - · Associated with ID, hepatic disorders, cataracts.
  - ○ Congenital hypothyroidism
    - · Causes growth retardation of brain and bone, ID (irreversible if not treated within first 6 weeks of life), and over time all the other symptoms of insufficient thyroid hormone.
    - · Requires life-long replacement therapy.
    - · Thyroid levels must be monitored to adjust to periods of increased need, such as during ages 3 to 4 and adolescence.

C. **Genetic disorders.** A variety of genetically based syndromes have been associated with ID (e.g., Down syndrome or trisomy 21). These disorders typically have predictable physical attributes, physiology, behavior, pathology, and associated medical and neurologic complications. (see Table 15.2) Individual variations in all the syndromes occur—so extensive variation should be expected in presenting symptoms, response to medications, and complications from secondary conditions. As more children are put in the mainstream of the educational system and more intensive corrective and supportive therapies are instituted early in life, individuals with ID and known syndromes can be expected to have improved functional outcomes. These therapeutic interventions necessarily change the predictive accuracy of previously described syndromes and the developmental and health issues for the person through their lifespan. With proper supports, people with ID can be expected to contradict published prognoses.

D. **Autistic spectrum disorders.** Autistic spectrum syndromes are of heightened concern given the apparent increased incidence and associated disability. Most individuals with autism have some degree of ID although this is not universally true and is not true of individuals with Asperger syndrome. The hallmark of autistic spectrum disorders (except for Asperger syndrome) is delayed speech and

TABLE 15.2   Recognized Genetic Syndromes Presenting with Intellectual Disabilities

Down syndrome:
Approximately 7,000 infants are born annually with DS in the United States; this is a rate of 1:800 live births; the rate is independent of race or socioeconomic status. Life expectancy is variable, with some individuals living into their seventies; congenital cardiac malformations and complications from them contribute to earlier death; dementia in the fifties is reported in approximately 50%; thyroid problems and celiac disease are common medical comorbidities; atlantoaxial instability should be screened between 3 to 5 years of age and before participation in contact sports or Special Olympics.

Behavior: Characteristically placid and good-natured; although aggression, hyperactivity, and impulsivity are seen pretty regularly. Increased sociability and decreased self-injurious behavior is typical. Some clinicians report people with DS have an increased ability for imitation, which may contribute to having better acceptance in social situations. Given the high rate of hypothyroidism, thyroid functions should be investigated whenever there has been a recent change in cognition, behavior, or mood.

Cognitive Profile: Highest developmental scores are typically in infancy, with progressive slowing of cognitive development relative to normal-aged peers. Developmental language delay is present, with expressive language more affected than receptive; language pragmatics are good, with poorer grammatical abilities. Visual processing tends to be better than auditory processing; there may be deficits in short-term memory and delayed recall on formal testing.

Fragile X syndrome (Fra-X):
This syndrome is caused by massive expansion of CGG triplet trinucleotide repeats in the 5'-untranslated region of the Fragile X mental retardation-1 gene (FMR-1). Affected subjects have more than 200 repeats; phenotypically normal carriers have 43 to 200 repeats on the X chromosome at Xq27.3. Fra-X is the most common known cause of inherited intellectual disability. The prevalence in men is about twice that in women. The frequency of the permutation and mutation may be variable in different populations because of founder effects for those populations. Although prenatal testing by chorionic villus sampling can be done, the optimum time for determination of genetic risk is before pregnancy to determine genetic risk, clarification of carrier status, and availability of prenatal testing.

Physical characteristics are present from birth: Elongated face, large protruding ears, protruding jaw, hyperextensible joints, and enlarged testes in men after puberty.

Rett syndrome:
Most common cause of profound ID in women; prevalence is 1:10,000 to 1:12,000 in girls. Inherited as X-linked dominant condition, usually a single occurrence within a family. Prenatal testing is available if the MECP2 mutation has been identified in a family member. Early development is normal, with deceleration of head growth between 5 months and 4 years of age, loss of previously acquired hand use, communication dysfunction, and social withdrawal. It is categorized as a pervasive developmental disorder in DSM-IV-TR. It is complicated by secondary medical conditions of seizures, breath-holding episodes, hyperventilation, dystonia, spasticity, scoliosis, and peripheral vasomotor problems.

Behavior: Stereotypic midline hand movements of wringing, tapping, clapping, mouthing of hand and fingers are seen, as purposeful hand movements are lost. Ataxia of the trunk and gait appears in first 4 y of life; expressive and receptive language is severely impaired; psychomotor retardation is common. By age 5 to 7 y the social withdrawal is less pronounced. Gait and motor coordination deteriorates progressively, necessitating a wheelchair. Gaze remains a vital method of communicating with the world around them; interest may be shown by increased activity of the purposeless midline hand movements.

Lesch-Nyhan disease:
Lesch-Nyhan disease is a sex-linked recessive condition caused by an inborn error of (purine nucleotide) metabolism, with a prevalence rate of 1:380,000. (With each pregnancy the mother will have a 25% chance of having an affected male, a 25% chance of having a carrier female, and a 50% chance of having an unaffected child.) Occurrence in women is extremely rare. Prenatal testing is available.

(continued)

TABLE 15.2   (Continued)

Clinical Features: Overproduction of uric acid may vary from mild to severe; movement disorder; anemia and growth retardation; cognitive disability; behavioral disorder including self-injury. Self-biting may progress to deliberate self-harm, such as head banging, eye poking, pulling fingernails, persistent psychogenic vomiting. The severity of cognitive impairment reflects the severity of L-N variant. Severity of symptoms are correlated with uric acid levels and deficiencies in dopamine transport in basal ganglia structures, but at present are not fully explained at a biochemical level.

Prader-Willi syndrome:

PWS is the most common dysmorphic form of obesity because of the compulsive hyperphagia. It was identified as a syndrome of obesity, short stature, cryptorchidism, and intellectual disability. Hypotonia, hypogonadism, small hands and feet, and dysmorphic facies are also reported. It occurs in 1:10,000 to 1:22,000 live births; lifespan is dependent upon control of obesity and its secondary medical complications, especially diabetes, and heart failure. Over 90% of cases occur sporadically; paternal deletion of 15q11-q13, or maternal uniparental disomy of chromosome 15, or imprinting center mutation.

Behavioral Features: Compulsive food-hoarding, gorging, and seeking food; skin picking; irritability, anger, and low frustration tolerance; stubbornness. Depressive and anxiety symptoms are very common; 50% of children and adults with PWS have behavioral symptoms requiring specialized attention. Some test in the normal IQ range, while most are in the mild to moderate IQ range. Learning disabilities may be more severe than the individual IQ would suggest.

Angelman syndrome:

AS involves a defect on chromosome 15 in the same region as PWS of the chromosome inherited from the mother; the prevalence rate is 1:12,000 to 1:20,000 persons. Most cases are spontaneous sporadic mutations, though familial inheritance is reported. Typical physical features include a wide mouth, smiling, with a thin upper lip, pointed chin, prominent tongue, and wide-spaced teeth; head circumference is usually below 50%; approximately half have fair hair and skin; two third have strabismus. Motor milestones are delayed and truncal hypotonia is seen; many walk only between 3 and 4 y of age. Eighty percent have seizure disorders, with onset between 1.5 to 2 y of age; myclonic seizures and drop attacks are most common. Speech is much delayed.

Behavioral Features: AS often laugh inappropriately and frequently; hand flapping occurs with arousal; sleep is characteristically interrupted by frequent awakenings; hyperactivity interferes with concentration and socialization. Difficulties in speech and coordination contribute to underestimation of intellectual abilities, which are described as severely impaired. Comprehension is much better than expressive language.

Williams syndrome:

Williams, Barratt-Boyes and Lowe identified a syndrome that includes supravalvular aortic stenosis, peripheral pulmonary stenosis, intellectual disability, and characteristic facial appearance. It is a contiguous gene deletion disorder resulting from a hemizygous deletion of 1.5 Mb on one copy of chromosome 7 at 7q11.23. The facial features include broad forehead, medial eyebrow flare, depressed nasal bridge, stellate patterned iris, widely spaced teeth, and full lips (often described as "elfin-like"). Cognitive pattern is one of visuospatial difficulties, with strengths in auditory processing and in language. These school-based tasks remain seriously limited throughout the lifespan, though the capacity to understand what others are feeling and thinking has been demonstrated to approach normal function.

Behavioral Features: Often recognized by an overfriendly manner, excess sociability with strangers, high degree of empathy, attentional difficulties, and expressive language ability (better than IQ would lead one to expect). In some cases, perseverative behaviors, excessive anxiety, attention deficit disorder and sleep disorders are cause of dysfunction. Adaptive living skills are often impaired so that independent living in the community is feasible in <25%.

DS, down syndrome; PWS, prader-willi syndrome; AS, angelman syndrome; IQ, intelligence quotient.

language, impaired social skills ("social reciprocity"), and exaggerated interest or obsessions with a limited array of topics or objects. Autisticm spectrum disorders can be diagnosed by age 3, and associated clinical symptoms include poor eye contact, resisting cuddling, ritualistic behaviors of rocking and hand waving, obsession with order, late onset of talking, rhyming, or echolalic speech.

E. **Nonverbal learning disorders.** There are a group of children that may present with some degree of intellectual impairment, social awkwardness, and a variety of behavioral disturbances such as extremes of rage, poor attention, and poor organization. Formal neuropsychological assessment typically shows problems in several domains including graphomotor skills, reading comprehension, mechanical arithmetic, and mathematical reasoning/abstraction, and science. Interpersonal and behavioral problems may be evident in difficulties adapting to novel situations, awkward social interactions, and mood disturbances. This profile can make the individual appear intellectually more impaired than they are. A variety of terms have been used to describe these children including right hemisphere syndrome and the more common term nonverbal learning disorders (NVLD). The underlying pathophysiology of this disorder is not clear but is speculated to involve a developmental white matter disconnection syndrome, which affects the right hemisphere disproportionately.

F. **Exposure to medications/drugs/toxins.** Many prescribed drugs (e.g., antiepilepsy, antidepressants, antipsychotics, and antibiotics) can result in developmental abnormalities from facial midline variants to cardiac defects and even lack of cognitive and emotional control. Prevention is achieved by frank discussions with patients before pregnancy, planning to reduce medications to the lowest levels possible or discontinuation of medications, and supporting informed choices made by the patient. Drugs of abuse may cause direct harm, or may be associated with infectious diseases such as human immunodeficiency virus/acquired immunodeficiency syndrome (HIV/AIDS) or sexually transmitted diseases that cause ID. Among the most common and best recognized of this category are fetal alcohol syndrome (FAS) disorder and fetal alcohol effects (FAE) or alcohol, related neurodevelopmental disorders (ARND), and lead exposure.

Exposure to high levels of blood alcohol throughout pregnancy produces physical hallmarks of growth deficiency, short palpebral fissures, flat midface, short upturned nose, and smooth, or long philtrum; optic nerve hypoplasia often causes ocular disorders.

Allelic differences in both the mother and fetus alcohol dehydrogenase may account for much of the phenotype variation seen in FAS/FAE. Brain development is also widely and variably affected by alcohol. Some of the neurologic problems associated with FAS/FAE include:

- Microcephaly
- Tremors
- Hyperactivity
- Fine or gross motor problems
- Attentional deficits

- Learning disabilities, especially impaired generalizing of learning
- Intellectual disabilities (25% of cases)
- Seizures
- Central auditory dysfunction
- Poor abstract reasoning
- Emotional lability (anger and impulsivity)

Often their excellent verbal fluency is mistaken as sophisticated comprehension—making them extremely vulnerable to direct and indirect forms of abuse.

Early life exposure to lead increases risk for brain damage, ID, hepatic damage, anemia, decreased hearing, hyperactivity, renal disorders, and behavioral disturbance. Sources of environmental lead include lead-based paint, dust, soil, water (plumbing and lead solder), and certain ceramics. It is critical to keep children away from these sources and to enforce washing of hands and face before eating. Repeatedly testing lead levels through early childhood, especially at 12 and 24 months is indicated if the individual is felt to be at risk. If initial results are borderline, retesting within 6 months to verify decreasing serum level should be done. Normal is <10 mg per dL; >45 mg per dL is severely toxic; >70 mg per dL is a medical emergency. Emergency treatment is chelation therapy and supportive measures.

References

1. Luckasson R, Borthwick-Duffy S, Buntinx WHE, et al. *Mental retardation: Definition, classification, and systems of supports*, 10th ed. Washington, DC: American Association on Mental Retardation; 2002.
2. APA. *Diagnostic and statistical manual of mental disorders -IV-TR*, 4th ed. Text Revision. Washington, DC: American Psychiatric Association Press; 2000.
3. Yeargin-Allsopp M, Murphy CC, Cordero JF, et al. Reported biomedical causes and associated medical conditions for mental retardation among 10-year-old children. Metropolitan Atlanta, 1985–1987. *Dev Med Child Neurol.* 1997;39:142–149.
4. Harris JC. *Intellectual disability: Understanding its development, causes, classification, evaluation, and treatment*, 1st ed. New York: Oxford University Press; 2006.
5. Pary RJ, ed. Psychiatric problems in older persons with developmental disabilities. In: Fletcher RJ, Gardner WI, eds. *NADD monogram series*. Kingston, NY: NADD Press; 2002.
6. Dosen A, Day K, eds. *Treating mental illness and behavior disorders in children and adults with mental retardation*. Washington, DC: American Psychiatric Press; 2001.
7. Tymchuk AJ, Lakin KC, Luckasson R, eds. *The forgotten generation. The status and challenges of adults with mild cognitive limitations*. Baltimore, MD: Paul H. Brookes Publishing Co.; 2001.
8. Drews CD, Yeargin-Allsopp M, Decoufle P, et al. Variation in the influence of selected socio-demographic risk factors for mental retardation. *Am J Public Health.* 1995;85:329–334.
9. Nelson CA, Luciana M, eds. Handbook of developmental cognitive neuroscience. In: Johnson M, Pennington B, eds. *Developmental cognitive neurosciences*, 1st ed. Cambridge, MA: MIT Press; 2001:662.

10. Ferrell R, Wolinsky EJ, Kauffman CI, et al. Neuropsychiatric syndromes in adults with intellectual disability: Issues in assessment and treatment. *Curr Psychiatry Rep.* 2004;6:380–390.

IV. MANAGEMENT

A. **Principles of management**
1. **Diagnostic process.** It is important to characterize the degree and profile of ID. Reliance on simple IQ measures is rarely sufficient. It is usually desirable to have a full neuropsychological profile to outline the cognitive strengths and weaknesses and to help in the following:
   • Document abilities for functioning within standard educational systems.
   • Identify a characteristic pattern of cognitive strengths and weaknesses for an individual (e.g., strong visuospatial abilities, or mathematical learning disorder, etc.) to facilitate an individualized learning program tailored to their needs.
   • Establish an "objective" baseline of cognitive function to permit later comparison after gains, or after new injury and illness. (e.g., in evaluation of dementia or pseudodementia).
   Point of emphasis: As noted in the preceding text, IQ does not predict social functioning very well, nor risk for future illness or disease, nor realistic expectations of an individual's life course. Therefore in addition to the formal cognitive assessment it is helpful to include the following:
   • Clinical evaluations, school and work records, history, as described in the subsequent text.
   • Assessment of pragmatic ability in social and real-life situations, appropriate to age and experience (adjust for children and adults).
   The clinician must establish a differential diagnosis by excluding primary communication disorders, which mimic lowered IQ functioning (e.g., deafness, blindness, cerebral palsy), and disorders, which may be less evident as barriers to performance (e.g., learning disability, communication disorder). The differential includes medical and metabolic causes of psychiatric and behavioral changes, especially if there is a history or evidence of recent cognitive or functional decline. It is important to factor in whether the individual has had opportunities to experience trial and error, or the lack thereof. People who are significantly deprived of social interaction demonstrate a severe paucity of social reciprocity and have poor test-taking behavior and skills.
   • Address comorbidity: Concomitant medical conditions affect behavior and communication. For example, pain creates a serious need to communicate pleas for assistance, including agitated or aggressive behavior. Obesity and sleep apnea can cause profound fatigue, decreased attention, and poor initiative. Impaired attention and poor recall of events may be caused by partial seizures.

- Engage the assistance of a support team in making a valid assessment: The clinician needs multiple sources of accurate observations, particularly because this is a population that is somewhat limited in the ability to give accurate history. Any treatment will depend upon the support system to assure that the identified patient receives the intended therapy. Increased collaboration with the team enhances the likelihood of making the correct diagnosis and being able to implement effective treatment.

2. **Laboratory evaluations**
   - Causes of disordered communication and motor functioning in children and adults (beyond ID) must be looked for. Genetic screening in first few days of life for metabolic disorders and known genetic syndromes is important. Most states support a limited panel, but parents may request comprehensive screening (lead, PKU, galactosemia, thyroid, etc.). One should assure that proper immunizations occurred. Auditory and visual screenings for sensory disorders, using electrophysiology techniques, are often helpful.
   - Genetic studies are warranted when physical examination and history cannot explain the observed symptoms. Adults may also be referred for screening, as genetic testing has improved in sensitivity and specificity. Common findings may include Rett syndrome, Prader-Willi syndrome (PWS), Angelman syndrome (AS), Down syndrome (DS), Williams syndrome, and so on. The most commonly overlooked condition that can be diagnosed with genetic studies is Fragile X. Referral to a dysmorphology specialist is warranted when screening did not occur during infancy. The predictive power of the test must be considered when choosing to use genetic screening (e.g., CAG repeats for Huntington disease vs. apoE4 for Alzheimer disease).

3. **History and evaluation must be comprehensive.** As with any complex disorder, sequential information about pregnancy, delivery, and early development (milestones for motor, sensory, and cognition development) should be obtained. Patterns of development within the family of origin can assist the clinician in estimating whether the observed development is characteristic for the identified patient; later on the comparisons are useful for understanding differences and similarities between family members. The neuropsychiatric evaluation must be done *in person*. Often the clinic examination room is a safe and neutral enough place to perform a comprehensive examination of physical and mental capabilities. When anxiety is too severe, when physical handicaps prevent adequate evaluation, when behavior is radically different at the clinician's office as compared with other locations, then the evaluator must compile his or her opinion from examination(s) he/she performs in different settings. Constraints in a busy practice often preclude making such observations on short notice, but typical work/school/sports/home

settings can be visited to understand and evaluate the impact of these different settings on an individual.

Most times, the evaluation will take two or three meetings to form an adequate impression of current symptoms and past experiences to be able to formulate a diagnostic hypothesis. When verbal communication is very limited in an individual, the clinician must be very careful to make hypothesis-based clinical reasoning the foundation of all therapeutic interventions. Comprehensive notes at the outset and after each intervention strategy must serve as resource material for reexamination of the clinical impressions and treatment efforts/effects.

4. **Psychiatric diagnosis.** As severity of ID increases, the relative amount and severity of psychiatric illness increases. Psychiatric disorders occur roughly 2 to 4 times more frequently in ID than in the general population. For example, the general population rate for schizophrenia is approximately 1%, and the rate of schizophrenia among people with ID is reported as 2% to 3%. Some studies report psychotic illnesses most frequently, while others note that anxiety spectrum disorders are the most frequent. Relative rates of common psychiatric disorders are summarized in Table 15.3. Clinical practice using standard diagnostic labels (International Classification of Diseases [ICD] and DSM) has increased the validity and reliability of diagnostic recognition of psychiatric illness in people with ID. Threshold conditions for disorders listed within these diagnostic schemes should be applied to people with ID, making appropriate modification for the individual's handicaps. For example, verbal expression of mood is not an absolute requirement: Motor speed, degree of sustained interest, nonverbal communications, eye contact, and body language are common expressions of mood in addition to affect. Attention and concentration can be evaluated through consistency in completing tasks of differing durations, as well as through the evident thought process that a person follows when making decisions or reacting to people's dialogue around them. Judgment and insight may be assessed through relevant activity in the person's daily life, rather than

TABLE 15.3   Rates of Mental Health Disorder in People with ID

Disorder	%
Anxiety disorders	10–35
PTSD	22 [range 19–72]
Psychosis	2–5
Depression	0.6–30
Personality disorder	~3
Substance abuse	0.2–20

PTSD, post-traumatic stress disorder.

hypothetical artificial constructs. Suicidal ideation and intent should be taken seriously. If a person with ID makes a nonlethal attempt to kill or injure himself/herself, the individual's understanding of the possible and intended consequences of action should be considered (not how lethal was the attempt). An important modification of effort by the examiner is to differentiate between phrases that are being repeated by a person with ID because they have been heard or because they have elicited attention, and phrases that express their own experiences.

Clinicians are advised to find the most parsimonious explanation for altered behavior. Conversely, use caution to not miss exceptions that indicate more than one clinical difficulty. People with more severe forms of ID, as a rule, have less variety in their repertoire of expressions of distress (e.g., agitation may express dislike, fear, depression, lack of comprehension, pain, disagreement, being misunderstood, or frustration). More than one Axis I diagnosis may be the focus of treatment, and may occur simultaneously with more than one Axis II diagnosis. Having ID/MR does not prevent an individual from developing personality disorder. Dementia may be seen at earlier ages than in the general population. For example, the rate of Alzheimer disease is increased in persons with DS in their fifth and sixth decade. This disorder must be differentiated from depression and other reversible medical conditions, especially in younger individuals.

Substance abuse and dependence is becoming a greater clinical problem for people with ID as they live more fully in the community. Social expectations for fitting in, especially during adolescence and early adulthood, make it hard for many people to resist drinking alcohol. Often, people with ID do not have the economic means to buy illicit drugs. However, they may be the vulnerable people who are sent to deliver illicit drugs and are manipulated by others in maintaining chemical dependency. The diagnostic challenge of detecting such abuse and dependence is further challenged by the lack of treatment resources that are adapted to provide substance abuse rehabilitation for people with cognitive limitations.

V. TREATMENT

A. **Optimize the physical health.** The least intrusive and least toxic treatment support should be offered. Restoring nutritional deficits, removing toxic exposure, providing necessary immunizations, and assuring appropriately interesting environments will maximally assist the development of the child's intellectual, motor, social, and emotional well-being. It is critical to carefully assess for new or recurrent medical causes of newly noted changes in behavior such as infections, pain, medication reactions and so on.

B. **Optimize the environment.** A comprehensive assessment of environmental influences and factors can be summarized in a good environmental assessment. This is not usually immediately available to neuropsychiatric clinicians—hence the importance of delving into these questions during the initial history and on return visits. Some trained professionals, such as behavior therapists, will incorporate a study of environmental factors into their assessment of the individual psychological characteristics and responses of a person with ID. It is important to collect information about the individual's living situation including the following:

- Specifics about safety, noise, privacy, autonomy, access to necessary or desired services, the physical layout and aesthetic aspects of their abode.
  - Activity during the day, from school, work or day habilitation must be reviewed.
  - How many people does the individual encounter? Are these the people with whom the person with ID interacts, or are they just viewed from a distance?

Unfortunately, abuse is quite common in this vulnerable population. If abuse is suspected, or it is clear that a patient is not safe, the clinician must notify the authorities to investigate the situation and assure the patient's safety. The local agencies include child protective services, adult protective services, protection and advocacy agencies, and the police.

Sensory disabilities that interfere with reception from, perception of, and interaction with the immediate environment must be suspected first and rectified if possible. Because of developmental plasticity of neurons, interventions geared at training and improving the functional repertoire of children with ID must be pursued aggressively and consistently.

C. **Somatic treatments.** Most individuals with ID do not require psychotropic medications. However, if the first two steps are not effective, then psychotropic agents may be indicated. Pharmacotherapy should be hypothesis driven, and therefore open to revision by the clinician with the input of all other members of the patient's team (e.g., the patient, family, guardians, staff, teachers, and other therapists). Paradoxical responses to an individual medication, or to a class of medication, are common. If this occurs in childhood (such as an activating response to diphenhydramine, instead of the sedation expected) and there is an indication for a specific medication, it warrants a repeated, cautious trial in adulthood. All reactions to medications should be documented and carried forward in the person's medical record so that repeated trials of ineffective medications are not carried out. Reiss and Aman provide a review of pharmacologic studies in people with ID across many diagnoses. As people with ID get older, past combinations of medications and behavioral interventions will need to be reevaluated and adapted to changes in their abilities (improvements and degenerations). Drug–drug interactions should be evaluated with the onset of maladaptive behavior, changes in sleep or appetite, changes in interest or initiative.

D. **Complementary and alternative medicines.** Complementary and alternative medicines (CAM) cover a wide range of ancillary and alternative therapeutic interventions. For example, acupuncture has a long-standing well-documented literature that supports its rigorous methodology and provides objective evaluation of outcome; particularly useful for musculoskeletal pain and migraines. Other treatments may represent current fads with little proven benefit. Relaxation methods provide decreased stress, improved sleep, and improved sense of well-being that are tangible results affecting neuropsychiatric complaints.

Advocates for people with ID (e.g., parents, relatives, and staff) will often try teas, poultices, and other over-the-counter remedies on the advice of family members, on hearing of one good report, or an advertisement. It is difficult to say categorically that these are good or bad for the identified patient. Many are innocuous. Some herbal treatment is therapeutic—especially in individuals who are particularly sensitive to higher dosages of medications. For example, treatment with valerian root may restore sleep to a person who has restless sleep and becomes hung-over with traditional sedative-hypnotics. The clinician must create an environment where the patients (and/or representatives) will not fear or hesitate to disclose the other substances that are being given to the patient. "Natural" supplements (from ginseng to caffeine and sugar) can be the source of altered behavior, changes in sleep or appetite. Extra dosages of vitamins can be necessary supplements (such as need for carnitine) or can build up to toxicity (particularly for the fat-soluble vitamins). Acupressure, acupuncture, and massage are established treatments for chronic pain, and some acute pain syndromes. Agitation and worry can be greatly reduced by reassuring physical treatment, such as a weighted vest, or by deep tissue pressure. Sensory integration therapy is advocated for the integration of multiple sensory inputs, particularly in individuals with autism, and seems to be very effective for some individuals with this diagnosis. A moderate and inquisitive approach to all modalities is encouraged, as many of these therapies work in similar ways to allopathic medicines, but through less direct access into the nervous system.

E. **Informed consent.** Every patient must have a full understanding of the purpose for which they are taking medication. Depending upon their intellectual capabilities, this understanding may reside fully within themselves (own guardian), fully within another person (a full treatment guardian), or in some mix of legal and pragmatically derived supporters and advisors.

If the person with ID is unable to make fully independent treatment decisions, then at least assent must be obtained. When working with a treatment guardian or legal guardian (such as parents of a child), full exploration of intended effects, possible deleterious effects and potentially lethal effects has to be made within a context. A description of the symptoms that are the focus of treatment efforts and alternative therapeutic interventions must be reviewed and discussed. There are aspects to everyone's behavior that will not be changed through medications, psychotherapy, or wishful thinking—and that, too, must be acknowledged. A critical piece of effective pharmacotherapy is a regular review that the medication is having beneficial effect as intended, and is still indicated.

An individual (or their representative) has the right to refuse treatment and to withdraw from the treatment at any time. Discussing safe ways to do this is important to communicate with all people involved in the patient's care, especially when they are dependent upon others for accuracy in total amount taken, description of side effects, timing of doses during the day, and communication of clinical efficacy (e.g., many staff members are not aware of the differences in withdrawal from anticonvulsants, benzodiazepines, antidepressants, or antibiotics—all are pills, antisomething). The clinician must review the status of understanding about medications with the patients and their caregiver at every opportunity. Beyond affirming understanding, this dialogue enhances communication and elicits information about the effects medications are having on the individual's functioning.

References
1. Reiss S, Aman MG, eds. *Psychotropic medication and developmental disabilities: The international consensus handbook.* Columbus, OH: Ohio State University Nisonger Center; 1998.
2. King BH. Pharmacological treatment of mood disturbances, aggression and self-injury in persons with pervasive developmental disorders. *J Autism Dev Disord.* 2000;30:439–445

VI. APPROACH TO SPECIFIC SYNDROMES

A. **Cognitive enhancement.** As in the normal population, individuals with ID can develop dementing disorders. Some conditions, such as DS carry an increased risk for early onset of Alzheimer disease. Medications to enhance cognitive function have been tried in small series of cases. As with other cases of dementing illnesses, drugs (such as donepezil or Aricept) will decrease the rate of decline in cognitive abilities. Clinicians have to be assured that they are contributing to improved quality of life and preventing loss of useful functioning in the individual with intellectual/developmental disabilities (I/DD). No medication will reverse the underlying developmental intellectual disorder, but medications may play a role in reversible causes of intellectual decline (such as depression and early phases of dementia). The number of patients requiring such therapy is likely to increase as the patient population ages and has a longer survival rate.

Treatment strategies include ensuring that all underlying general medical and neurologic disorders have been optimally treated, including comprehensive, and adequate pain management. The promotion of exercise and reestablishing a regular sleep–wake cycle is essential for sufficient rest to promote optimal cognitive function. Caregivers should be instructed in *behavioral management* of the patient's behavioral problems, including prevention and modification of the adverse behaviors. *Psychotherapeutic interventions* should also be considered, including individual (particularly cognitive-behavioral therapy), group (including formal support groups), and family therapy, although the efficacy of such treatments has not been formally studied. There are no U.S. Food and Drug Administration-approved somatic treatments for degenerative cognitive disorders in people with I/DD. There are no typical recommendations as the studies are preliminary. The decision to start medicines like deprenyl needs to be made for preservation of cognitive functioning, employment, daily living skills, and so on. In general, cognitive decline is slowed by 6 months to a year, in studies of elderly persons in the general population.

Reference

1. Reiss S, Aman MG, eds. *Psychotropic medication and developmental disabilities: The international consensus handbook.* Columbus, OH: Ohio State University Nisonger Center; 1998.

B. Mood disorders. The clinical background of depression and/or manic-depressive illness requires changes in diurnal biorhythms of at least 2 weeks' duration by standard criteria such as DSM or ICD. The rate of depression is 6% to 30%. Disappointment or elation over recent events reflects short-term responsivity, rather than fundamental change in mood. Untreated, depression may persist for 2 to 3 years before remitting; or a pattern of learned helplessness may create persistent depressed mood and behavior. Medical disorders that frequently cause depressive-like symptoms and depression include pain, thyroid disorders, gastrointestinal (GI) disorders, and conditions that cause shortness of breath.

Treatment should be directed at evaluation of the underlying general medical and neurologic disorders and comprehensive adequate pain control. Assure that the patient's environment and lifestyle are optimized, with promotion of exercise, regular sleep–wake cycle, and meaningful daily activities. Environmental supports include appropriate training of caregivers to provide therapeutic support for behavioral management of problematic or dangerous behaviors. Psychotherapy interventions from individual to group/family and art/music therapy should be offered to provide safe, structured opportunities for patients to express their feelings, to explore alternative solutions for dealing with problems, and to increase their understanding of themselves and their motivations.

Medications such as antidepressants of the selective serotonin reuptake inhibitor (SSRI) -type are frequently used for improvement of mood, reduction of anxiety, stabilization of sleep, reduction of repetitive thoughts or behaviors, and decreased reactivity. If one drug in this class does not work, others should be tried to find a better biologic match. Increases of serotonin in children can produce a sudden and severe worsening of depressive symptoms, including hallucinations. Some people with ID, whether children or adults, may experience similar responses. In general, starting with SSRI at a low dose (sometimes at half the lowest available pill) to demonstrate no unintended side effects and increasing the dose at weekly intervals (at 3 days if the situation is urgent and longer intervals if there is a lot of fear of potential side effects) allows for careful observations of general behavior related to the medication to be differentiated from daily variations in behavior.

There are no typical medications or doses to start treatment. Concomitant medical conditions, medications, and symptom profile will determine the choice. It is useful to start with half the typical starting dose, assure there are no detrimental side effects and increase at several days to 1 week intervals. For example, sertraline at 12.5 mg daily for 3 days, 25 mg daily for 4 days, 50 mg daily for 1 week, 75 mg daily for 1 or 2 weeks and so on. The time of day the dose is taken is determined by whether the patient is sedated (given at bedtime) or made more alert and motivated (given upon awakening). Medication trials should be for at least 4 to 6 weeks at a reasonably therapeutic dose before switching.

After three SSRIs have been tried to at least normal therapeutic dosage without benefit, mixed drugs such as venlafaxine (Effexor) or bupropion (Wellbutrin) should be considered; if trouble with sleep, nightmares, or excessive anxiety predominate the clinical picture, tricyclic antidepressants are indicated. The advantage of the latter is that serum levels can be monitored and the risk of overdose is minimized if the individual does not manage their own medications. SSRIs and serotonin-norepinephrine reuptake inhibitor (SNRIs) may induce akasthisia (see subsequent text), which may present with agitation and aggression.

References
1. Reiss S, Aman MG, eds. *Psychotropic medication and developmental disabilities: The international consensus handbook.* Columbus, OH: Ohio State University Nisonger Center; 1998.
2. King BH. Pharmacological treatment of mood disturbances, aggression and self-injury in persons with pervasive developmental disorders. *J Autism Dev Disord.* 2000;30:439–445

C. **Psychotic disorders.** The prevalence of psychosis is increased in people with ID, in proportion with other psychiatric illness, but remains much less common than thought of 40 years ago. Schizophrenia is diagnosed at approximately 1% to 1.5% of the general population, putting its prevalence to approximately 3% in the population with ID. Because a person is taking antipsychotic medication, the clinician should not assume that a psychotic disorder is present—the medication could be used for aggression, as a sleep aid, as adjunctive treatment of depression or mania, or to treat involuntary movements. Clinical diagnosis of schizophrenia or other psychosis must be made on the basis of psychotic symptoms; careful documentation of clinical symptoms and response to treatment should be maintained and kept up-to-date in records so that duplicative diagnostic trials do not occur. Medical conditions, adverse response to other drugs, and ingestion of drugs of abuse must be looked for and treated comprehensively before a diagnosis of psychotic disorder can be established.

Antipsychotic medications are indicated for the treatment of psychosis, intractable mood disorder, severe agitation (such as sometimes occurs in dementia or autism), and as adjunctive therapy when the severity and persistence of clinical symptoms warrant. Although antipsychotics have recently been associated with increased risk of death in elderly dementing patients, it is unclear that this mortality risk applies equally to other vulnerable populations.

Side effects of typical and atypical antipsychotics help determine drug of choice for a given clinical situation: High anticholinergic effects help treat rapid GI emptying and increase sedation (e.g., chlorpromazine); atypical antipsychotics like olanzapine may contribute to a metabolic syndrome, but may also counterbalance anorexic effects of some antiseizure medication. A limited number of antipsychotics come in injectable form; most are very long acting, with the exception of olanzapine (Zydis) and droperidol. Size of the tablet, availability in liquid form, color, and frequency of administration are factors that influence the patient's willingness to take medication on a regular basis. A typical way to start a trial is to choose a nonsedating atypical medication, such as risperidone at 0.5 to 1 mg daily and increase the dose after 2 weeks. Acute side effects might comprise drooling or excess stiffness, including cogwheel rigidity that are likely to respond to 0.5 or 1 mg of benztropine given either once or twice daily. The neuropsychiatrist will keep alert to potential side effects, such as involuntary movements, excess sedation, akasthisia, GI problems, and so on, that cause distress and motivation to stop the medication. Clinical trials of antipsychotics require at least 8 weeks at therapeutic dose with no improvement or change before they can be considered to be ineffective.

When patients report symptoms, they often have trouble telling that it is related to the medication, so the clinician must keep an alert ear to distinguish that voicing changes in current functioning may be because of the prescribed medication. All antipsychotic medications (typical>atypical) put people at risk for developing tardive dyskinesia. Because of the increased frequency of involuntary movements and mannerisms in people with ID, it is not clear that the use of antipsychotics increases the rate of movement disorders. In people with ID and schizophrenia, there is no increased risk for tardive dyskinesia.

Screening for involuntary movements should be done before initiating antipsychotic medication, monthly at times of major dose changes, and less frequently thereafter—probably annually for someone who is taking medication long term.

Akasthisia, a perception of unremitting internal restlessness and expressed as an inability to sit still, may be induced by antipsychotics, SSRI antidepressants, or idiosyncratically. It must be differentiated from agitation, as both of these conditions involve a perception of pressure to move the body. Agitation is often improved by increased dosage, whereas akasthisia is often worsened by an increased dose.

References
1. Reiss S, Aman MG, eds. *Psychotropic medication and developmental disabilities: The international consensus handbook.* Columbus, OH: Ohio State University Nisonger Center; 1998.
2. Duggan L, Brylewski J. Effectiveness of antipsychotic medication in people with intellectual disability and schizophrenia: A systematic review. *J Intellect Disabil Res.* 1999;43:94–104

D. **Anxiety disorders.** Anxiety symptoms are normal physiologic responses. Disorders of anxiety occur because of too many overwhelming experiences (such as trauma), lack of learning how to cope with uncertainty (too sheltered from life experiences), and physiologic disorders (e.g., panic attack, or thyroid storm). Including post-traumatic stress disorders (PTSD), anxiety disorders are the most prevalent disorders in people with ID (10% to 70%). They are also the most amenable to treatment. Factors to look for in the course of assessment include time of day, predictability of exacerbations, mitigating factors, physiologic arousal (piloerection, dilatation of pupils, shortness of breath, rapid pulse, and increased blood pressure), repetitive behavior (purposeful or purposeless), and report of increased or persistent worry. The efficacy in reducing anxiety is determined by integrating three factors: Etiology for the anxiety, perception of the "danger," and personal response to "danger."

Treatment of anxiety, from severe normal anxiety to anxiety disorders and anxiety concomitant with other psychiatric illness is often incomplete. Normal anxiety responses require reassurance and cognitive-behavioral approaches to assessment and coping. Pharmacologic management of anxiety includes benzodiazepines, SSRI and tricyclic antidepressants, antipsychotics, antiepileptics/mood stabilizers, β-blockers, α-blockers, narcotics, and opioid-blockers. No single pharmacologic treatment will suit all situations; side effects of medications may make the meanings attributed to internal perception and behavioral responses worse, for example, benzodiazepines may make a person disinhibited and more likely to impulsively lash out at people who come near them; constipation because of anticholinergic effects may make a person become irritable, and/or have headaches, etc.). There are a number of strategies for a choice of first drug. If a patient has panic attacks, some anxiety, and difficulty sleeping, for example, then imipramine is at the top of the list of drugs of choice. More routine anxiety could be effectively treated with low dose benzodiazepine. Alprazolam 0.5 mg several times per day is often effective and can be used short term or long term on an as-needed basis. More persistent anxiety might respond better to citalopram or escitalopram starting at 10 mg daily and increasing only after 2 or 3 weeks with no evident change in symptoms. As with other medications, a trial at a standard therapeutic dosage (for citalopram at least 40 mg daily) for 4 to 6 weeks must demonstrate lack of clinical efficacy.

Reference
1. Reiss S, Aman MG, eds. *Psychotropic medication and developmental disabilities: The international consensus handbook.* Columbus, OH: Ohio State University Nisonger Center; 1998.

E. **Sleep disorders.** Sleep disorder investigation requires questions about diet, exercise, sleep hygiene, possible current abuse, past abuse, nightmares, toileting needs, medications, medical conditions (pain, GERD, seizures, etc.), mood, perceptual disorders, and safety. Nonaddictive forms of sedative-hypnotics should be tried preferentially, as they can be used long term (e.g., trazodone from 25 to 400 mg per night). Assuring regular sleep is critical to preventing mood and affective lability, decreasing irritability, improving attention, and concentration, and motor performance. Because tricyclic antidepressants suppress rapid eye movement (REM) sleep they may be particularly effective for PTSD-induced nightmares. Over-the-counter antihistamine, herbal tea, and relaxation techniques may be as effective as medication and are to be recommended for long-term treatment. Short-acting benzodiazepine (e.g., lorazepam) may assist with falling asleep better than a traditional sedative, such as Restoril or Ambien. Trazodone as mentioned in the preceeding text is well tolerated by most people and can be used without developing tolerance (biologic or behavioral) to its effects. During times of stress people may require an increase, which subsequently may be lowered to a routine dose; some drugs increase or decrease its metabolism and may necessitate increased or decreased dosing.

Reference
1. Reiss S, Aman MG, eds. *Psychotropic medication and developmental disabilities: The international consensus handbook.* Columbus, OH: Ohio State University Nisonger Center; 1998.

F. **Self-injurious behavior.** Self-injury may occur in any condition; the treatment must be directed at the underlying psychological or medical condition. A few genetic conditions are associated with self-injurious behavior (SIB), namely Lesch-Nyhan with increased self-biting. Because there is no uniform agreement on what constitutes self-injury, the literature is broad and opinion is diverse. Prevalence data is misleading because of inclusion of untreated anxiety conditions, limited physical environments (institutional settings), and lack of comprehensive diagnostic evaluations. Head-banging may be a response to overstimulation in a child with autism or expression of headache in another child or adult without other means to communicate their distress. Environmental assessment is extremely important in proper evaluation of antecedents and meaning of SIB.

There are no diagnosis-specific medications for SIB or violent behavior. A combination of clinical trials to reduce unpredictable arousal, decrease impulsivity, increase mental flexibility, and increase comprehension of the surrounding environment must be tried. β-blockers (e.g., propranolol 40 to 420 mg per day) and α-blockers (e.g., clonidine 0.05 to 0.3 mg three times daily) often effectively decrease arousal which increases the opportunity for an individual to comprehend a change in his/her environment. Individuals with autism are prone to extreme expressions of distress and rage when sensory cues are overwhelming and intrusive to them, such as noises, changes in routine, and disruption of an object from its normal place. Controlling the environment may be the most appropriate treatment. Anticonvulsant medications may reduce impulsivity or rage and may reduce pain (e.g., valproic acid 125 to 1,250 mg b.i.d. to q.i.d., carbamazepine 100 to 400 mg b.i.d. to t.i.d., gabapentin 200 to 1,200 mg b.i.d. to q.i.d., etc.). The idea that there could be a typical strategy for SIB pharmacotherapy stretches treatment algorithm aficionados—there is none. Clinical evaluation of the cause and meaning of the SIB, including triggers, responses, secondary gain, and underlying medical conditions is the essential guidepost for starting any additional medication. Sometimes, sedation is required quickly and giving benzodiazepines with anticonvulsants may work. An example would be 2 mg lorazepam and 500 mg valproic acid. Antipsychotics tend to take longer to take effect. When anxiety is a strong component of the trigger for SIB, clonidine, or propranolol (mentioned in the preceding text) can be administered; the clinical effect is usually rapid within a day or two and doses can be increased every several days as long as the blood pressure is not dropping too low. Propranolol is slower to take action and several weeks at a dose over 160 mg per day is needed before feeling reasonably sure that it is not clinically effective.

References
1. Reiss S, Aman MG, eds. *Psychotropic medication and developmental disabilities: The international consensus handbook.* Columbus, OH: Ohio State University Nisonger Center; 1998.
2. King BH. Pharmacological treatment of mood disturbances, aggression and self-injury in persons with pervasive developmental disorders. *J Autism Dev Disord.* 200;30:439–445
3. Aman MGPD, De Smedt GMD, Derivan AMD, et al. Double-blind, placebo-controlled study of risperidone for the treatment of disruptive behaviors in children with subaverage intelligence. *Am J Psychiatry.* 2002;159:1337–1346.

VII. CONCLUSIONS

A. Health is a state of complete physical, mental, and social well-being. For most people with ID, physical and mental health concerns are similar to those of the general population. Medical care should be provided within settings appropriate for the medical condition.

B. IDs have a wide range of etiologies, many of which are unknown. Neuropsychiatric manifestations need to be addressed carefully and thoughtfully. These techniques require direct clinical examination, comprehensive historical information, and integration of expert information from multiple disciplines. The neuropsychiatrist must be prepared to insist upon proper evaluations being completed by other disciplines as well as from his/her own.

C. Disorders that are first diagnosed in childhood will continue into adult life, and will interact with health concerns of a normal lifespan and life experience. Psychiatric disorders will present about two to three times more frequently than the general population.

   Diagnostic criteria for mental illness need to be recognized. Treatment should be targeted at diagnostic symptoms in ways that increase the patient's functional abilities. Underlying medical and genetic conditions will have lifelong effects on the development of secondary medical and psychiatric conditions and responses to therapeutic interventions.

D. Self-determination is an important concept for all individuals. People with ID should have the opportunities to choose health care providers, to participate in making health-related decisions, and to express their opinions and experiences of treatment. Advocating for full participation in health care by the person with ID will increase the collegial role of the clinician in the entire system of supports for the patient.

E. Developmental plasticity of the nervous system is an underrecognized factor in predicting the course of chronic neurodevelopmental conditions. IDs present a field within neuropsychiatry that is largely unexplored. New research and clinical information is needed to extend our understanding of the individual developmental interactions between experience, environment, genetics, and meaning at the neuronal and conceptual levels.

References

1. Roizen NJ, Patterson D. Down's syndrome. *Lancet.* 2003;361: 1281–1289.
2. Hagerman RJ, Cronister AC, eds. *The fragile X syndrome: Diagnosis, treatment, and research,* 2nd ed. Baltimore, MD: Johns Hopkins University Press; 1996.
3. Hagberg B, Aicardi J, Dias K, et al. A progressive syndrome of autism, dementia, ataxia, and loss of purposeful hand use in girls: Rett's syndrome: Report of 35 cases. *Ann Neurol.* 1983;14:471–479.
4. Shretlen DJ, Harris JC, Park KS, et al. Neurocognitive functioning in Lesch-Nyhan disease and parital hypoxanthine-guanine phosphoribosyltransferase deficiency. *J Int Neuropsych Soc.* 2001;7: 805–812.
5. Prader A, Labhart A, Willi H. Ein syndrom von adipositas, kleinwuchs, kryptorchismus und oligophrenie nach myatonieartigem zustand in neugeborenenalter. *Schineizerishce Medizinishce Wochenschrift.* 1956;86:1260–1261.
6. Williams JCP, Barratt-Boyes BG, Lowe JB. Supravalvular aoritc stenosis. *Circulation.* 1961;24:1311–1318.

Chapter 16

AGITATION AND AGGRESSION*

Jonathan M. Silver, Stuart C. Yudofsky,
Karen E. Anderson

BACKGROUND

1. Consistent with the biopsychosocial model of understanding human emotions and behavior, agitation, aggression, and violence are most often the result of a complex matrix of neurobiology (including genetics and neuropathology), life experience (including the unconscious sequelae of neglect and/or abuse), and the social context, in which these feelings and behaviors occur. When such signs and symptoms occur in people with brain disorders, they constitute a major source of disability to individuals so affected, as well as being a significant source of stress to their families.

2. Agitation and aggression may emerge during the acute stages of recovery from brain injury, where such behaviors can endanger the safety of the patients and their caregivers. Agitation that occurs in the hospital after traumatic brain injury (TBI) may also be predictive of longer lengths of stay and decreased cognition, with low frustration tolerance and explosive behavior being elicited by minimal provocation. These episodes may range in severity from mild irritability to outbursts that result in significant damage to property and physical trauma to others. Not infrequently, people who suffer aggressive outbursts, because of central nervous system (CNS) lesions must be relegated for prolonged periods of time to highly restrictive environments—such as state psychiatric facilities—for the protection of themselves and of others.

---

*This Chapter is an adaptation of Chapter 14 in the Textbook of Traumatic Brain Injury, American Psychiatric Publishing, Inc., 2005. Revised and used with permission of the Publisher.

Prevalence

OVERVIEW

1. The prevalence of agitation and aggression related to neurologic disorders varies widely based on the specific condition and study. This variability depends on the nature of the population being studied (e.g., in acute general hospital settings vs. rehabilitation and outpatient settings), the age and gender of the sample, whether there was a high prevalence of preexisting personality disorders in the sample, and so on. For example, aggressive behavior during a seizure is infrequent and, when it occurs is most random and not directed. During the immediate postictal phase, agitation and aggression occur when the patient is confused, suffers delirium, and often is directed toward caregivers.

2. Alzheimer disease, the most common type of dementia, often causes behavioral changes along with memory loss. Several studies, surveying individuals in homes and chronic care residences, have indicated that agitation was the most common and the most persistent symptom; agitation and physical aggression were both likely to increase in prevalence over time. Studies of the emotional and psychiatric syndromes associated with epilepsy have documented an increase in hostility, irritability, and aggression interictally. In individuals with temporal lobe epilepsy, aggressive behavior was associated with early onset of seizures, a long duration of behavioral problems, and male gender. Those patients who have mental retardation and require institutionalization frequently exhibit aggressive behaviors. Forty percent of residents in institutions for mentally retarded individuals, have disruptive behaviors or injure themselves or others, or damage property.

3. Mood lability, irritability, agitation, and aggression are common and often highly disabling after TBI, and this common condition offers an excellent paradigm and prototype for the prevalence, neurobiology, pathophysiology, and treatment of these symptoms and behaviors across the entire neuropsychiatric spectrum of disorders. Therefore, in the remainder of this chapter, the authors will focus largely upon agitation and aggression following TBI wherein the facts and principles presented can be generalized to other neuropsychiatric illnesses.

PREVALENCE OF AGITATION AND AGGRESSION IN PATIENTS WITH TBI

During the acute recovery period, 11% to 96% of individuals with brain injury exhibit agitated behavior.[1] After the acute recovery phase, irritability or bad temper is common. Studies of mild TBI have evaluated individuals for much briefer periods of time: 1-year estimates from these studies range from 5% to 70%. Prediction of who will develop aggressive behavior after brain injury is challenging. Risk factors may include the presence of major depression, frontal lobe lesions, poor preinjury social functioning, irritability, impulsivity, and a preinjury history of aggression, and a history of alcohol and substance abuse; neuropsychological test performance does not consistently predict propensity toward violence in those who have suffered brain injury.

Characteristics of Aggression after Brain Injury

In the acute phase after brain injury, patients often experience a period of agitation and confusion, which may last from days to months. In rehabilitation facilities, these patients are described as "Confused, Agitated" (a Rancho Los Amigos Scale score of 4), and have characteristics similar to those with delirium. Agitation usually appears in the first 2 weeks of hospitalization and resolves within 2 weeks. Restlessness may appear after 2 months and may persist for 4 to 6 weeks. In our clinical experience, after the acute recovery phase has resolved, continuing aggressive outbursts have typical characteristics (see Table 16.1). These episodes may occur in the presence of other emotional changes or neurologic disorders that occur secondary to brain injury, such as mood lability or seizures.

Neuroanatomy of Aggression

Many areas of the brain are involved in the production and mediation of aggressive behavior, and lesions at different levels of neuronal organization can elicit specific types of aggressive behavior, but especially those in the frontotemporal region. Certain behavioral syndromes have been related to damage to specific areas of the frontal lobe. The orbitofrontal syndrome is associated with behavioral excesses (e.g., impulsivity, disinhibition, hyperactivity, distractibility, and mood lability). Outbursts of rage and violent behavior occur after damage to the inferior orbital surface of the frontal lobe and anterior temporal lobes. The current diagnostic category in Diagnostic and Statistical Manual of Mental Disorders, 4th edition text revision (DSM-IV-TR) is "personality change due to a general medical condition".[2] Patients with aggressive behavior would be specified as "aggressive type," whereas those with mood lability would be specified as "labile type."

Neurotransmitters in Aggression

Many neurotransmitters are involved in the mediation of aggression. Among the neurotransmitter systems, serotonin, norepinephrine, dopamine, acetylcholine,

TABLE 16.1   Characteristic Features of Aggression after Brain Injury

Reactive	Triggered by modest or trivial stimuli
Nonreflective	Usually does not involve premeditation or planning
Nonpurposeful	Aggression serves no obvious long-term aims or goals
Explosive	Buildup is not gradual
Periodic	Brief outbursts of rage and aggression; punctuated by long periods of relative calm
Ego-dystonic	After outbursts, patients are upset, concerned, and/or embarrassed, as opposed to blaming others or justifying behavior

and the γ-aminobutyric acid (GABA) systems have prominent roles in influencing aggressive behavior. It is often difficult to translate studies of aggression in various species of animals to a complex human behavior. Multiple neurotransmitter systems may be altered simultaneously by an injury that affects diffuse areas of the brain, and it may not be possible to relate change in any one neurotransmitter to a specific behavior, such as aggression. In addition, different transmitters affect one another, and frequently the critical factor is the relationship among the neurotransmitters. There is the most data focusing on the serotonergic and noradrenergic systems in mediating aggressive behavior.

ASSESSMENT

Differential diagnosis

Individuals who exhibit aggressive behavior or agitation associated with neuropsychiatric disorders require a thorough assessment. Multiple factors may play a significant role in the production of aggressive behaviors in these patients.

1. For people who suffer from TBI or severe stroke that leads to coma, during the time period of emergence from coma, agitated behaviors can occur because of delirium. The usual clinical picture is one of restlessness, confusion, and disorientation.
2. For patients who become aggressive after stroke, TBI or other CNS insults, it is important to assess systematically the presence of concurrent neuropsychiatric disorders, because this may guide subsequent treatment. Therefore, the clinician must diagnose psychosis, depression, mania, mood lability, anxiety, seizure disorders, and other concurrent neurologic conditions.
3. When aggressive behavior or agitation occurs during later stages of recovery from an acute insult to the brain, after confusion and posttraumatic amnesia have resolved, the clinician must determine whether the aggressivity and impulsivity of the individual antedated, was caused by, or was aggravated by the brain injury. For example, patients who have suffered a TBI or stroke may have a history of neuropsychiatric problems including learning disabilities, attentional deficits, behavioral problems, or personality disorders.
4. Drug effects and side effects commonly result in disinhibition or irritability (see Table 16.2). The most common drug associated with aggression is alcohol, during both intoxication and withdrawal. Stimulating drugs, such as cocaine and amphetamines, as well as the stimulating antidepressants, may produce severe anxiety and agitation in patients with or without brain lesions. Many other drugs may produce confusional states, especially anticholinergic medications that cause agitated delirium.
5. Patients with TBI, stroke, and other neuropsychiatric conditions with acute onset are susceptible to developing other medical disorders that may increase aggressive behaviors (see Table 16.3). The clinician should not, *a priori*, assume that the brain injury, *per se*, is the cause of the aggressivity, but should assess the patient for the presence of other common etiologies of aggression. Because patients with neurologic disorders are

TABLE 16.2   Medications and Drugs Associated with Aggression

Alcohol: Intoxication and withdrawal states
Hypnotic and antianxiety agents (barbiturates and benzodiazepines): Intoxication and withdrawal states
Analgesics (opiates and other narcotics): Intoxication and withdrawal states
Steroids (prednisone, cortisone, and anabolic steroids)
Antidepressants: Especially in initial phases of treatment
Amphetamines and cocaine: Aggression associated with manic excitement in early stages of abuse and secondary to paranoid ideation in later stages of use
Antipsychotics: High-potency agents that lead to akathisia
Anticholinergic drugs (including over the counter sedatives) associated with delirium and central anticholinergic syndrome

---

more susceptible to accidents, falls, and other sources of brain disorders, a neurologic disorder may be the "underlying condition" that leads to the traumatic injury. In addition, when there are exacerbations or recurrences of aggressive behavior in a patient who has been in good control, an investigation must be completed to search for other etiologies, such as medication effects, infections, pain, or changes in social circumstances.

6. Psychosocial factors are important in the expression of aggressive behavior in patients with neuropsychiatric disorders. For example, those who have suffered TBI may be acutely sensitive to changes in their environment or to variations in emotional support. Social conditions and support networks that existed before the injury affect the symptoms and course of recovery. Certain patients become aggressive only in specific circumstances, such as in the presence of particular family members. This relation suggests that there is some maintained level of control over aggressive behaviors, and that the level of control may be modified by behavioral therapeutic techniques. Most families require professional support to adjust to the impulsive behavior of a violent relative with organic dyscontrol of aggression. Frequently, efforts to avoid triggering a rageful or violent episode often lead families to withdraw from a patient. This can result in the paradox that a way that the patient learns to gain attention by being aggressive. Therefore, the unwanted behavior is unwittingly reinforced by familial withdrawal.

TABLE 16.3   Common Etiologies of Aggression in Individuals with TBI

Medications, alcohol, and other abused substances, and over the counter drugs
Delirium (hypoxia, electrolyte imbalance, anesthesia and surgery, uremia, and so on)
Alzheimer disease
Infectious diseases (encephalitis, meningitis, pneumonia, urinary tract infections)
Epilepsy (ictal, postictal, and interictal)
Metabolic disorders: Hyperthyroidism or hypothyroidism, hypoglycemia, vitamin deficiencies

Documentation of Aggressive Behavior

1. Before therapeutic intervention is initiated to treat violent behavior, the clinician should document the baseline frequency of these behaviors. There are spontaneous day-to-day and week-to-week fluctuations in aggression that cannot be validly interpreted without prospective documentation. Aggression—like certain mood disorders—may have cyclic exacerbations. It is essential that the clinician establishes a treatment plan, using objective documentation of aggressive episodes to monitor the efficacy of interventions and to designate specific time frames for the initiation and discontinuation of pharmacotherapy of acute episodes and for the initiation of pharmacotherapy for chronic aggressive behavior.

2. The Overt Aggression Scale is an operationalized instrument of proved reliability and validity that can be used to easily and effectively rate aggressive behavior in patients with a wide range of disorders[3-5] (see Figure 16.1). The scale consists of items that assess verbal aggression, physical aggression against objects, physical aggression against self, or physical aggression against others. Each category of aggression has four levels of severity that are defined by objective criteria. An aggression score can be derived, which equals the sum of the most severe ratings of each type of aggressive behavior over a particular time course. Aggressive behavior can be monitored by staff or family members using the Overt Aggression Scale. Documentation of agitation can be objectively rated with the Overt Agitation and Severity Scale[6] (see Figure 16.2).

TREATMENT

Principles

1. Aggressive and agitated behaviors may be treated in a variety of settings, ranging from the acute brain injury unit in a general hospital, to a "neurobehavioral" unit in a rehabilitation facility, to outpatient environments including the home setting. A multifactorial, multidisciplinary, collaborative approach to treatment is necessary in most cases. The continuation of family treatments, psychopharmacologic interventions, and insight-oriented psychotherapeutic approaches is often required.

2. We recommend utilizing the Consensus Guidelines for the Treatment of Agitation in the Elderly with Dementia, as a framework for the assessment and management of agitation and aggression in patients with neuropsychiatric illness.[7]

3. In establishing a treatment plan for patients with agitation or aggression, the overarching principle is that diagnosis comes before treatment (see preceding text). The history of the development of symptoms in a biopsychosocial context is usually the most critical part of the evaluation. It is essential to determine the mental status of the patient before the agitated or aggressive event, the nature of the precipitant, the physical and social environment in which the behavior occurs, the ways in which the event

Overt Aggression Scale

Stuart Yudofsky, M.D., Jonathan Silver, M.D., Wynn Jackson, M.D., and Jean Endicott, Ph.D.

Identifying Data

Name of patient	Name of rater
Sex of patient: 1 male 2 female	Date / / (mo/d/y) Shift: 1 night 2 day 3 evening

☐ No aggressive incident(s) (verbal or physical) against self, others, or objects during the shift (check here).

Aggressive Behavior (check all that apply)

Verbal aggression	Physical aggression against self
☐ Makes loud noises, shouts angrily	☐ Picks or scratches skin, hits self, pulls hair (with no or minor injury only)
☐ Yells mild personal insults (e.g. "You're stupid!")	☐ Bangs head, hits fist into objects, throws self onto floor or into objects (hurts self without serious injury)
☐ Curses viciously, uses foul language in anger, makes moderate threats to others or self	☐ Small cuts or bruises, minor burns
☐ Makes clear threats of violence toward others or self (I'm going to kill you.) or requests to help to control self	☐ Mutilates self, makes deep cuts, bites that bleed, internal injury, fracture, loss of consciousness, loss of teeth

FIGURE 16.1 The Overt Aggression Scale (OAS). (Reprinted with permission from Yudofsky SC, Silver JM, Jackson W, et al. The overt aggression scale for the objective rating of verbal and physical aggression. *Am J Psychiatry.* 1986;143:35–39.)

Physical aggression against objects

- ☐ Slams door, scatter clothing, makes a mess
- ☐ Throws objects down, kicks furniture without breaking it, marks the wall
- ☐ Breaks objects, smashes windows
- ☐ Sets fires, throws objects dangerously

Physical aggression against other people

- ☐ Makes threatening gesture, swings at people, grabs at clothes
- ☐ Strikes, kicks, pushes, pulls hair (without injury to them)
- ☐ Attacks others, causing mild to moderate physical injury (bruises, sprain, welts)
- ☐ Attacks others, causing severe physical injury (broken bones, deep lacerations, internal injury)

Time incident began ____ : ____ AM/PM   Duration of incident: ____ : ____ hours/minutes

Intervention (check all that apply)

- ☐ None
- ☐ Talking to patient
- ☐ Closer observation
- ☐ Holding patient

- ☐ Immediate medication given by mouth
- ☐ Immediate medication given by injection
- ☐ Isolation without seclusion (time out)
- ☐ Seclusion

- ☐ Use of restraints
- ☐ Injury requires immediate medical treatment for patient
- ☐ Injury requires immediate treatment for other person

Comments

FIGURE 16.1   (continued)

Overt Agitation Severity Scale

Stuart C. Yudofsky, M.D. and Heather Kopecky, Ph.D.

Intensity (I)	Behavior	Frequency (F)					Severity score (SS) (I × F = SS)
		Not Present	Rarely	Some of the time	Most of the time	Always present	
A.	**Vocalizations and oral/facial movements**						
1.	Whimpering, whining, moaning, grunting, crying	0	1	2	3	4	= ___
2.	Smacking or licking of lips, chewing, clenching jaw, licking, grimacing, spitting	0	1	2	3	4	= ___
3.	Rocking, twisting, banging of head	0	1	2	3	4	= ___
4.	Vocal perseverating, screaming, cursing, threatening, wailing	0	1	2	3	4	= ___
B	**Upper torso and upper extremity movements**						
1.	Tapping fingers, fidgeting, wringing of hands, swinging or flailing arms	0	1	2	3	4	= ___
2.	Task perseverating (e.g., opening and closing drawers, folding and unfolding clothes, picking at objects, clothes, or self)	0	1	2	3	4	= ___
3.	Rocking (back and forth), bobbing (up and down), twisting or writhing of torso, rubbing or masturbating self	0	1	2	3	4	= ___
4.	Slapping, swatting, hitting at objects or others	0	1	2	3	4	= ___
C	**Lower extremity movements**						
1.	Tapping toes, clenching toes, tapping heel, extending flexing, or twisting foot	0	1	2	3	4	= ___
2.	Shaking legs, tapping knees and/or thighs, thrusting pelvis, stomping	0	1	2	3	4	= ___
3.	Pacing, wandering	0	1	2	3	4	= ___
4.	Thrashing legs, kicking at objects or others	0	1	2	3	4	= ___
						Total OASS	= ___
						Subtract baseline OASS	= ___
						Revised OASS	= ___

FIGURE 16.2 Overt Agitation Severity Scale (OASS). (Reprinted with permission from Yudofsky SC, Kopecky HJ, Kunik ME, et al. The overt agitation severity scale for the objective rating of agitation. *J Neuropsychiatry Clin Neurosci.* 1997;9:541–548.)

Instructions for completing form

Step one: For each behavior, circle the corresponding frequency.

Step two: For every behavior *exhibited*, multiply the intensity score (I) by the frequency (F) and record as the severity score (SS).

Step three: For the Overt Agitation Severity Score (OASS), total all severity scores and record as total OASS.

Step four: Does this patient have a neuromuscular disorder (i.e., Parkinson's disease, tardive dyskinesia) affecting total OASS? Yes   No

Step five: If yes, please establish a baseline OASS in non-agitated state and subtract from above total OASS for revised OASS.

Comments:

Diagnosis: _____   Name of rater: _____

Sex of patient: Male _____   (1)   Female (2) _____   Time of observation: _____

Age: _____   Date:: _____

Current medications:

Name: Dose: Frequency:

Name: Dose: Frequency:

Name: Dose: Frequency:

Name: Dose: Frequency:

Name: Dose: Frequency:

FIGURE 16.2 (continued)

is mitigated, and the primary and secondary gains related to agitation and aggression.

4. After appropriate assessment of the possible etiologies of these behaviors, treatment is focused on the occurrence of comorbid neuropsychiatric conditions (depression, psychosis, insomnia, anxiety, delirium) and whether the treatment is in the acute (hours to days) or chronic (weeks to months) phase, and the severity of the behavior (mild to severe).

5. Although there is no medication that is approved by the U.S. Food and Drug Administration (FDA) specifically for the treatment of aggression associated with neuropsychiatric disease, medications are widely used (and commonly misused) in the management of patients with acute or chronic aggression. The reported effectiveness of these medications is highly variable, as are the reported rationale for their prescription. Some of these medications are offered to inhibit excessive activity in temporolimbic areas (e.g., as with anticonvulsants), to reduce "hyperactive" limbic monoaminergic neurotransmission (e.g., noradrenergic blockade with propranolol, dopaminergic blockade with haloperidol), or to augment orbitofrontal and/or dorsolateral prefrontal cortical activity with monoaminergic agonists (e.g., amantadine, methylphenidate, and perhaps buspirone), or increase serotonergic input (selective serotonin reuptake inhibitors [SSRIs]). Unfortunately, there is a paucity of rigorous double-blind, placebo-controlled studies (i.e., "Level I" studies) or even prospective cohort studies (i.e., "Level II" studies) to guide clinicians in the use of pharmacologic interventions. The International Brain Injury Association has assembled a task force on reviewing the literature pertaining to the neurobehavioral consequences of TBI (in progress). The clinician must be aware that patients may not respond to just one medication, but may require combination treatment, similar to the pharmacotherapeutic treatment for refractory depression.

6. Table 16.4 summarizes our recommendations for the use of various classes of medication in the treatment of chronic aggressive disorders associated with TBI.

   a. Acute aggression may be treated by using the sedative properties of antipsychotic medications or benzodiazepines.

   b. Chronic aggression

      (i) In treating aggression, the clinician, when possible, should diagnose and treat underlying disorders and use, when possible, antiaggressive agents specific for those disorders.

      (ii) When there is partial response after a therapeutic trial with a specific medication, adjunctive treatment with a medication with a different mechanism of action should be instituted. For example, a patient with partial response to β-blockers can have additional improvement with the addition of an anticonvulsant.

Acute Aggression

ANTIPSYCHOTIC DRUGS

In patients with brain injury and acute aggression, we recommend starting an atypical antipsychotic medication such as risperidone at low dosages of 0.5 mg

TABLE 16.4   Pharmacotherapy of Agitation

- Acute agitation/severe aggression
  High-potency antipsychotic drugs (haloperidol, risperidone)
  Benzodiazepines (lorazepam)
- Chronic agitation

Drug	Primary Indication
Atypical antipsychotics (risperidone, olanzapine, quetiapine, clozapine)	Psychosis
VPA, CBZ, Gabapentin	Seizure disorder, severe aggression
Serotonergic antidepressants (SSRI, trazodone)	Depression, mood lability
Buspirone	Anxiety
β-blockers	Aggression without concomitant neuropsychiatric sequelae (i.e., anxiety, depression, etc.)

orally with repeated administration every hour until control of aggression is achieved. If, after several administrations of risperidone, the aggressive behavior of the patient does not improve, the hourly dose may be increased until the patient is so sedated that he or she no longer exhibits agitation or violence. Once the patient is not aggressive for 48 hours, the daily dosage should be decreased gradually (i.e., by 25% every day) to ascertain whether aggressive behavior reemerges. In this case, consideration should then be made about whether it is best to increase the dose of risperidone and/or to initiate treatment with a more specific antiaggressive drug. Other atypical antipsychotic medications such as olanzapine, quitiepine (which has few extrapyramidal symptoms [EPS]), or ziprasidone may be used, although there is no published experience.

Recent studies have suggested that there is an increased risk of stroke when antipsychotic medications are prescribed for agitation in elderly patients with dementia. For this reason, a careful benefit/risk analysis must be made before prescribing antipsychotic medications under these circumstances. This involves the severity and dangerousness of the agitation, as well as potential risks from the medication.

SEDATIVES AND HYPNOTICS
There is an inconsistent literature on the effects of the benzodiazepines in the treatment of aggression. The sedative properties of benzodiazepines may be helpful in the management of acute agitation and aggression. Paradoxically, several studies report increased hostility, aggression, and the induction of rage in patients treated with benzodiazepines. However, these reports are balanced by the observation that this phenomenon is rare. Benzodiazepines can produce amnesia, and preexisting memory dysfunction can be exacerbated by the use of benzodiazepines. Patients with brain injury may also experience increased problems with coordination and balance with benzodiazepine use. For this reason, we prefer not to use benzodiazepines in the treatment of acute aggression in patients with TBI.

Chronic Aggression

If a patient continues to exhibit periods of agitation or aggression beyond several weeks, the use of specific antiaggressive medications should be initiated to prevent these episodes from occurring. Because no medication has been approved by the FDA for treatment of aggression, the clinician must use medications that may be antiaggressive but that have been approved for other uses (e.g., seizure disorders, depression, hypertension)[8].

ANTIPSYCHOTIC MEDICATIONS

If, after thorough clinical evaluation, it is determined that the aggressive episodes result from *psychosis*, such as paranoid delusions or command hallucinations, then antipsychotic medications will be the treatment of choice. There have been double-blind placebo-controlled studies of risperidone showing efficacy in the treatment of agitation in elderly patients with dementia, as well as children with autism and serious behavioral problems. Olanzapine appears to be more sedating, and quitiepine may have fewer EPS than does risperidone. Quitiepine appears to be the antipsychotic medication (except for clozapine) least likely to produce extrapyramidal effects in vulnerable populations, such as those with Parkinson disease. Clozapine may have greater antiaggressive effects than other antipsychotic medications. However, the increased risk of seizures must be carefully assessed.

Antipsychotics are the most commonly used medications in the treatment of aggression. Although these agents are appropriate and effective when aggression is derivative of active psychosis, the use of neuroleptic agents to treat chronic aggression, especially secondary to TBI, is often ineffective and the patient may develop serious complications. Usually, it is the sedative side effects rather than the antipsychotic properties of antipsychotics that are used (or misused) to "treat" (or mask) the aggression. Often, patients develop tolerance to the sedative effects of the neuroleptics and, therefore, require increasing doses. As a result, extrapyramidal and anticholinergic-related side effects occur. Paradoxically (and frequently) because of the development of akathisia, the patient may become more agitated and restless as the dose of neuroleptic is increased, especially when a high-potency antipsychotic such as haloperidol (Haldol) is administered. The akathisia is often mistaken for increased irritability and agitation, and a vicious cycle of increasing neuroleptics and worsening akathisias occur. There is some evidence from studies of injury to motor neurons in animals that have found that haloperidol decreases recovery. This effect was only seen when animals actively participated in a behavioral task and not when the animals were restrained after drug administration. It is possible that the effect on decreasing dopamine and inhibiting neuronal function, which may be the mechanism of action to treat aggression, may have other detrimental effects on recovery. Whether this finding is generalizable to recovery in brain injury and with the "atypical antipsychotics" remains unclear. However, the finding raises important potential risk/benefit issues that must be considered before antipsychotic drugs are used to treat aggressive behavior in patients with neuronal damage.

ANTICONVULSANT MEDICATIONS

1. The anticonvulsant carbamazepine has been shown to be effective for the treatment of bipolar disorders and has also been advocated for the

control of aggression in both epileptic and nonepileptic populations. Open studies have indicated that carbamazepine may be effective in decreasing aggressive behavior associated with developmental disabilities, schizophrenia, and patients with a variety of other organic brain disorders.[8]

2. In our experience and that of others, the anticonvulsant valproic acid may also be helpful to some patients with aggression that is secondary to neurologic disorders. There have been limited number of open case reports published on patients with TBI. Gabapentin may be beneficial for the treatment of agitation in patients with dementia. Doses have ranged from 200 to 2400 mg per day. For patients with aggression and epilepsy whose seizures are being treated with anticonvulsant drugs such as phenytoin and phenobarbital, switching to carbamazepine or to valproic acid may treat both conditions. Oxcarbazepine may be an alternative to carbmazepine, although there are no published reports at this time.

ANTIDEPRESSANTS

1. The antidepressants that have been reported to control aggressive behavior are those that act preferentially (amitriptyline) or specifically (trazodone, sertraline, and fluoxetine) on serotonin. Trazodone has also been reported to be effective in the treatment of aggression that occurs with organic mental disorders.[8] Fluoxetine, a potent serotonergic antidepressant, has been reported to be effective in the treatment of aggressive behavior in a patient who suffered brain injury as well as in patients with personality disorders and depression, and adolescents with mental retardation and self-injurious behavior.[8] We have used SSRI with considerable success in aggressive patients with brain lesions. The dosages used are similar to those for the treatment of mood lability and depression.

2. We have evaluated and treated many patients with emotional lability that is characterized by frequent episodes of tearfulness and irritability, and the full symptomatic picture of neuroaggressive syndrome. These patients, who would be diagnosed under DSM-IV as "Personality Change, Labile Type, Due to Traumatic Brain Injury" have responded well to SSRI antidepressants (see Chapter 11).

ANTIMANIC MEDICATIONS

Although lithium is known to be effective in controlling aggression related to manic excitement, many studies suggest that it may also have a role in the treatment of aggression in selected, nonbipolar patient populations, including individuals with mental retardation who exhibit self-injurious or aggressive behavior, children and adolescents with behavioral disorders, prison inmates, and those with other organic brain syndromes.[8]

Individuals with brain injury have increased sensitivity to the neurotoxic effects of lithium. Because of lithium's potential for neurotoxicity, we limit the use of lithium in those patients whose aggression is related to manic effects or recurrent irritability related to cyclic mood disorders.

ANTIANXIETY MEDICATIONS

In several neurologic disorders, it has been shown that anxiety is a coexisting disorder with agitation and aggression. Serotonin appears to be a key neurotransmitter in the modulation of aggressive behavior. In preliminary open case studies, buspirone, a 5-HT 1A agonist, has been reported to be effective in the management of aggression and agitation for patients with TBI, as well as dementia, and developmental disabilities and autism. In rare instances, we have found that some patients become more aggressive when treated with buspirone. We recommend that buspirone be initiated at low dosages (i.e., 7.5 mg b.i.d.) and increased to 15 mg b.i.d. after 1 week. Dosages of 45 to 60 mg per day may be required before there is improvement in aggressive behavior, although we have noted dramatic improvement within 1 week.

Clonazepam may be effective in the long-term management of aggression, although evidence is restricted to case reports. We use clonazepam when pronounced aggression and anxiety occur together, or when aggression occurs in association with neurologically induced tics and similarly disinhibited motor behaviors. Doses should be initiated at 0.5 mg b.i.d. and may be increased to as high as 2 to 4 mg b.i.d., as tolerated. Sedation and ataxia are frequent side effects.

ANTIHYPERTENSIVE MEDICATIONS: β-BLOCKERS

1. Since the first report of the use of β-adrenergic receptor blockers in the treatment of acute aggression in 1977, over 25 articles have appeared in the neurologic and psychiatric literature reporting experience in using β-blockers with over 200 patients with aggression.[8] Most of these patients had been unsuccessfully treated with antipsychotics, minor tranquilizers, lithium, and/or anticonvulsants before treatment with β-blockers. The β-blockers that have been investigated in controlled prospective studies include propranolol (a lipid-soluble, nonselective receptor antagonist), nadolol (a water-soluble, nonselective receptor antagonist), and pindolol (a lipid-soluble, nonselective β- receptor antagonist with partial sympathomimetic activity). This literature suggests that β-adrenergic receptor blockers are effective agents for the treatment of aggressive and violent behaviors, particularly those related to neurologic disorders.

2. Guidelines for the use of propranolol are listed in Table 16.5 When a patient requires the use of a once-a-day medication because of compliance difficulties, long-acting propranolol (i.e., Inderal LA) or nadolol (Corgard) can be used. When patients develop bradycardia that prevents prescribing therapeutic dosages of propranolol, pindolol can be substituted, using one tenth the dosage of propranolol. Pindolol's intrinsic sympathomimetic activity stimulates the β- receptor and restricts the development of bradycardia. The major side effects of β-blockers when used to treat aggression are lowering of blood pressure and pulse rate. Because peripheral β- receptors are fully blocked in doses of 300 to 400 mg per day, further decreases in these vital signs usually do not occur even when doses are increased to much higher levels. Despite reports of depression with the use of β-blockers, controlled trials and our experience indicate that it is a rare occurrence.[9] Because the use of propranolol is associated with significant increases in plasma levels of thioridazine, which has an absolute dosage ceiling of 800 mg per day, the combination of these two medications should be avoided whenever possible.

TABLE 16.5   Clinical Use of Propranolol

1. Conduct a thorough medical evaluation
2. Exclude patients with the following disorders: Bronchial asthma, chronic obstructive pulmonary disease, insulin-dependent diabetes mellitus, congestive heart failure, persistent angina, significant peripheral vascular disease, and hyperthyroidism
3. Avoid sudden discontinuation of propranolol (particularly in patients with hypertension)
4. Begin with a single test-dose of 20 mg/day in patients for whom there are clinical concerns with hypotension or bradycardia. Increase dose of propranolol by 20 mg/day every 3 days
5. Initiate propranolol on a 20 mg t.i.d. schedule for patients without cardiovascular or cardiopulmonary disorder
6. Increase the dosage of propranolol by 60 mg/day every 3 days
7. Increase medication unless the pulse rate is reduced below 50 bpm, or systolic blood pressure is <90 mm Hg
8. Do not administer medication if severe dizziness, ataxia, or wheezing occurs. Reduce or discontinue propranolol if such symptoms persist
9. Increase dose to 12 mg/kg body weight or until aggressive behavior is under control
10. Doses of >800 mg are not usually required to control aggressive behavior
11. Maintain the patient on the highest dose of propranolol for at least 8 weeks before concluding that the patient is not responding to the medication. Some patients, however, may respond rapidly to propranolol
12. Use concurrent medications with caution. Monitor plasma levels of all antipsychotic and anticonvulsive medications

Reprinted from Yudofsky SC, Silver JM, Schneider SE. Pharmacologic treatment of aggression. *Psychiatric Ann.* 1987;17:397–407. Used with permission.

Psychotherapeutic Treatments of Aggression and Agitation Associated with Neuropsychiatric Conditions

Agitation and aggression are often caused and influenced by a complex matrix of neurobiologic, psychological, and environmental factors. Because of the dangerous and unpredictable nature of aggression, caregivers, both in institutions and at home, have intense and sometimes injudicious reactions to aggression when it occurs. Psychosocial interventions and psychotherapies of several varieties (most often in single-case design studies) have been shown to be highly effective in treating patients with aggression secondary to brain injury and may be useful when combined with pharmacotherapy. Most studies are single-case design, when specific behavioral interventions are instituted. Behavioral treatment strategies include those designed to replace aggression with more productive behaviors and decelerative techniques[10] provide details about these interventions. Two replacement strategies include assertiveness training, which is most appropriate for patients who become angry when their needs are not met, and differential reinforcement schedules, where the rate of previolent behaviors are targeted. Decelerative techniques include social extinction (useful for the patients who are previolent and respond to social reinforcers), contingent observation (provides the opportunity for violent responders to model self-control from peers), self-controlled time-out, overcorrection, and contingent constraint (last resort option). A full exegesis of the important role of behavioral treatments and psychosocial interventions for aggression, irritability, and agitation is beyond the scope of this chapter.

CONCLUSIONS

Aggressive and agitated behavior, associated with neuropsychiatric disorders, is common and can be highly disabling. Aggression often significantly impedes appropriate rehabilitation of a patient and his or her reintegration into family, occupational, educational, and community settings. There are many psychosocial and neurobiologic factors that can lead to or aggravate aggressive behavior in association with neuropsychiatric conditions. After appropriate evaluation and assessment of possible etiologies and contributing factors, treatment begins with the documentation of the aggressive episodes. Psychopharmacologic strategies differ according to whether the medication is for the treatment of acute aggression or the need to prevent episodes in the patient with chronic aggression. Although the treatment of acute aggression involves the judicious use of sedation, the treatment of chronic aggression is guided by underlying diagnoses and symptomatologies. Behavioral strategies and psychosocial interventions remain an important component in the comprehensive treatment of patients with agitation and aggressions, and are often used to complement pharmacologic treatment regimens.

References
1. Silver JM, Yudofsky SC, Anderson KA. Aggression. In: Silver JM, McAllister TW, Yudofsky SC, eds. *Textbook of traumatic brain injury.* Washington, DC: American Psychiatric Publishing; 2005.
2. American Psychiatric Association: Diagnostic and Statistical Manual of Mental Disorders, Text Revision, 4th Edition. Washington, DC, American Psychiatric Association, 2000.
3. Silver JM, Yudofsky SC. The overt aggression scale: Overview and clinical guidelines. *J Neuropsychiatry Clin Neurosc.* 1991;3(Suppl):S22–S29.
4. Yudofsky SC, Silver JM, Jackson W, et al. The Overt Aggression Scale for the objective rating of verbal and physical aggression. *Am J Psychiatry* 1986;143:35–39.
5. Yudofsky SC, Silver JM, Schneider SE. Pharmacologic treatment of aggression. *Psychiatric Annals* 1987;17:397–407.
6. Yudofsky SC, Kopecky HJ, Kunik ME, et al. The Overt Agitation Severity Scale for the Objective Rating of Agitation. *J Neuropsychiatry Clin Neuroscience* 1997;9:541–548.
7. Alexopoulos GS, Silver JM, Kahn DA, et al. *The expert consensus guideline series: Treatment of agitation in older persons with dementia. Postgraduate medicine, A special report.* 1998.
8. Yudofsky SC, Silver JM, Hales RE. Treatment of agitation and aggression, in Textbook of Psychopharmacology, 2nd Edition. Edited by Schatzberg AF, Nemeroff CB. Washington, DC, American Psychiatric Press, 1998.
9. Yudofsky SC. β-blockers and depression: The clinician's dilemma. *JAMA.* 1992;267:1826–1827.
10. Corrigan PW, Bach PA. In: Silver JM, McAllister TW, Yudofsky SC, eds. *Behavioral treatment in textbook of traumatic brain injury.* Washington, DC: American Psychiatric Publishing, Inc.; 2005:661–678.

FORENSIC NEUROPSYCHIATRY*

James R. Merikangas

I. DEFINITION

Forensic neuropsychiatry is a subspecialty that applies to legal issues, a scientific and clinical understanding of the behavioral manifestations of brain disease.

II. BACKGROUND

Psychiatrists and neurologists are frequently involved with the legal system in a variety of ways; either as the attending physician, giving medical information about one's own patient through records or personal testimony, or as a consultant not actually treating the person in question. A doctor examining a patient for the purpose of rendering an opinion, rather than for treatment, is said to be performing an *Independent Medical Examination* (IME). A forensic neuropsychiatric evaluation is of use to give a diagnosis and prognosis in a legal setting, for purposes of rating disability, determining competence to make decisions, or determining civil or criminal responsibility. The court (the judge), or lawyers on either side of the question in litigation, may request the physician to explain in layman's language the relevant medical facts or opinions. Forensic neuropsychiatry may also refer to forensic specialists who practice within the penal or correctional system, working as treating physicians in prisons or hospitals for

---

*There are five primary sources for the laws, rules, and regulations that apply to mental health professionals, and these vary from state to state. Laws come from the state and federal constitutions; the legislatures; administrative rules and regulations; rules of court promulgated by the state supreme court; and the state and federal court cases that apply, interpret, and construe the existing state law. The different professions are treated differently by these rules, and each profession has its own ethical rules set out by their individual governing boards. Therefore, this overview is only a guide, and not a substitute for legal advice or the actual statutes involved.

the criminally insane, or determining competence or insanity for the court. Forensic fellowships are available in a number of training sites, and most psychiatric residency programs include some background in the basics of commitment procedures and competency determination.

III. THE ADVERSARY SYSTEM

A. Courts in the United States use the adversary system in an attempt to establish facts and render decisions in torts and criminal cases. Each side of a dispute will present an argument and evidence to support it, and through cross-examination either side will attack the testimony of witnesses, including expert witnesses. The same process is used in a number of other venues, including arbitration, or simply reviews by insurance providers or medical boards.

B. In many countries outside the United States, in the criminal court, a panel of court approved or appointed experts may be employed to reach a consensus regarding the question of sanity or criminal responsibility. This procedure is more efficient than a trial and avoids "a battle of the experts." This unseemly contest of disputing experts may only serve, in the eyes of the public, to discredit the medical profession and the scientific method in general.

IV. SCIENTIFIC EVIDENCE

A. It is important for courts to evaluate the scientific basis of testimony and the credentials of "experts" before they are presented to the juries or the boards. This process is largely at the discretion of the judge in a case, but is guided by a number of decisions and rules, which have been evolving recently. The *Daubert rule* is the most important of these regarding the admissibility of scientific evidence. In the past it has sufficed for an expert to simply express an opinion on the basis of his or her own experience or review of the literature, but now one must show that an opinion is the generally accepted view of specialists in a particular field, and that the relevant peer-reviewed literature will support that position. Daubert versus Merrell Dow Pharmaceuticals, 92–102, 509 U.S. 579 (1993), is the case that set the standard for scientific testimony in court. It is the basis of the federal rule for scientific testimony, but is gaining wider acceptance in state courts across the country. Daubert states that scientific evidence is inadmissible unless the technique is "generally accepted" as reliable in the scientific community, rests on a reliable foundation, and is relevant to the question at hand. The judge has the task of determining whether the method and reasoning is scientifically valid. The Daubert decision superseded Frye versus United States, 54 App. D.C. 46, 293 F. 1014, which required "general acceptance."

V. EXPERT WITNESS

A. If the physician is to give an opinion about a patient he has not been treating, he is then referred to as an *expert witness*. He may be conducting an IME of a patient, or simply testifying to a review of facts of a case in question. It is mandatory for doctors giving testimony to facts or opinion to understand the purpose of their testimony and to be precise regarding the facts in question.

B. In an attempt to improve their expertise in dealing with the legal system, and to bolster their credibility with the courts, some physicians seek to be certified as experts through various "boards" offering forensic credentials. These boards include the American Board of Psychiatry and Neurology, which offers subspecialty certification in Forensic Psychiatry. A physician becomes an *expert* witness by presenting his or her credentials and qualifications to the court and being accepted by the judge. Therefore, expert witnesses should be experienced in the field of knowledge in question and be armed with the applicable peer-reviewed scientific literature. They must be prepared to outline their reasoning in a way that judge and jury can follow and understand. It is not enough to have the proper credentials and to express an opinion on the basis of personal experience; one must be able to prove the point and stand up to cross-examination by a well-prepared lawyer. Compensation is based on an hourly rate, including record review, examination of the patient, and time for depositions or courtroom testimony.

VI. DEGREE OF CERTAINTY

Despite the Daubert rule, there will remain many areas where the medical/scientific literature is unclear, insufficient, or vague, and the clinical material may be subject to several interpretations. Even something as apparently concrete as the reading of an x-ray is subject to interpretation and clinical judgment, a fact that may be lost on a judge or jury. An expert must, therefore, be careful to admit the level of certainty to which an interpretation of clinical opinion may be held even if it is undisputed. In some cases opinions must be expressed "to a reasonable degree of medical certainty" (90% to 100%), a rather high standard, but one to which a clinician adheres in medical practice. For medical causation the opinions may be "to a reasonable degree of medical probability" (>50% likelihood, or "more likely than not"), a much lower standard. These definitions may vary from state to state, and may differ depending on the court. Unfortunately, the outcome of such apparently imprecise measures may be expressed in an all-or-none decision or finding of fact.

VII. TORTS

A. A *Tort* is a claim of wrong, due to another person, for which a legal remedy (usually money) is sought. Torts may involve persons or classes, individuals or corporations and are tried in civil, rather than criminal courts. Some examples of torts follow below.

B. **Malpractice**

1. Patients or their heirs may sue for malpractice if a treatment has a bad outcome, or if they feel that there was negligence, abuse (sexual, emotional, or physical), a violation of

confidentiality, or an adverse reaction to a medication or treatment. For a doctor to be liable, the patient must prove that a *duty* existed to provide proper treatment and there was *negligence*. The determining factor in such a case is whether it was a violation of *the standard of care.*

2. The standard of care is usually defined as that level of competence and care usually exercised by practitioners in the same specialty as the physician involved in the treatment. *Practice parameters* are published by the American Academy of Neurology, the Academy of Child and Adolescent Psychiatry, and the American Psychiatric Association. Although, these do not have the force of law, they are useful to assist in the determination of the standard of care. Of course, if the physician is doing something for which he lacks the training or expertise, it is undertaken at the risk of being held to the same standard as experts in that field. The standard of care is a national one; doctors in rural areas are held to the same standards as those in a university hospital. Interns are judged by the same standard as their attending physician.

3. For a case to prevail there must be *damages,* and there must be *causation.* Damages are the actual harm, which results from a deviation from the standard of care, and are not simply a death, emotional trauma or disfigurement, which in the normal course of events may be the natural outcome of disease or injury.

4. Expert testimony must state what constitutes the standard of care in a given situation, what the deviation was, and the cause-and-effect relationship of that deviation and the harm done. Often the experts for the defense and plaintiff have opposite opinions, and therefore, it is up to a jury to decide the case on the merits perceived, and the strength of the arguments presented by the competing lawyers. Unfortunately, in the case of complicated medical matters, the result may depend on the eloquence of the expert or the lawyer, rather than scientific basis of the opinions presented.

5. **Review boards.** A number of jurisdictions in the United States now require an evaluation by a screening board composed of doctors and lay people before a case of alleged medical malpractice may be brought to court or arbitration. This approach can be a valuable screening tool to prevent frivolous lawsuits from going forward, but also depends upon expert reports by an affidavit or a testimony.

6. **Who gets sued for malpractice?** In a malpractice suit it is common for plaintiff attorneys to sue everyone involved in the care of the patient, including those who have no culpability or only a remote connection to the incident in question. This action may be done as a fact-finding maneuver, because then subpoenas may be issued to take *depositions* (sworn testimony which may be used as evidence in court),

and the complete medical record may then be produced for review.

7.   **Do you need an attorney if you are sued?** Although the various insurance companies involved have attorneys to defend the physicians being sued, their interests may diverge from those of the doctor. Thus, it may be appropriate for the defendant doctor to retain an attorney to represent his interests, in case the insurance company wants to settle a case simply to avoid a trial, particularly when the physician is in fact not responsible for the perceived damages.

C.   **Toxic torts.** Dangerous chemicals in the environment may cause neurologic damage to the central or peripheral nervous system, with manifestations ranging from cancer, to dementia, or neuropathy. In some jurisdictions, including California, a legitimate fear of cancer from a toxic exposure is compensable. Claims of multiple chemical sensitivity, toxic mold and similar problems require careful environmental evaluations and rigorous adherence to scientific methods on the part of expert witnesses.

VIII. COMPETENCE

A.   Competence refers to the ability of a person to testify or make a decision. Competence is specific to the purpose, that is, to testify, to make a will or a contract, to refuse or permit treatment, to confess or give a statement, to be tried or executed, or to be employed in a sensitive area or occupation. These various types of competence have different standards, and it is essential that the physician understands the statutory requirements and limits for each type before expressing an opinion.

B.   The phrase, "being of sound mind and body" is often incorporated in a will. Witnesses to the will attest to that fact, but a lay observation is not the same as a legal determination based on neuropsychological testing. Therefore, if a person is demented, or psychotic, or so depressed that they do not care what happens, they may not be competent to make a will. To be competent to make a will requires only that the person knows what his estate consists of, and knows how he wishes to dispose of it. It does not require a detailed understanding or logical reasons, as long as the person making the will is not subjected to undue influence or delusions. This requirement will be spelled out in legal language, which may vary from jurisdiction to jurisdiction, and is a looser standard than that required for other purposes. Neuropsychiatric testimony based on a retrospective review of medical records and witness statements may be relied upon to make a determination of testamentary capacity of a deceased person.

C.   Competence to stand trial requires that the defendant *understand* the charges against him, the nature of the proceedings including the functions of judge, jury, prosecutor, witnesses, and his own attorney, and be able to *assist* his attorney by communicating with him and being able to confront witnesses or accusers. Clearly, this competence is a more complex question than that of being competent to make a will. A defendant found to be incompetent to stand trial will usually be remanded to a mental hospital to be treated to restore competence. Of course, in some cases of psychosis or dementia, either Alzheimer disease or from traumatic brain injury, incompetence may be permanent. In such cases charges may be dismissed and civil commitment proceedings may follow.

D. Competence to waive Fifth Amendment rights to remain silent when in police custody (which is not the same as being under arrest) or when given the "Miranda warning," may require expert testimony. If a defendant is mentally retarded or psychotic or suicidal they may not be able to avoid self-incrimination or a false confession. Expert testimony may then be required to throw out the confession or statement, which may have been extracted by deception or duress. The Fifth Amendment was devised to prevent gaining confessions through torture, because it was recognized that such confessions are not to be relied upon.

E. Competence to enter a guilty plea may also require expert evaluation and testimony in the case of a suicidal suspect or one incompetent for mental or physical reasons.

F. Competence to be executed requires that the convicted knows why he is being put to death, and to understand what death is, and that it is a punishment mandated by his having committed a crime. A psychotic person may lack such an understanding, and the Supreme Court has ruled that it is unconstitutional to execute children or those with mental retardation. It should be noted that it is unethical for a physician to participate in killing prisoners. An ethical physician will neither administer a lethal injection, nor testify that a prisoner is competent to be executed if the result is the killing of that person, even if that is what the law permits.

IX. INSANITY

Insanity is a legal concept, the definition of which varies between the various states, the federal government, and the military. The *M'Naghten* (also McNaughton, or McNaghten) *rule* was formerly the basis for most insanity statutes in the United States and Great Britain. This case involved the murder in 1843 of the secretary to the British Prime Minister by a Daniel McNaughton who was psychotic and delusional, thinking the Prime Minister was conspiring against him. He was found innocent by reason of insanity, despite the fact that he intended the murder and acted deliberately. Under the rule, a person was innocent by reason of insanity if by reason of a defect of mind or reason they did not know right from wrong. Formerly, under the *Durham rule* a defendant would be innocent by reason of insanity if the act was the product of a mental disease or defect, causing the ability to conform conduct to the requirement of law to be substantially impaired. Since the famous *Hinckley case* the federal rule for insanity removed the part of the rule regarding the ability to control one's actions, or to conform one's conduct, thereby reducing the standard to simply *not knowing right from wrong*. This change has in some courts led to the absurd idea that would suggest that a person who was psychotic and acting under a delusion would be guilty simply because they knew that they were firing a gun at a human being, regardless of delusion that they were acting in self-defense. Command hallucinations would not be acknowledged, and by the same lack of logic a child who could not distinguish right from wrong could be tried "as an adult." *Mens rea* means a guilty state of mind, a mental state that implies deliberation and intent. An alcoholic blackout or a state of delirium may arguably remove *mens rea* and be exculpatory. Although the "insanity defense" is rarely employed, and more rarely succeeds, an antimental illness trend has been carried to the extreme of totally eliminating insanity in the laws of some states, and eliminating mental illness as compensable under workers compensation in some other jurisdictions.

X. MITIGATION, EXTENUATION, AGGRAVATION

These terms are used in criminal sentencing procedures and have statutory definitions that vary from place to place. In general, *mitigating circumstances* include diminished capacity from mental illness or brain damage that may not reach the level of legal insanity, but which may allow for an alternative to jail or a reduced sentence. *Extenuating circumstances* are those factors that tend to excuse an action or diminish the culpability of a perpetrator without eliminating guilt. *Aggravation* refers to those things that make a crime more heinous or cruel, perhaps invoking the nonscientific concept of *evil*.

XI. FUTURE DANGEROUSNESS

A. In sentencing proceedings psychiatrists or psychologists may be asked to predict future dangerousness, or predict adaptation to prison life. This is an area where the potential to misuse speculation and opinion exists, because the Daubert rules do not exist in criminal court. Physicians must be wary of making statements that are unscientific or simply representative of personal bias.
B. The diagnosis of pedophilia or sexual sadism is not a defense in criminal court, despite a strong biologic basis for these conditions, but the possibility of antisex drive hormone treatment may be a consideration in ordering treatment at sentencing. Following the completion of prison time, commitment proceedings may sometimes be instituted to mandate inpatient hospitalization for dangerous sexual offenders, or outpatient treatment may be ordered as a condition of probation.
C. A "*duty to warn*" exists when a treating, or evaluating physician has the opinion that a patient presents an imminent risk of harming an identifiable individual or group. The physician is then obligated to warn that person directly or through the proper authorities of the risk, and is liable if harm results from failing to do so.

XII. DISABILITY DETERMINATIONS

A. *Disability* refers to the incapacity of a person to perform a specific activity and is contingent on the setting where a job or other activity is to be performed, not just on a diagnosis. Therefore a physician making a disability determination must take into consideration the purpose, as a person may be disabled as a roofer, but perfectly fit to operate a crane.

B. According to the Guides to the evaluation of Permanent Impairment, *impairment* is defined as, "a loss, loss of use, or derangement of any body part, organ system, or organ function." This volume provides the method of determining and quantifying impairments in a structured manner that is generally accepted and reproducible.

XIII. ENTITLEMENTS

A. The law provides for disabled or handicapped persons with a number of programs, which require medical information in order to be implemented. The one most frequently encountered in neuropsychiatric practice is Social Security (SSI). To obtain social security disability benefits, evidence of disability must be presented. This evidence includes records from treating physicians and special reports generated by consultants. A disability for social security purposes is, "the inability to do any substantial gainful activity by reason of any medically determinable physical or mental impairment which can be expected to result in death or which has lasted or can be expected to last for a continuous period of not less than 12 months." On occasion, an adversary proceeding before an administrative law judge must determine if a patient is eligible for payments.

B. Other entitlements include the right to education, the right to be free from discrimination, the right to accommodation, and the right to protection in a number of areas, including physical and mental health treatment in prison. Neuropsychiatric opinion may be required to establish the need for rehabilitation or treatment in a variety of settings, each of which will have statutory requirements spelled out in legal language. The consultant reports, therefore, must be tailored to the specific questions to be probative.

XIV. MOTOR VEHICLES

The rules for reporting impaired drivers vary form state to state. In some jurisdictions it is mandatory to report patients with epilepsy, and in others such disclosure is covered by strict privacy rules. Therefore, it is necessary to refer to local law before making a report regarding fitness to operate a motor vehicle. Although there are no upper age limits on the right to drive, physicians must judge whether elderly patients or those with dementia, should continue to have a license. Patients with movement disorders, visual field impairments, or other problems affecting judgment or coordination, may also be subject to reporting requirements.

XV. EMPLOYMENT

A. Job discrimination, sexual harassment, and workplace conditions are frequently the subject of disputes and claims of emotional stress. In torts involving workplace problems, the claim of emotional disturbance or post-traumatic stress disorder (PTSD) is common. As PTSD and acute stress disorder are defined as being due to an event involving threatened death or serious injury, these claims are more often made than proven.

B. There is little peer-reviewed research that would provide a basis for determining the degree of emotional harm from sexual harassment, but the onset of psychiatric illness and emotional disorders should be documented.

C. Several federal laws prohibit discrimination against the disabled in a number of settings including schools, the government, public accommodations, or by employers with 15 or more employees. Physicians need to be sure their offices and clinics are handicapped accessible. Determinations of disability or handicap may be required to assist patients in obtaining equal access to jobs and education.

XVI. BRAIN DEATH

A. Brain death determinations and removal of life support have specific requirements determined by ethics boards and state law. Demonstration of absent cerebral blood flow by angiogram or nuclear medicine scans is the gold standard. Electrocerebral silence by electroencephalography (EEG) under conditions of the absence of sedating medications may be utilized with other criteria. Explicit rules must be followed and documented in these cases to remove life support, including reference to advance directive and health care power of attorney documents.

B. Advance directives and living wills are available in outline form from state health departments and hospitals. Neuropsychiatrists and other physicians should provide these documents as part of the intake of new patients to make clear their wishes and to avoid emotionally wrenching disagreements when a terminal illness occurs without warning.

XVII. LIABILITY OF EXPERTS

Are forensic examinations the practice of medicine? This is an unresolved question. If there is no doctor–patient relationship, there cannot be malpractice, because no *duty* exists to provide treatment according to the standard of care. Various states have ruled, however, that the absence of a doctor–patient relationship does not necessarily immunize the forensic examiner from liability. The American Medical Association has taken the position that forensic activity *is* the practice of medicine and should be subject to peer review. *Witness immunity* protects testimony in court in a lawsuit, and witnesses cannot be sued for their testimony. There may be a limited degree of *quasi-judicial immunity* when performing examinations for court purposes. The expert has a duty to not injure the examinee, to tell the truth, and to inform the patient of a potentially serious medical problem. Certainly these examinations fall within the universal maxim of medical ethics, "first do no harm." Some states have regulations regarding who may testify in court in malpractice cases, requiring state residence, or limiting the percentage of income that may be derived from forensic versus medical practice. Experts must therefore check with the state medical board where they wish to testify to see if a license in that state is required, or if there is mandated limit on the percentage of income from forensic activity. A determination in writing from their malpractice carrier is also recommended. It is unethical for an expert witness to accept a contingency fee dependent on the outcome of a case.

XVIII. FORENSIC EVALUATIONS

A. The standard of care to be used by psychiatrists and neurologists when conducting a mental health evaluation includes the duty to do no harm, to properly diagnose, to tell the truth, and to maintain confidentially. Every medical school across the country teaches the same standards for the neuropsychiatric evaluation with perhaps only minor variations in techniques, but the approach and result will be consistent. The Diagnostic and Statistical Manual of Mental Disorders, 4th edition (DSM-IV) provides an outline for the method of psychiatric diagnosis, including the history, the physical examination, and laboratory tests in broad outline. A forensic examiner must be meticulously thorough and free of bias in the evaluation, with an emphasis on a differential diagnosis, as testimony under oath may be required. The examining doctor must never jump to a conclusion merely on the basis of signs or symptoms before him. A competent physician must consider all possible diagnoses and rule out those that are inapplicable.

B. In making a differential diagnosis one must distinguish between "organic" (i.e., secondary to a known cause) and "functional" basis for the psychiatric symptoms. The distinction is archaic, but unfortunately the lay public still does not fully appreciate that all behavior is the result of a biologic process. Any competent neuropsychiatric evaluation must include, as its absolute first step, differentiation between learned behavior or behavior which is the result of environmental influences, and those behaviors more directly "secondary to a given disease or lesion." An organic basis is a physical disability, either medical or neurologic. Almost any psychiatric or psychological symptoms can be the result of an organic cause. Therefore, every psychiatrist must be hyperalert to the possibility of a demonstrable metabolic or structural lesion or disease as the cause of the apparently psychological symptoms.

C. A "functional" basis conventionally is either psychological or psychosocial. Psychosocial means the cause is the result of major environmental stresses that may influence behavior. In criminal matters organic brain disorders can seriously affect "free will," volition, deliberation, understanding, and intent. DSM-IV makes this very clear. For example, a person who appears to have a personality disorder, including antisocial personality disorder, may have a clearly defined organic disease, which causes the psychiatric symptomatology, and eliminates the diagnosis of antisocial personality as a consideration.

D. A correct diagnosis of organic brain disease is particularly important in the forensic field, because in the legal setting and throughout society as a whole, it is much more convincing for a juror or anyone else to believe a person has mental health problems or is actually mentally ill if there is a demonstrable physical deficiency. For this reason, it is particularly important that forensic psychiatrists look to a neurologic examination first. A physical defect is a very strong arguing point for damages. This is so because when problems are the result of organic deficiencies it is easier for a forensic neuropsychiatrist to measure, or at least describe the way the organicity influences behavior. Brain imaging can be helpful to demonstrate areas of brain damage and reduced blood flow by single photon emission computed tomography (SPECT), or areas or altered glucose metabolism by positron emission tomography (PET). Care must be taken when interpreting these images to not mistake normal variation for disease, and to be aware that even "hysterical" or "functional" conditions may have changes by these methods. Functional magnetic resonance imaging (MRI) is gaining acceptance as a way to demonstrate the changes in brain function in dyslexia and other disorders of thought or emotion.

E. In the case of litigation, malingering must always be considered. Proper observation will often be the clue to feigning illness for gain, and video surveillance is not uncommon in disputed cases. Nonanatomic neurologic deficits may be malingered or may be the result of conversion disorders. A careful neurologic examination and observation of the patient when he performs an action, which would be impossible for a truly injured person, will be of help in suspicious situations. For instance, in the *Hoover test*, the examiner places his hands under the heels of the supine patient and asks him to lift each leg. If the "paralyzed" leg presses down when the "normal" leg is raised, it is not truly paralyzed. There are, however, no absolute tests for malingering, except for observations that a supposed lost function returns when the subject thinks he is not being observed. Tests that require *effort* may be mistakenly interpreted when the performance is poor because of depression, fatigue, or conditions such as myasthenia gravis or a subtle cerebrovascular accident (CVA).

F. A physician conforming to the nationally accepted standard of care for a neuropsychiatric evaluation will conduct an examination, which includes a thorough list of past illness, the origin of the claimed complaint, the course and treatment history, and the medical records of previous assessment and treatment. It is advisable to examine primary sources, including viewing MRI, computed tomography (CT) scan, and x-ray images, rather than relying simply on reports.

G. In addition, one must obtain a thorough family history and history of the individual's past life development, education, occupation, and marriage. The examiner for an IME should obtain employment records when possible.

H. To assess personality styles an Minnesota multiphasic personality inventory test (MMPI) may be useful, as histrionic presentations or inconsistencies may demonstrated. The MMPI is only one bit of data that may be considered, and is not a diagnostic instrument by itself. A traditional mental status examination, which tests the way the individual is functioning at the moment, such as current operations of perception, orientation, thought, feelings, and behavior, is not a substitute for a comprehensive neuropsychological examination by a qualified neuropsychologist to quantify brain damage. An assessment of mood, affect, hallucinations and delusions, impulse control, seizures, appetite, and sleep patterns is required for psychiatric diagnosis and for the evaluation of the functional impact of brain injury or disease.

I. A full general physical examination with detailed neurologic examination is basic to neuropsychiatric assessment, and if indicated, a complete blood and urine toxicology workup.

J. An electroencephalogram is indicated for episodic disorders. MRI of brain, spine, or other body parts may be indicated to demonstrate structural lesions. CT scans of the brain or spine are preferred for the people who cannot have MRIs because of contraindications such as metal fragments in the eyes or cardiac pacemakers, or when a bone problem is suspected. SPECT or PET scan (nuclear medicine procedures that measure regional brain metabolism, and therefore function) in cases of seizures or cognitive changes can provide diagnostic information.

K. Some findings that may mandate the need for further special testing include: Any history of neurologic difficulty or injury, including any blow to the head, particularly if there is an alteration of consciousness, a history of substance abuse, strokes or Alzheimer disease, or history of a variety of endocrinologic conditions, which may cause brain dysfunction. Infections like meningitis or encephalitis, or pseudotumor cerebri may mandate cerebrospinal fluid (CSF) removal and analysis of pressure, chemistry, immunology, and microscopic examination. For a more comprehensive outline refer Neuropsychiatric Approach to the Patient by Fred Ovsview in *Kaplan and Sadock's Comprehensive Textbook of Psychiatry.*

XIX. BRAIN AND BEHAVIOR

A. If an organic defect is discovered, there must be evidence of a clinical correlation before it may be concluded that it influences behavior by diminishing judgment, by increasing rage reaction, or by increasing the impetus to commit a violent act. Lesions of the frontal or anterior temporal lobes are more likely to be related to poor judgment or impulsivity that lesions in other locations, but a history of behavior before and after brain trauma is more compelling. Organic brain disorders make individuals more susceptible to the effects of drugs, alcohol, fatigue, and stress.

XX. CHILD CUSTODY

These examinations are fraught with potential difficulties. It is not enough to simply evaluate the mental and psychiatric condition of a child; each of the parents must be evaluated separately and with the child to make a judgment regarding the best interest of the child. Being mentally ill or mildly retarded may not render a parent unfit, whereas antisocial or narcissistic personality may be primary considerations.

XXI. MENTAL RETARDATION

The Supreme Court has recently ruled that it is unconstitutional to execute children or those with mental retardation, but this concession has not been extended to the mentally ill as of this date. Mental retardation has different definitions according to the DSM-IV or the American Association on Mental Retardation (AAMR), and developmental disability has a different legal meaning than the same intellectual level that may be the result of an acquired brain injury. One must consult the definition required by the setting where a neuropsychiatric opinion is being rendered. General intellectual functioning and adaptive functioning constitute a two-pronged test. Mental retardation is based on the following ranges of intelligence quotient (IQ): 50–55 to 70 (mild); 35–40 to 50–55 (moderate); 20–25 to 35–40 (severe); and below 20 or 25 (profound); but mere numbers are not sufficient for the diagnosis, which must be developmental in origin (e.g., onset before age 18).

XXII. COMMITMENT PROCEEDINGS

Each state has rules for the emergency involuntary hospitalization of persons who may, in the opinion of the police or a physician, be a danger to themselves or others, or may be unable to care for themselves by reason of mental illness. Physicians or the police may institute emergency certificates to take patients into custody and deliver them to hospital emergency departments. In some jurisdictions they may be committed if they "may fall prey to designing others." Probate court proceedings may determine if further deprivation of liberty and the right to self-determination is indicated after somebody has been committed. Others may petition probate court to force treatment on incompetent individuals with appropriate legal representation of the various parties involved. The role of the neuropsychiatrist is to provide a thorough evaluation to the court bearing on the questions of competence to make decisions, to care for one's self, or the risk of harmful behavior in the future. The report may be submitted in the form of an affidavit or by testimony at a court proceeding, or simply on the emergency commitment form.

XXIII. CONFIDENTIALITY

Since the time of Hippocrates ethics and law have protected doctor—patient communications. The most recent iteration of these is provided by the Health Insurance Portability and Accountability (HIPAA) Act of 1996 . These complex regulations require explicit releases for information even between referring doctors and hospitals, and mandate recording each release in a permanent record that may be examined by the government. The law provides for criminal penalties for unauthorized disclosure of information. Courts may subpoena neuropsychiatric records, but it is the obligation of physicians to insure that information about third parties or private information not relevant to the purpose of the court action be redacted. Legal advice is recommended in questionable circumstances.

References
1. American Psychiatric Association. *Diagnostic and statistical manual of mental disorders*, 4th ed. Washington, DC: American Psychiatric Association; 1994.
2. Appelbaum PS, Gutheil TG. *Clinical handbook of psychiatry and the law*, 2nd ed. Baltimore, MD: Williams & Wilkins; 1991.
3. Cocchiarella L, Andersson GBJ, eds. *Guides to the evaluation of permanent impairment*, 5th ed. Chicago: American Medical Association Press; 2001.
4. Edlund W, Gronseth G, So Y, et al. *American academy of neurology clinical practice guideline process manual*, 2004 ed. www.aan.com, Accessed September 1, 2005.
5. Gunn J, Taylor PJ. *Forensic psychiatry: Clinical, legal & ethical issues.* Oxford: Butterworth-Heinemann; 1993:48, 88.
6. Haerer AF. *DeJong's the neurological examination*, 5th ed. Philadelphia, PA: JB Lippincott Co; 1992.
7. Jennett B, Teasdale G. *Management of head injuries.* Philadelphia, PA: FA Davis Co; 1981.
8. Latham PS, Latham PH. Selected legal issues. In: Coffey CE, Brumback RA, eds. *Pediatric neuropsychiatry.* Philadelphia, PA: Lippincott Williams & Wilkins; 2006:715–727.
9. Lishman WA. *Organic psychiatry*, 3rd ed. Oxford: Blackwell Science; 1998.
10. Sadock BJ, Sadock VA, eds. *Kaplan & Sadock's comprehensive textbook of psychiatry*, 8th ed. Philadelphia, PA: Lippincott Williams & Wilkins; 2005.
11. Schaumberg HH, Albers JW. Pseudoneurotoxic disease. *Neurology.* 2005;65:22–26.
12. Spar JE. Competency and related forensic issues. In: Coffey CE, Cummings JL, eds. *Geriatric neuropsychiatry.* Washington, DC: American Psychiatric Press; 2000:945–963.

Chapter 1

RATIONAL APPROACH TO BRAIN IMAGING AND ELECTROPHYSIOLOGY

Robin A. Hurley, Nash N. Boutros, Katherine H. Taber

BACKGROUND

The first step in the evaluation of a patient with a neuropsychiatric disorder is a thorough history and physical examination. After gathering this information, the clinician can make an informed decision if brain imaging or electrophysiology is warranted in the assessment process. These diagnostics may improve the care of patients with neuropsychiatric disorders. The information obtained from such studies may help clarify diagnosis, estimate prognosis, or improve the treatment plan. In this chapter, we discuss principles of test ordering in the clinical setting, review the main brain imaging and electrophysiologic modalities, and provide case examples of their application in neuropsychiatry.

PRINCIPLES OF ORDERING AND INTERPRETATION

Brain Imaging

Brain imaging can contribute information for diagnosis, prognosis, and treatment planning, as noted in the preceding text. The research into each of these contributions is limited not only by the complexities of functional anatomy, but also by our ability to design studies that would separate out these contributions. As a diagnostic aid, imaging can help identify pathologies that produce clinical symptoms. This, in turn, informs both prognosis and treatment planning. These are interdependent factors in formulating patient management.

   In general, it is employed to *confirm* the presence of focal brain pathology in a patient with findings from the history or examination which suggest such pathology. Patients with *focal sensory or motor changes referable to the brain*, or with obvious brain disease (stroke, epilepsy) or injury, are the traditional domains of neurologists. In these patients the indications for brain imaging are reasonably clear and straightforward. The importance of imaging in patients with *dementia or significant cognitive change* is also well established. Imaging of the cognitively impaired patient may assist in the differential diagnosis of Alzheimer disease (AD), multi-infarct dementia, or cognitive decline due to another cause.[1]

More challenging are those patients presenting with behavioral, emotional, or cognitive changes, the domain of neuropsychiatrists. Findings suggestive of focal brain pathology in these patients include atypical symptoms or symptom presentations, and focal deficits on neuropsychiatric examination (see Table 18.1). Specific examples of such indications include subsyndromal cognitive deficits, unusual age at symptom onset, unusual symptom evolution, personality changes, accompanying neurologic signs/symptoms, unusual symptoms (symptoms outside clinical norms), and sustained confusion/delirium.[2] In addition, neuroimaging is recommended if there is a history of poison or toxin exposure including severe alcohol abuse with significant cognitive/social impairments, or brain injury (traumatic or "organic").

Erhart et al. found that treatment was changed in 15% of nondemented patients because of magnetic resonance imaging (MRI) findings.[2] As an example, neuroimaging for differential diagnostics may clarify directions for treatment of cognitive impairment. Acetylcholinesterase inhibitors are helpful in the management of early stage cognitive impairment. Finding brain lesions can alert the clinician to avoid psychotropic agents suspected to slow neuronal repair (e.g., typical neuroleptics) or those agents documented to increase confusion in the patient with brain injury (e.g., lithium or strongly anticholinergic agents).[3] If periventricular white matter abnormalities are present on imaging, then small

TABLE 18.1   Clinical Indications for Imaging in Psychiatric Patients

Medical Conditions or Working Diagnoses
Traumatic brain injury (including sudden deceleration or blast injuries)
Significant alcohol abuse
Seizure disorders with psychiatric symptoms
Movement disorders
Autoimmune disorders
Eating disorders
Poison or toxin exposure
Delirium

Clinical Factors
Psychiatric symptoms outside ''clinical norms'' or with any unusual presentation or
  course
New-onset mental illness after age 50
Presentations at an atypical age for the working diagnosis
Initial psychotic break
Focal neurologic signs
Catatonia
Dementia or cognitive decline
Sudden personality changes

vessel hypertensive disease (poorly controlled blood pressure) may be present. A more aggressive control of blood pressure is then indicated.

Electrophysiology

Unusual presentations and atypical age of onset are the main "red flags" indicating the need for more extensive investigations. Inui et al. emphasized the atypicality of the clinical presentation as the most important factor for initiating an electroencephalograph (EEG) evaluation.[4] They found the frequency of epileptiform discharges (including controversial waveforms) to be significantly higher among patients with mood-incongruent psychotic mood disorder (33%) and schizophreniform disorder (30%) as compared with nonpsychotic mood disorder (3.2%) and schizophrenia (0%).

BRAIN IMAGING AND ELECTROPHYSIOLOGIC MODALITIES

Definitions

1. *Tomography* is the creation of a two-dimensional (2-D) image or section (from the Greek *tomos* [a cutting or slice] and *grapho* [to write]).
2. *Computed tomography* (CT), *computer-assisted tomography* uses computer processing to assemble information from multiple x-ray images into a 2-D cross-sectional image.
3. *Spatial resolution* determines the level of detail that can be seen in a two- or three-dimensional (2- or 3-D) image. It is defined by the number of *pixels* (picture elements) the image contains in each dimension and their individual size. A related concept is *voxel* (volume element).
4. *Slice thickness* is the width of tissue included in each image.
5. *Signal-to-noise* is the ratio of the desired information (signal) to the accompanying background activity (noise).
6. *Plane-of-section* describes the orientation of a cross-sectional image. The *coronal* plane divides the body into front (anterior) and back (posterior) portions. The *sagittal* plane divides the body into right and left portions. The *axial* or *horizontal* plane divides the body into upper and lower portions.
7. A *contrast agent* is any substance that is introduced into the body to make an anatomic structure more visible on images.
8. *Background activity* is the dominant ongoing EEG rhythm. The term usually refers to the background activity during resting wakefulness. Under normal conditions, this activity is dominated by alpha rhythms. This activity is characterized by waxing and waning and readily attenuates when the person open his/her eyes or begins to concentrate.
9. *Beta, alpha, theta, and delta* are the traditional EEG frequency bands. Recent advances in EEG analysis have blurred the boundaries between these traditional ranges—beta (>13.5 Hz), alpha (8.5 to 13.5 Hz) (Fig. 18.5B), theta (4 to 8 Hz) (Fig. 18.5C), delta (0.5 to 3.5 Hz).
10. *Spike-and-sharp waves* are paroxysmal (i.e., occur suddenly and are distinct from the ongoing background activity) events and usually are indicative

of an epileptic process. The difference between a spike and a sharp wave is a matter of the duration of the discharge. Spikes are <70 ms in duration and sharp waves are between 70 and 200 ms in duration. This difference could be a reflection of the depth of the focus from the surface. The term *spike-and-wave complex* refers only to the presence of a prominent wave after each spike, likely reflecting an inhibitory process after the excitatory spike (Fig. 18.5D).

Structural Brain Imaging

COMPUTED TOMOGRAPHY
CT uses photons and a collecting detector to record tissue density. On standard CT, air (the least dense) is black and bone (the most dense) is white. All other tissues are a shade of gray (see Table 18.2). Conventional CT uses several rings of detectors to acquire several images simultaneously. A computer translates the detections into a 2-D picture. This is either displayed on a computer monitor or printed onto x-ray film. Radiation exposure is clinically insignificant (approximately 5 rads). For extra protection, scans are angled to avoid the lens of the eye. If urgently needed in pregnancy, lead aprons are worn. The recent introduction of spiral CT further reduces the radiation exposure, and provides true 3-D imaging. An advantage of 3-D imaging is that no areas are missed between slices.

Modern CT scanners can generate brain images that range from 0.5 to 10 mm in thickness, with 3 to 5 mm used most commonly. The slice thickness of a CT image is an important variable in clinical scanning. Thinner slices allow visualization of smaller lesions. However, the thinnest sections have less contrast (i.e., the signal intensity difference between gray and white matter is less) because the signal/noise is lower. It also takes longer to complete the examination because more slices must be acquired. Therefore, there is more chance of patient movement degrading the images. The longer scan time also decreases the number of patients that can be examined in a day. Thicker sections (or slices) have greater contrast but smaller lesions may be missed. There is also greater artifact due to increased volume averaging. This is particularly true in the base of the skull and may obscure brain stem and mesial temporal structures.

TABLE 18.2   Relative Image Intensity on Computed Tomography (Noncontrast)

Tissue Type	Image Intensity
Air	Black
Water, cerebrospinal fluid	Very dark gray
White matter of brain	Medium gray
Gray matter of brain	Light gray
Clotted blood[a], calcified tissue, bone	White

[a]Clot becomes isointense to brain by 1 to 2 weeks after onset.

MAGNETIC RESONANCE IMAGING

MRI is based on manipulating the small magnetic field around the nucleus of the hydrogen atom (proton), a major component of water in soft tissue. To take an MRI of a patient's soft tissues, the patient must be placed inside a large magnet. The strength of the magnet is measured in tesla (T). Most clinical systems have a field strength of 1.5 T, although 3.0 T systems are becoming more available for clinical work. (More powerful systems are often used in research settings.) A

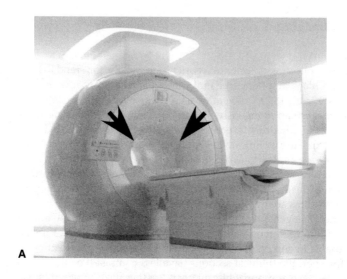

A

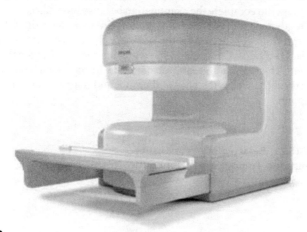

B

FIGURE 18.1   Magnetic resonance imaging equipment. **A:** Standard clinical magnetic resonance scanners are enclosing, with a relatively small opening (*arrows*) (Achieva, picture courtesy of Phillips Medical Systems). **B:** An open design lowers the likelihood of claustrophobia and provides better access to the patient (Panorama 0.6 T, picture courtesy of Phillips Medical Systems).

midfield system is generally 0.5 T, and low-field units range from 0.1 to 0.5 T. The greater signal available with 1.5 and 3.0 T systems allows higher resolution images to be collected. However, this increased detail is costly because high-field systems are more expensive than mid- or lowfield systems. Also, many patients feel uncomfortable while lying inside these huge enclosing magnets (see Fig. 18.1A). Open design magnets are now available that provide less feeling of confinement to the patient (Fig. 18.1B).

To create an MRI, the patient's hydrogen atoms are exposed to a carefully calculated series of radio frequency (RF) pulses while the patient is within the scanner's magnetic field. These RF pulses change the magnetization of the hydrogen atoms, generating tiny electric signals that are picked up by a receiver placed close to the area being scanned (the imaging coil). A head coil that encloses the head, allowing maximum signal pickup, is used to obtain brain images. The magnetic field gradients needed to acquire the image are created by huge coils of wire embedded in the magnet, driven with large current audio amplifiers similar to those used for musical concerts. These can create a great deal of noise during the scan, and may distress the unprepared patient.

In MRI there are a wide variety of image types possible, each sensitive to a different physical aspect of tissue. This is quite different from CT, where the images reflect a single parameter, the density of tissue. The pulse sequence used to acquire the MRI (the combination of RF and magnetic field pulses used by the computer to create the image) determines the unique information the image will contain. Clinical MRI most commonly uses the spin echo (SE) or the fast spin echo (FSE) sequences. The expected appearances of tissues using the most common SE imaging methods are summarized in Table 18.3. T1-weighted images are traditionally considered best for displaying anatomy, whereas T2-weighted images are best for displaying pathology. However, both pathology and cerebrospinal fluid (CSF) will appear bright, making it difficult to visualize pathology near the ventricles. A variation on the T2-weighted scan has been developed (called *fluid attenuated inversion recovery* [FLAIR]) where CSF is dark, making pathology near CSF-filled spaces much easier to see. FLAIR MRI is extremely useful in neuropsychiatry (see Fig. 18.2).

Two other methods that are useful in clinical imaging are gradient echo (GE) or gradient refocused echo (GRE) and diffusion-weighted (DW) MRI. GE imaging (also called *susceptibility weighted imaging*) is very sensitive to anything in the tissue causing magnetic field inhomogeneity, such as hemorrhage or calcium. These images have artifacts at the interfaces between tissues with very different magnetic susceptibility, such as bone and brain. The artifacts at the skull base are sometimes severe. DW MRI is sensitive to the speed of water diffusion, and may be able to visualize areas of ischemic stroke in the critical first few hours after onset. It is also showing potential in the imaging of other conditions, including neurodegenerative conditions and traumatic brain injury (TBI).

COMPUTED TOMOGRAPHY VERSUS MAGNETIC RESONANCE IMAGING

CT is more widely available and is less expensive than MRI (see Table 18.4). Several types of pathology, particularly calcification, acute hemorrhage, and bone injuries, are better imaged with CT. Otherwise, MRI is preferred because it has a much higher resolution, can provide images in any plane of section, does not have artifacts near bone, and is sensitive to more types of pathology. CT has limited contraindications surrounding contrast agent administration: Allergy to iodine,

TABLE 18.3 Relative Image Intensity on Magnetic Resonance Imaging (Noncontrast)

Tissue Type	Image Intensity		
	T1 Weighted	T2 Weighted	Spin Density Weighted
Air	Black	Black	Black
Water, cerebrospinal fluid	Black	White (black on FLAIR)	Gray
White matter of brain	Light gray	Dark gray	Medium gray
Gray matter of brain	Medium gray	Medium gray	Light gray
Bone	Black	Black	Black
Calcified tissue	Variable, usually gray	Variable, usually gray	Variable, usually gray
Pathology (not blood)	Gray	White	White
Blood—acute	Dark gray	Black	Light gray
Blood—subacute	White	White	White

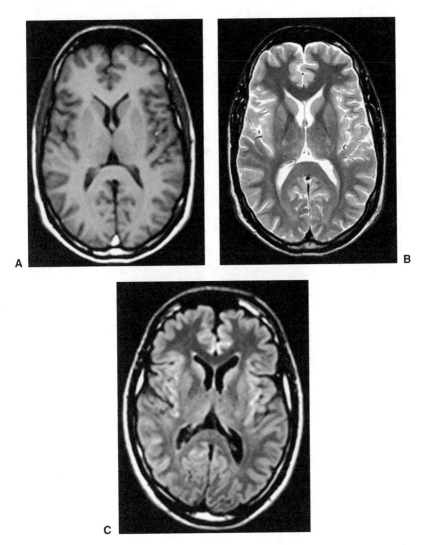

FIGURE 18.2   Magnetic Resonance Imaging. Axial magnetic resonance images of a normal adult brain (Achieva, pictures courtesy of Phillips Medical Systems). **A**: T1-weighted (T1W) magnetic resonance image. **B**: T2-weighted (T2W) magnetic resonance image. **C**: Fluid attenuated inversion recovery (FLAIR) image.

contrast dyes, or shellfish, creatinine ≥1.5 mg per dL, or metformin administration on the day of contrast scan. Contraindications to MRI include magnetic metals in the body, history of welding without screening x-rays, or implanted electrical, mechanical, or magnetic devices.

CONTRAST-ENHANCED STRUCTURAL IMAGING
Structural brain images can be acquired either with or without intravenous administration of a contrast agent. These intravascular agents normally do not

TABLE 18.4   Factors to Consider When Choosing an Imaging Modality

Clinical Considerations	CT	MRI
Availability	Universal	Limited
Sensitivity	Good	Superior
Resolution	0.5 mm	1.5 mm
Average examination time	1 min	30–45 min
Plane of section	Axial only	Any plane of section
Conditions for which it is the preferred procedure	Screening examination	All subcortical lesions
	Acute hemorrhage	Poison or toxin exposure
	Calcified lesions	Demyelinating disorders
	Bone injury	Eating disorders
		Examination requiring anatomic detail, especially temporal lobe or cerebellum
		Any condition best viewed in nonaxial plane
Contraindications	History of anaphylaxis or severe allergic reaction (contrast-enhanced CT)	Any magnetic metal in the body, including surgical clips and sutures
	Creatinine ≥1.5 mg/dL (contrast-enhanced CT)	Implanted electrical, mechanical, or magnetic devices
		Claustrophobia
	Metformin administration on day of scan (contrast-enhanced CT)	History of welding (requires skull films before MRI)
		Pregnancy (legal contraindication)
Cost to patient per scan without contrast medium[a]	~$230	~$550
Cost to patient per single dose of contrast medium[a]	~$60 nonionic	~$110

[a]Costs are regionally variable. Please consult imaging sources in your area for current figures.
CT, computed tomography; MRI, magnetic resonance imaging.

penetrate into the brain, as they cannot pass through an intact blood–brain barrier (BBB). If this barrier is disrupted, the contrast agent leaks into surrounding tissue and changes its appearance on imaging. Conditions where the BBB may open include tumors, inflammatory or autoimmune conditions such as lupus or multiple sclerosis, and infectious processes. Other conditions where a contrast agent is useful include evaluation of suspected aneurysms, arteriovenous malformations, or other vascular processes (e.g., temporal arteritis).[5–7]

ORDERING THE EXAMINATION

The neuroradiologist needs very clear clinical information on the imaging request form (not just "rule out pathology" or "new-onset mental status changes"). If a lesion is suspected in a particular location, the neuroradiologist should be informed of this or give enough clinical data for selection of the best imaging method and parameters to view suspicious areas. The neuroradiologist and technical staff also need information on the patient's current condition (e.g., delirious, psychotic, easily agitated, or paranoid). This may eliminate difficulties with patient management during the scan.

Metabolic Brain Imaging

Regional cerebral blood flow (rCBF) and regional cerebral metabolic rate (rCMR) provide indirect measures of brain activity. Neuronal activity consumes oxygen and metabolites, and there is a close coupling between neuronal activity, rCBF and rCMR. If acquired under resting conditions, both rCMR and rCBF provide a way to assess overall state of brain areas. This is particularly useful for identification of "hidden" lesions, areas that are dysfunctional but do not look abnormal on structural imaging. In addition, functional imaging techniques are available to measure various neurotransmitter receptor systems. In general, patients whose clinical symptoms do not fit the classic historical picture for the working diagnosis should be considered for some form of functional imaging.[1,6,8–12]

SINGLE PHOTON EMISSION COMPUTED TOMOGRAPHY

Single photon emission computed tomography (SPECT) is based on imaging the distribution of a blood-borne radiotracer. A gamma camera collects the data used by the computer to reconstruct a tomographic image, similar to the procedure for standard CT. Resolution is heavily dependent on the age and sophistication of the equipment. Older systems had limited detectors and produced lower quality images. The newer multiple-head cameras provide a resolution of approximately 6 to 7 mm. SPECT is much more widely available than positron emission tomography (PET) (another functional imaging technique). Although other types of radiotracers are available, most SPECT studies measure rCBF. The most commonly used SPECT brain blood flow tracer remains ^{99m}Tc-hexamethylpropylene amine oxine (HMPAO) followed by 1,1-ethyl cysteinate dimer (ECD).

SPECT is the preferred functional imaging modality for identification of the seizure focus in epilepsy (ictal imaging examination). It is also very useful in the evaluation of dementia. Hypoperfusion in temperoparietal cortex is suggestive of AD, although a similar pattern of perfusion loss may be seen in patients with Parkinson disease who have dementia. SPECT may also be useful in distinguishing AD from other forms of dementia (vascular, frontotemporal [Pick], or Lewy body

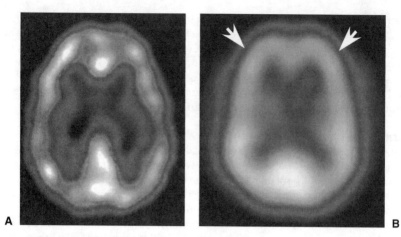

A   **B**

FIGURE 18.3   Single photon emission computed tomography (SPECT). Axial cerebral blood flow SPECT images. **A**: In a normal individual all of the cerebral cortex has a relatively high (as indicated by—orange–white color) rate of blood flow (see color insert—picture courtesy of CTI). **B**: In this patient with a traumatic brain injury (TBI) there are areas of lower than expected perfusion in several regions (*arrows*).

dementia). SPECT can be used to look for evidence of TBI in patients with neurobehavioral symptoms after an injury and a normal structural scan (see Fig. 18.3).

POSITRON EMISSION TOMOGRAPHY

PET is based on imaging the distribution of an intravenously administered short-lived radioactive tracer. The object to be imaged (the head) is surrounded by rings of detector pairs. The pixel size, and therefore the resolution of the image, is determined by the center-to-center spacing of these detectors. The present limit for spatial resolution is approximately 2.5 mm. In most clinical studies a single set of PET images is acquired, providing a "snap shot" of the state of the brain at a single point in time. Less often a series of image sets are acquired, providing a dynamic view of the state of the brain over time. The most commonly used tracer is 18-fluoro-2-deoxyglucose ($[^{18}F]$-FDG). It is taken up into cells similarly to glucose and undergoes metabolism to fluorodeoxyglucose-6-phosphate. At this point it does not undergo further metabolism and is trapped within cells, providing a measure of rCMR for glucose. Other radiotracers provide measures of rCBF, neurotransmitter transporter binding, and neurotransmitter receptor binding.

PET is used in the evaluation of many neurologic conditions, particularly epilepsy (interictal seizure focus localization), central nervous system malignancies (both detection and grading), head trauma (lesion detection), and cerebrovascular disease (evaluation of transient ischemia and cerebral vascular reserve). PET is also useful in helping differentiate between different dementing disorders. The ability of PET to detect perfusion changes consistent with AD may be superior to that of SPECT, with studies reporting sensitivity of 87% to 94% and specificity of 85% to 96% (see Fig. 18.4).

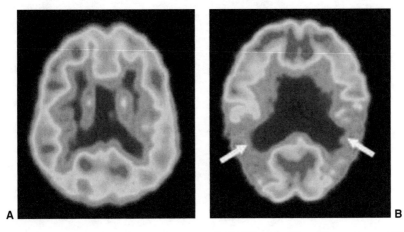

FIGURE 18.4   Positron emission tomography (PET). Axial fluorodeoxyglucose PET images of cerebral energy metabolism (pictures courtesy of CTI). **A:** In a normal individual all of the cerebral cortex has a relatively high (as indicated by—orange–red color [see color insert]) metabolic rate. **B:** In this patient with Alzheimer disease there are clear areas of reduced metabolism bilaterally (*arrows*).

Electroencephalography

EEG refers in general to recording of the electrical activity of the brain whether from the scalp, cortex, or depth recording from electrodes implanted within the brain (see Fig. 18.5A). The term *Standard EEG* (or routine EEG) is used to denote the visual (non–computer-assisted) interpretation of the scalp-recorded EEG. Routine EEG is a widely available and a relatively inexpensive test. Therefore, clinicians should have a rather low threshold for ordering an EEG when the presenting clinical picture is atypical. It is crucial, for EEG to be useful, that the clinician ordering the test be familiar with the limitations of the test and with the general implications of the different abnormalities that can be detected through an EEG. It is equally important that the electrophysiologist be familiar with EEG abnormalities that commonly occur in psychiatric disorders.[13] Two types of EEG abnormalities are commonly indicative of underlying pathology: Paroxysmal activity indicating episodic and unpredictable abnormal neuronal discharges (Fig. 18.5D) and/or slowing of the normal rhythms of the brain (Fig. 18.5C). Both patterns can occur diffusely or focally. A diffuse pattern suggests a more generalized pathologic process; whereas a focal pattern suggests a localized pathologic process.

In the early years of electrophysiology, a number of EEG waveforms were described that were thought to have possible epileptic significance. These controversial waveforms were subsequently shown to have little, if any, association with epilepsy but were repeatedly noted to be more prevalent in psychiatric populations. Controversial waveforms include the fourteen and six positive spikes (14 and 6 PS), the small sharp spikes (SSS), the rhythmic midtemporal discharges (RMTD), and the six per second spike and waves (6/s Sp and W). The exact clinical correlates of these waveforms have not been thoroughly examined. The electroencephalographer should be familiar with these controversial discharges and the

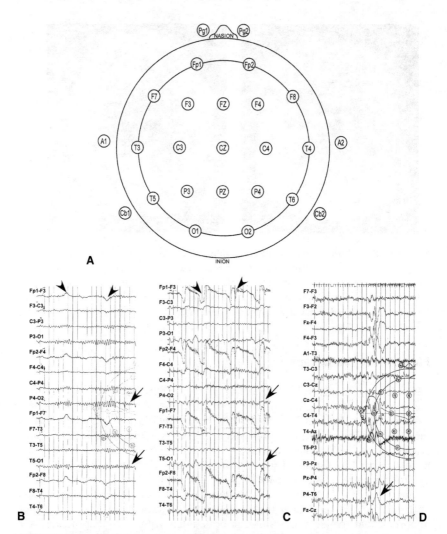

FIGURE 18.5   Electroencephalography (EEG). **A:** Diagram of the standard placement and nomenclature for the surface electrodes used to record EEG. **B:** Normal EEG activity obtained from an awake relaxed adult with eyes closed. The alpha activity (characteristic of this state) can be seen most clearly in the posterior regions (*arrows*). Artifacts due to eye movements can be seen in the anterior regions (*arrowheads*). **C:** This tracing was obtained from a patient with psychosis. The background rhythm is slow (theta, 4 to 5 Hz, *arrows*) indicating a diffuse encephalopathic process. The frontal leads reflect excessive eye movements (*arrowheads*). **D:** This tracing was obtained from an adolescent with mild mental retardation and aggressive episodes. It shows a normal background with superimposed spike-and-wave discharges which seem to originate from the right frontal/temporal region (*arrow*).

importance of their evaluation in psychiatric patients. However, these discharges require the patient to have fallen asleep during the recording, so evaluation may not be possible in all psychiatric patients. In a busy laboratory, it is often challenging for psychiatric patients to relax sufficiently to sleep. Insomnia during the study will render it "incomplete and unsatisfactory." Referring neuropsychiatrists should bear in mind that documentation of controversial waveforms can vary. If these are noted in the EEG report, then the neuropsychiatrist should investigate further or seek consultation regarding the clinical implications of such findings.[14]

Polysomnography

Polysomnography (PSG) is the recording of physiologic variables during sleep. A thorough PSG study provides data on sleep continuity, sleep architecture, rapid eye movement (REM) sleep physiology, sleep-related respiratory impairments, oxygen desaturation, cardiac arrhythmias, and periodic limb movements. Other specific measures can also be added such as nocturnal penile tumescence for the evaluation of erectile dysfunction. The term *all-night EEG* indicates a limited recording of data that allows the examination of the EEG signal and sleep architecture (EEG, eye movement, electromyography) without recording other physiologic parameters (e.g., breathing patterns, oxygen saturation, electrocardiogram) as is done in more routine PSG.

Evoked Potentials

Evoked potentials (EPs) are measured by signal averaging techniques, where the potentials elicited by repeated stimulation are superimposed. This enhances the stimulus-specific response (i.e., EP), and causes the background activity to be averaged out. The degree to which the background noise is averaged out is called *signal-to-noise ratio*. EPs can be classified on the basis of the stimulus inducing the response (visual, somatosensory, or auditory), or on the time since stimulation and response characteristics (early-, mid-, and long-latency responses). These are automatic responses, have little cognitive or psychological correlates, and are difficult to manipulate with laboratory-based paradigms. EPs are extremely useful when axonal injury is suspected (e.g., in multiple sclerosis). The early responses (initial waveform from stimulus onset to 20 to 30 ms) tests the integrity of the pathway the stimulus has to travel to reach the higher cortical centers. The midlatency responses occur between 30 and 250 ms. These responses are also automatic and reflect the sensory pathway of the specific stimulus (auditory, visual, or somatosensory). Although these responses have been shown to be abnormal in many psychiatric conditions, clinical utility is yet to be demonstrated. If a patient reports a sensory deficit (e.g., hemianesthesia, deafness) and the EPs are normal, the clinician should consider a psychologically based illness (see Fig. 18.6A).

Future Brain Diagnostic Techniques for Clinical Care

The following neurodiagnostic techniques are primarily available in tertiary medical centers and used more often in neuropsychiatric research, but have

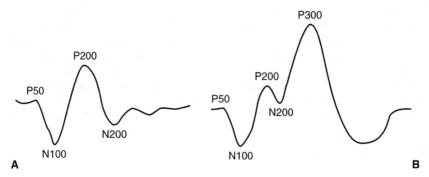

FIGURE 18.6   Evoked potentials and event-related potentials. **A:** The tracing demonstrates the automatic response evoked by an auditory stimulus (auditory evoked potential). The major components, P50, N100, P200 and N200, are labeled. **B:** The tracing demonstrates, in addition to the automatic responses, the P300 component that is generated when the subject attends to a target stimulus.

some current clinical neuropsychiatric applications. However, they are quickly becoming more commonplace in the broader clinical care setting. The challenge remains to clarify/establish their uses for the individual patient. Their applications to understanding the emotion/memory/behavioral circuitry from a basic science standpoint and for development of normative databases are well established. Other techniques such as magnetic resonance spectroscopy, functional MRI, and Xenon-enhanced CT are not discussed in this chapter, as they are largely research techniques with regard to patients with psychiatric symptoms.

QUANTIFIED ELECTROENCEPHALOGRAPHY
Quantified electroencephalography (Q-EEG) is the analysis of EEG data utilizing computer capabilities. The most common of these, spectral analysis, is a computer-based method of analyzing the EEG frequency spectrum over time. It allows for the determination of the relative predominance or power of any frequency band. It takes advantage of the analytic power of the computer and its ability to translate an enormous quantity of background EEG frequency data into concise parameters by a method called the *fast Fourier transform*. Other approaches include period-amplitude analysis and coherence analysis (synchrony of activity between different locations). It is impossible for the electroencephalographer to appreciate or analyze, unaided, all of the time-dependent changes in frequency content of an EEG, particularly when the number of recording electrodes is large (64 to 256). Often, electroencephalographic parameters are assigned a visual analog, such as color, which allows formation of topographic maps. However, the transformation of extremely complex data into a simple image can distort the underlying data. Therefore, interpretation of Q-EEG studies requires a highly experienced electroencephalographer.

Identification of the brain source of electrical activity recorded from the scalp is termed *the inverse problem*. Many solutions to this problem have been suggested over the years. One such method is called *low resolution electromagnetic tomography* (LORETA). LORETA has gained wide use and is progressively being applied to clinical situations (see Fig. 18.7). This method offers a 3-D tomography of

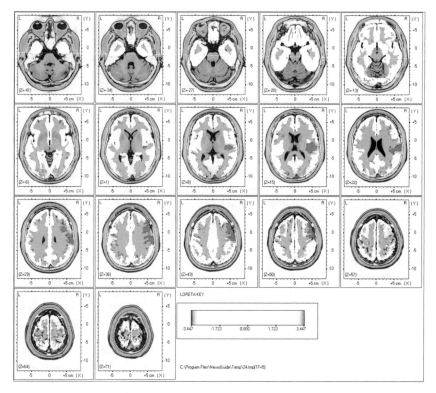

FIGURE 18.7   Quantified electroencephalography (Q-EEG). This EEG data was obtained as part of the evaluation and diagnosis of a middle-aged man with traumatic brain injury. The patient was hit on the right side of his head by a bat. He had symptoms of memory loss, spatial disorientation, depression, word finding problems and erratic mood. In comparison to data from an age matched normative database, the patient shows a focal abnormality of excessive theta activity (Z > 3 standard deviations at 5 Hz, red [see color insert]) in the right temporal and right frontal lobes (i.e., right inferior temporal and superior temporal lobes and the right middle frontal gyrus, Brodmann areas 8 and 42 were maximally deviant from normal). NeuroGuide analysis software was used to generate the Low Resolution Electromagnetic Tomography (LORETA) images (courtesy of Dr. Robert Thatcher).

brain activity using a dense grid (corresponding to a spatial resolution of 7) restricted to the cortical gray matter and the hippocampus. The grid is based on the digitized Talairach Atlas (provided by the Brain Imaging Center, Montreal Neurological Institute). LORETA images represent either the electrical activity (actually the square magnitude of the computed current density), or the *t*-values of voxel-by-voxel statistical comparison of electrical activity.[15]

EVENT-RELATED POTENTIALS

The late or event-related potentials (ERPs) are of special interest to psychiatry. ERPs are generated in response to a cognitive or specific information-processing event. Commonly studied ERPs include the P300 and the mismatch negativity (MMN) responses. The P300 is the most studied ERP in psychiatry. To date, there are almost 50 replications of a lowered amplitude of the P300 response in patients with schizophrenia.[16] The P300 is a positive wave occurring approximately 300 ms following the recognition of an odd stimulus imbedded among more regular visual, auditory, or somatosensory stimuli (Fig. 18.6B). The MMN is a negative wave that is generated when an unexpected stimulus is imbedded among more common stimuli. Although both are evoked by similar stimuli, the MMN is thought to reflect an automatic and preattentive process of detection of deviance. Currently available studies suggest that although ERPs may not be able to support a specific diagnosis, they can provide useful data regarding the information-processing capacity of a particular patient. It remains up to the clinician to integrate ERP data with the clinical picture just as results of neuropsychological or psychological testing are integrated into the case formulation. Standardization of technology and the development of test-retest reliabilities for the different measures may increase the clinical utility of ERPs.

MAGNETOENCEPHALOGRAPHY

Magnetoencephalography (MEG) is the recording of the magnetic fields generated by the brain (principally reflecting intraneuronal electric current). The MEG signal, which is a billion-fold weaker than the earth's magnetic field, can be conceptualized as the magnetic counterpart of the EEG or EP signal. MEG is more accurate than EEG in detecting deep-brain sources of neuronal activity. It can detect tangential current sources (e.g., neurons in the sulci whose axial orientation is parallel to the scalp). The recent availability of large-array superconducting biomagnetometer systems has made MEG a feasible diagnostic test, particularly in the workup of treatment-resistant patients with epilepsy who may benefit from resective surgery.

Magnetic source imaging, which combines MEG with MRI, has been used to produce neuromagnetic maps of somatosensory and auditory EPs in healthy subjects. The principal disadvantage of MEG is that the magnetometer must contend with a low signal-to-noise ratio, necessitating the use of expensive shielding to eliminate ambient magnetic noise. Therefore, MEG remains largely a research tool in neuropsychiatry.

APPLICATION OF BRAIN IMAGING AND ELECTROPHYSIOLOGY TO SELECTED CLINICAL PROBLEMS

As noted in the preceding text, common reasons to obtain these examinations in neuropsychiatry include clarification of diagnosis, assistance with treatment planning, and/or to gather prognostic information. Examples of conditions where imaging or EEG can be clinically useful are described in the following text. The imaging discussion is presented as case examples. The EEG discussion is organized by symptoms. It is prudent for the clinician to be mindful that brain imaging is only one part of clinical evaluation and treatment planning. Good clinical judgment must always be exercised in evaluating the significance of diagnostic findings in the clinical formulation of a case.

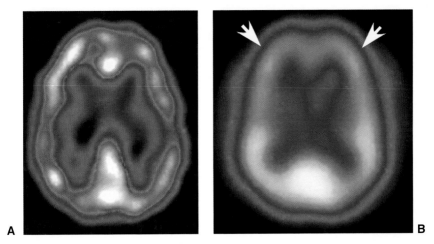

FIGURE 18.3 Single photon emission computed tomography (SPECT). Axial cerebral blood flow SPECT images. **A:** In a normal individual all of the cerebral cortex has a relatively high (as indicated by—orange–white color) rate of blood flow (picture courtesy of CTI). **B:** In this patient with a traumatic brain injury (TBI) there are areas of lower than expected perfusion in several regions (*arrows*).

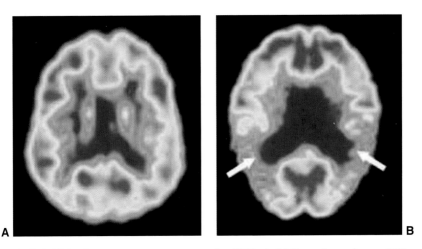

FIGURE 18.4 Positron-emission tomography (PET). Axial fluorodeoxyglucose PET images of cerebral energy metabolism (pictures courtesy of CTI). **A:** In a normal individual all of the cerebral cortex has a relatively high (as indicated by—orange–red color) metabolic rate. **B:** In this patient with Alzheimer disease there are clear areas of reduced metabolism bilaterally (*arrows*).

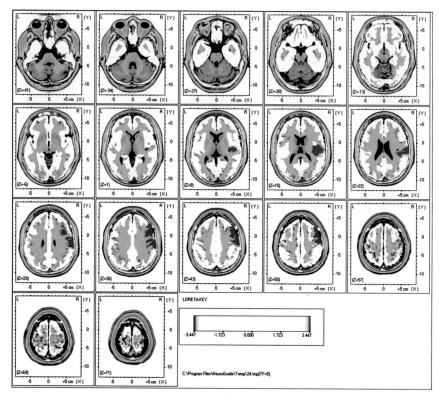

FIGURE 18.7 Quantified electroencephalography (Q-EEG). This EEG data was obtained as part of the evaluation and diagnosis of a middle-aged man with traumatic brain injury. The patient was hit on the right side of his head by a bat. He had symptoms of memory loss, spatial disorientation, depression, word finding problems and erratic mood. In comparison to data from an age matched normative database, the patient shows a focal abnormality of excessive theta activity (Z > 3 standard deviations at 5 Hz, red) in the right temporal and right frontal lobes (i.e., right inferior temporal and superior temporal lobes and the right middle frontal gyrus, Brodmann areas 8 and 42 were maximally deviant from normal). NeuroGuide analysis software was used to generate the Low Resolution Electromagnetic Tomography (LORETA) images (courtesy of Dr. Robert Thatcher).

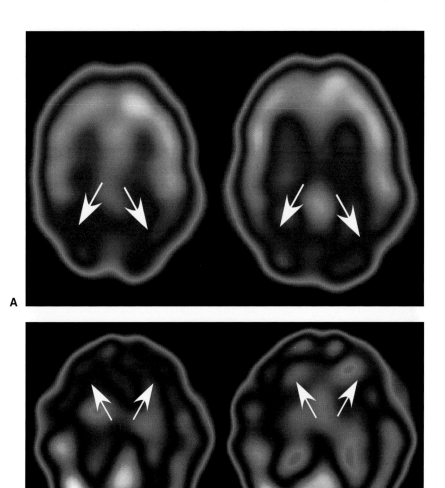

FIGURE 18.12 Using metabolic imaging for clarification of diagnosis. **A:** Mild memory loss suggested possible early Alzheimer disease (AD). Minimal diffuse atrophy identified by magnetic resonance imaging was not sufficient to make the diagnosis. Single photon emission computed tomography (SPECT) imaging of reduced blood flow in the parietal and occipital cortices (*arrows*) with preservation of blood flow in the frontal and temporal regions confirmed the diagnosis. Courtesy of Ronald Fisher, MD, PhD, Baylor College of Medicine. **B:** The symptoms were clinically atypical. SPECT imaging of reduced blood flow in the frontal lobes (*arrows*) supported a diagnosis of frontal temporal dementia (FTD, Pick) rather than AD or dementia with Lewy Bodies (DLB). Courtesy of Ronald Fisher, MD, PhD, Baylor College of Medicine.

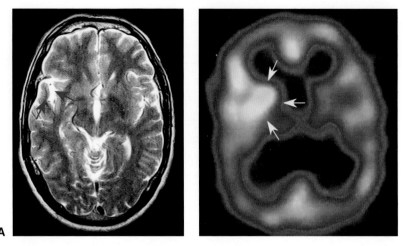

A   **B**

FIGURE 18.13 Using metabolic imaging to change the treatment plan. Depression unresponsive to antidepressant treatment and new-onset stuttering. Magnetic resonance imaging **(A)** revealed mild enlargement of the lateral sulcus on the right (*arrows*). **B:** Single photon emission computed tomography imaging revealed an area of increased blood flow in the right temporal lobe, findings consistent with the presence of an epileptic focus.

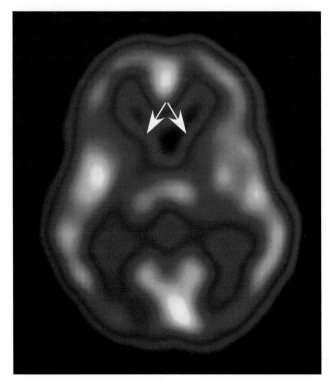

FIGURE 18.14 Using metabolic imaging to obtain prognostic information. Although magnetic resonance imaging was normal, the symptoms in this patient with Huntington disease were becoming more severe. Single photon emission computed tomography imaging showed that there was very little blood flow to the caudate nuclei (*arrows*), indicating progressing functional impairment.

Structural Imaging

CLINICAL INDICATION: CHANGE IN PREVIOUS PSYCHIATRIC SYMPTOMS

A man (in his late forties) presented with new-onset visual hallucinations, wandering from the home confused, and picking at his clothing. There was a history of mild to moderate alcohol dependence with mild cognitive slowing and intermittent auditory hallucinations in the past. He had been abstinent for several years. Extensive questioning of the family revealed a fall from a short ladder 1 month earlier with no apparent injury. MRI examination revealed a right mesial temporal lesion (see Figs. 18.8A–C). This led to a change in diagnosis from worsening alcohol-induced psychosis to partial complex (nongeneralizing) seizures from mesial temporal sclerosis secondary to the traumatic fall. Treatment for the seizures was initiated and the patient's mental status cleared.

CLINICAL INDICATIONS: NEW-ONSET PSYCHIATRIC SYMPTOMS AND DIAGNOSIS OF HEAD INJURY

A man (in his mid-thirties) presented to the emergency room due to continual nausea/vomiting. He had mild confusion and abnormal electrolytes. Inpatient medicine admission for intravenous electrolyte replacement was initiated. While on the inpatient unit, the patient began to touch staff inappropriately, had

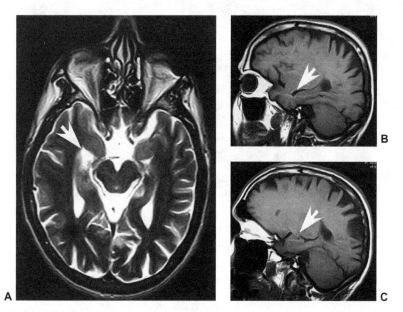

FIGURE 18.8   Using structural imaging for clarification of diagnosis following a change in symptoms. The final diagnosis in the case was changed to mesial temporal sclerosis secondary to a traumatic fall with partial complex (nongeneralizing) seizures when dilation of the tip of the right temporal horn (**A, B** *arrows*) was found upon magnetic resonance imaging examination (**A**, axial T2 weighted, **B** and **C**, sagittal T1 weighted). The normal appearance of this area is shown for comparison (**C**, *arrow*).

intermittent confusion, and exhibited bizarre behavior. A complete psychiatric evaluation confirmed these new behavioral changes and revealed a history of assault years earlier. MRI revealed a large left frontal traumatic lesion that spanned all of the prefrontal circuits (i.e., dorsolateral, orbitofrontal, cingulate) (see Figs. 18.9A,B). EEG revealed frontal status epilepticus (nongeneralizing). Diagnosis was established to be Mental Disorder Not Otherwise Specified (NOS) due to brain trauma and seizure disorder. Treatment was initiated accordingly.

CLINICAL INDICATIONS: UNUSUAL AGE OF ONSET AND COGNITIVE DECLINE
A woman (in her mid-forties) presented with new-onset mania. Specific symptoms included grandiose delusions, auditory hallucinations, rapid speech, agitation, erratic behavior, lability, disorganized thoughts, and poor insight/judgment. Initial

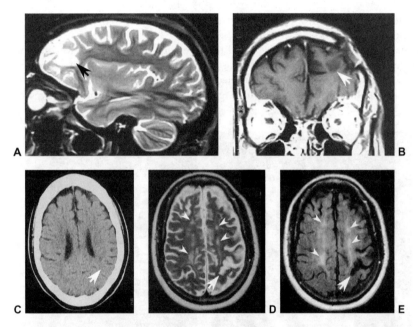

FIGURE 18.9   Using structural imaging for clarification of diagnosis with new-onset psychiatric symptoms. **A and B:** Sudden onset of bizarre behaviors. The final diagnosis in the case was established to be Mental Disorder NOS due to brain trauma and seizure disorder because of imaging and electroencephalography (EEG) findings. A large traumatic lesion was found in the left frontal lobe (**A, B** *arrows*) on imaging examination. Frontal status epilepticus was found on EEG examination. Note that the lesion is more easily identified on the T2-weighted (**A**, sagittal) than the T1-weighted (**B**, coronal) image. **C to E:** Atypical cognitive deficits. Initial imaging with computed tomography (**C**) identified an area of reduced white matter in the parietal lobe (*arrow*). Multiple areas of demyelination were present on magnetic resonance imaging examination (**D, E** *arrowheads*) in addition to the parietal atrophy (**D, E** *arrows*). The diagnosis of multiple sclerosis was confirmed by neurologic examination and lumbar puncture. Note that the lesions and atrophy are more easily identified on the fluid attenuated inversion recovery (FLAIR) (**E**, axial) than the T2-weighted (**D**, axial) image. NOS, not otherwise specified.

treatment with mood stabilizers cleared the presenting symptoms. Relapse occurred quickly. Rehospitalization revealed cognitive deficits in the presence of mania, an atypical presentation for a previously very high functioning individual. CT examination revealed an area of reduced white matter (Fig. 18.9C) and recommendation for MRI was made. Diffuse demyelination consistent with multiple sclerosis was found on MRI (Figs. 18.9D, E). A more extensive neurologic examination and lumbar puncture confirmed the diagnosis to be a pure neuropsychiatric presentation of multiple sclerosis.

CLINICAL INDICATION: SYMPTOMS OUTSIDE CLINICAL NORMS

A man (in his early forties) presented to his outpatient psychiatrist over several months with repeated reports of memory problems, auditory hallucinations, and racing thoughts. The patient had over 20 years of alcohol abuse and solvent inhalation. He was sober and stable in an outpatient alcohol rehabilitation program. The examination did not demonstrate any clinical evidence to support his reports. The patient's medications included fluoxetine, trifluroperazine, benztropine, trazodone, lithium, and famotidine. Owing to the patient's persistent reports of the symptoms mentioned in the preceding text, he was imaged. The MRI revealed significant diffuse atrophy consistent with prolonged alcohol abuse (see Fig. 18.10). The severity of the atrophy led to discontinuation of the lithium, trifluroperazine, and benztropine. The symptoms cleared. A new treatment plan was created that included very minimal doses of psychotropic medications. When required, such medications were to be dispensed in doses more closely resembling those for geriatric patients with severe dementia.

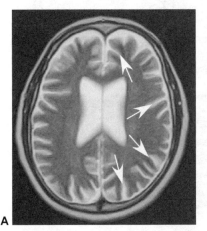 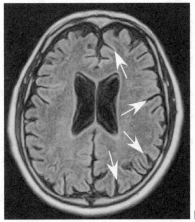

A   B

FIGURE 18.10   Using structural imaging to change the treatment plan. Incongruity between clinical examination and patient report of symptoms. Magnetic resonance imaging revealed diffuse atrophy consistent with the patient's history of alcohol abuse. Medications were modified based on the presence of these findings. Note that the atrophy is more easily identified by widening of sulci throughout cortex (*arrows*) on the fluid attenuated inversion recovery (FLAIR) (**B**, axial) than on the T2-weighted (**A**, axial) image. The ventricles are also enlarged, another indication of cortical atrophy.

CLINICAL INDICATION: PROGRESSION OF SYMPTOMS

A man (in his late forties) who was in treatment for metachromatic leukodystrophy exhibited a gradual worsening of symptoms, including disinhibition, depression, and increasing difficulties with activities of daily living. A repeat MRI was obtained to assess progression of demyelination to aid in long-term planning. The examination revealed significant worsening of the demyelination (see Fig. 18.11). Patient and family were informed.

Metabolic Imaging

CLINICAL INDICATION: COGNITIVE DECLINE

A man (in his mid-seventies) presented with mild memory loss. He was given a diagnosis of "possible early AD" and prescribed galantamine. The MRI revealed minimal diffuse atrophy. SPECT imaging revealed a pattern of hypoperfusion consistent with AD (classic bilateral parietal–occipital decreases with frontal and temporal regions intact) (see Fig. 18.12A). Case courtesy of Ronald Fisher, MD, PhD, Baylor College of Medicine.

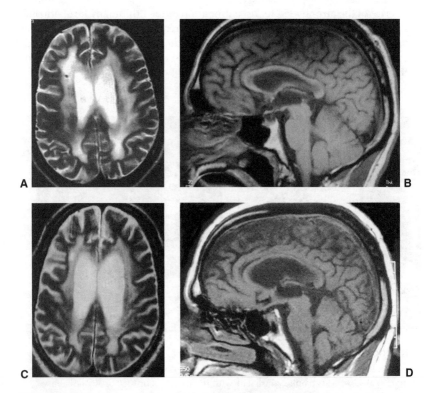

FIGURE 18.11   Using structural imaging to obtain prognostic information. Imaging examinations obtained 4 years apart from a patient with metachromatic leukodystrophy were used to assess progression. Comparison of early (**A,B**) and late (**C,D**) scans indicated significant increases in demyelination, atrophy, and ventricular enlargement.

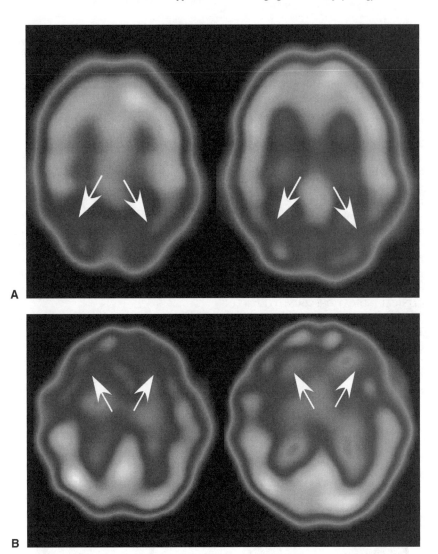

FIGURE 18.12   Using metabolic imaging for clarification of diagnosis. **A:** Mild memory loss suggested possible early Alzheimer disease (AD). Minimal diffuse atrophy identified by magnetic resonance imaging was not sufficient to make the diagnosis. Single photon emission computed tomography (SPECT) imaging of reduced blood flow in the parietal and occipital cortices (*arrows*) with preservation of blood flow in the frontal and temporal regions confirmed the diagnosis. Courtesy of Ronald Fisher, MD, PhD, Baylor College of Medicine. **B:** The symptoms were clinically atypical. SPECT imaging of reduced blood flow in the frontal lobes (*arrows*) supported a diagnosis of frontal temporal dementia (FTD, Pick) rather than AD or dementia with Lewy Bodies (DLB) (see color insert). Courtesy of Ronald Fisher, MD, PhD, Baylor College of Medicine.

CLINICAL INDICATION: COGNITIVE DECLINE

A woman (in her early fifties) presented with progressive memory loss over 1 year. Additional symptoms included increasing irritability and personality change. SPECT imaging revealed a pattern of hypoperfusion of the frontal lobes prototypic for frontal temporal dementia (Pick disease) (Fig. 18.12B). Case courtesy of Ronald Fisher, MD, PhD, Baylor College of Medicine.

CLINICAL INDICATION: SYMPTOMS OUTSIDE CLINICAL NORMS AND HEAD INJURY

A man (in his mid-forties) suffered blunt trauma to the lateral aspect of his head while working in a construction site. The patient was slightly dazed, but able to drive home. Over the next year, the patient developed a progressively more severe depression that did not respond to antidepressants. Additional symptoms included intermittent suicidal ideations and new-onset stuttering. MRI revealed a mild enlargement of the lateral sulcus of the right temporal lobe (see Fig. 18.13A). SPECT imaging revealed a greatly increased perfusion within the deep temporal lobe (right side), indicating a probable seizure focus (Fig. 18.13B). EEG did not reveal a spike-and-wave pattern (probably due to the depth of the focus). Aggressive anticonvulsant treatment cleared the mood instability and stuttering.

CLINICAL INDICATION: COGNITIVE DECLINE

A man (in his early twenties) had Huntington disease confirmed by genetic testing. The patient developed worsening of his symptoms including the aggression, depression, and choreoform movements. MRI was normal. A SPECT examination revealed minimal blood flow to the caudate nuclei, indicating significant functional impairment was present (see Fig. 18.14). The patient had a subsequent rapid deterioration over the next 3 years.

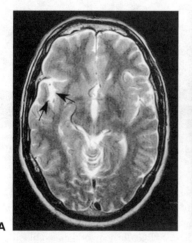 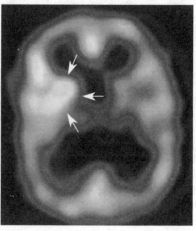

A   B

FIGURE 18.13   Using metabolic imaging to change the treatment plan. Depression unresponsive to antidepressant treatment and new-onset stuttering. Magnetic resonance imaging **(A)** revealed mild enlargement of the lateral sulcus on the right (*arrows*).
B: Single photon emission computed tomography imaging revealed an area of increased blood flow in the right temporal lobe, findings consistent with the presence of an epileptic focus (see color insert).

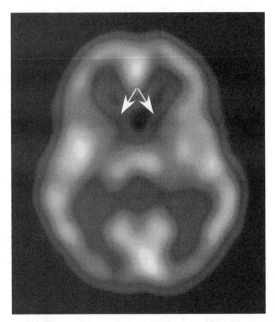

FIGURE 18.14   Using metabolic imaging to obtain prognostic information. Although magnetic resonance imaging was normal, the symptoms in this patient with Huntington disease were becoming more severe. Single photon emission computed tomography imaging showed that there was very little blood flow to the caudate nuclei (*arrows*), indicating progressing functional impairment (see color insert).

Electroencephalography

1. **Seizures (Epilepsy).** Patients with a history of epilepsy or of episodic behavioral changes suggestive of epilepsy should have thorough neurologic and EEG evaluations. The latter group includes patients with episodic dyscontrol as well as patients suffering from dissociative disorders with features resembling complex partial seizures. EEG examination is also warranted if there is a strong family history of epilepsy or if symptoms of temporal lobe syndromes exist. These include mood lability, viscosity, hyper-religiosity, episodic rage and anger, hyposexuality, and verbosity. These symptoms are frequently present in the interictal phase of temporal lobe epilepsy.

2. **Cognitive Impairment (Dementia vs. Pseudodementia).** Patients with advanced dementia rarely have a normal EEG (with the exception of frontotemporal dementia), so presence of a normal EEG can play an important role in diagnosing cases of pseudodementia (dementia secondary to depression or psychosis). In addition, the degree of EEG abnormality may be inversely related with clinical response to antidepressants when dementia and depression coexist.

3. **Acute Confusion or Disorganization.** EEG can be helpful in the acutely agitated delirious patient and can indicate whether the alteration in

consciousness is due to a diffuse encephalopathic process, a focal brain lesion, or continued epileptic activity without motor manifestations. Most often, patients with delirium have a toxic-metabolic encephalopathy. In general, with the progression of the encephalopathy there is diffuse slowing of the background rhythms from alpha (8 to 13 Hz) to theta (4 to 7.5 Hz) activity (Fig. 18.5C). Delta (<3.5 Hz) activity usually does not become prominent until the patient approaches nonresponsiveness. The major exception to the rule mentioned in the preceding text is seen during withdrawal from alcohol or during *delirium tremens.* Excessive fast activity (rather than slowing) dominates the EEG in patients with alcohol withdrawal delirium. Patients in alcohol withdrawal who are not delirious can have a normal EEG. Low-voltage fast activity can also be induced by benzodiazepines. This is essential to consider when interpreting EEGs.

4. **Episodic, Impulsive or Aggressive Behavior.** There is an increased occurrence of EEG abnormalities in borderline personality disorder patients compared with other groups of psychiatric patients (e.g., epileptic discharges over one or both temporal regions, bilateral frontal, temporal, or frontotemporal slowing, bilateral spike-and-wave discharges, paroxysmal EEG activity particularly posterior sharp waves, 14 and 6 positive spikes).[17] The prevalence of abnormal EEGs in clinic populations range widely from as low as 6.6% in patients with rage attacks and episodic violent behavior to as high as 53% in patients diagnosed with antisocial personality disorder.[18] Patients diagnosed with antisocial personality disorder also frequently harbor organic brain pathology that can be assessed with help of the EEG along with other neuro-evaluative tools. There is evidence that increased levels of violence are associated with frontotemporal asymmetry, with a greater level of delta power on the left compared with the right, as well as higher incidence of EEG and CT abnormalities. The presence of EEG abnormalities may be associated with a favorable therapeutic response to anticonvulsant medications for the treatment of aggression in mental illness. However, contrary evidence exists and this issue awaits larger, better controlled, prospective studies. Until definitive studies are available, current standard of practice is that a trial of anticonvulsant should be performed when an EEG proves to be abnormal, particularly focally and paroxysmally.

5. **Rapidly Changing Mood States (Rapid-Cycling Bipolar Disorder).** Studies have indicated that bipolar disorder and convulsive disorders may overlap.[19] Clinicians are encouraged to evaluate the EEGs of mood disorder patients for possible sharp waves and epileptiform activity. Patients presenting with a rapid-cycling bipolar disorder may exhibit epileptiform discharges (sharp waves) on EEG.[20] This may explain the reported efficacy of anticonvulsants for bipolar disorder. Similarly, some authors have described patients with "subictal" mood disorders as having paradoxical reactions to some mood-altering medications (lithium and antidepressants), with better response to anticonvulsants. These disorders are a compilation of other DSM-IV mood disorders outside of pure DSM-IV bipolar.

CONCLUSION

As the role of diagnostic testing expands, it is more and more crucial that clinicians develop the ability to evaluate the clinical utility of a diagnostic test. The field of evaluating the usefulness of diagnostic tests is indeed evolving in all branches of medicine.[21] In brief, for a test to be considered useful, a balance between the information it yields, the degree of invasiveness and discomfort associated with it, and its cost has to be evaluated. Issues of sensitivity of the test (i.e., the test's ability to detect an abnormality when one exists), specificity (the possibility of a negative test when an abnormality does not exist), and reliability (the presence of the abnormality in repeated testing), are factors that contribute to the value of the information the test provides. In the ideal world no test would be disseminated for wide clinical use until these three factors are known. Once these factors are established and a standardized method for performing the test is developed, then the value of the information yielded should be balanced against the cost and degree of invasiveness of the test. A test that yields some information (e.g., gives prognostic data without greatly influencing management) may still be worth performing if it is relatively noninvasive and of a reasonable cost. Here the judgment of a knowledgeable clinician becomes crucial. In contrast, a test that yields life saving information (e.g., cardiac catheterization) is usually recommended although the degree of invasiveness is considerable and the cost is substantial. It follows from the above that if an alternative test with either less invasiveness or lower cost can be developed to provide the same or comparable information, such an alternative should be seriously considered. Standards for reporting diagnostic tests were recently published and should serve as guides for evaluating the evidence provided in the literature for clinical applications of new or already available technology.[22]

ACKNOWLEDGMENTS

This work was supported in part by the VHA Mid-Atlantic Mental Illness, Research, Education and Clinical Center (RAH, KHT), and K24 DA000520 (NNB).

References
1. Warwick JM. Imaging of brain function using SPECT. *Metab Brain Dis.* 2004;19:113–123.
2. Erhart SM, Young AS, Marder SR, et al. Clinical utility of magnetic resonance imaging radiographs for suspected organic syndromes in adult psychiatry. *J Clin Psychiatry.* 2005;66:968–973.
3. Silver JM, Arciniegas DB, Yudofsky SC. Psychopharmacology. In: Silver JM, McAllister TW, Yudofsky SC, eds. *Textbook of traumatic brain injury.* Washington, DC: American Psychiatric Publishing, Inc.; 2005:609–639.
4. Inui K, Motomura E, Okushima R, et al. Electroencephalographic findings in patients with DSM-IV mood disorder, schizophrenia and other psychotic disorders. *Biol Psychiatry.* 1998;43:69–75.
5. Hurley RA, Hayman LA, Taber KH. Clinical imaging in neuropsychiatry. In: Yudofsky SC, Hales RE, eds. *The American psychiatric press textbook of neuropsychiatry,* 4th ed. Washington, DC: American Psychiatric Press; 2002:245–283.
6. Gupta A, Elheis M, Pansari K. Imaging in psychiatric illness. *Int J Clin Pract.* 2004;58:850–858.
7. Symms M, Jäger HR, Schmierer K, et al. A review of structural magnetic resonance neuroimaging. *J Neurol Neurosurg Psychiatry.* 2004;75:1235–1244.

8. Frankle WG, Laruelle M. Neuroreceptor imaging in psychiatric disorders. *Ann Nucl Med*. 2002;16:437–446.
9. Parsey RV, Mann JJ. Applications of positron emission tomography in psychiatry. *Semin Nucl Med*. 2003;33:129–135.
10. Dougall NJ, Bruggink S, Ebmeier KP. Systematic review of the diagnostic accuracy of 99mTc-HMPAO-SPECT in dementia. *Am J Geriatr Psychiatry*. 2004;12:554–570.
11. Anderson KE, Taber KH, Hurley RA. Functional imaging. In: Silver JM, McAllister TW, Yudofsky SC, eds. *Textbook of traumatic brain injury*. Washington DC: American Psychiatric Press; 2005:107–133.
12. Newberg AB, Alavi A. The role of PET imaging in the management of patients with central nervous system disorders. *Radiol Clin North Am*. 2005;43:49–65.
13. Struve F, Boutros NN. Somatic implications of generalized and/or focal slowing in psychiatric patients. *Clin EEG Neurosci*. 2005;36:171–175.
14. Boutros NN, Struve F. Electrophysiological assessment of neuropsychiatric disorders. *Semin Clin Neuropsychiatry*. 2002;7:30–41.
15. Zumsteg D, HungerBühler H, Wieser H. *Atlas of adult electroencephalography*. Bad Honnef, Germany: Hippocampus-Verlag; 2004.
16. Jeon YW, Polich J. Meta-analysis of P300 and schizophrenia: Patients, paradigms, and practical implications. *Psychophysiology*. 2003;40:684–701.
17. Boutros NN, Torello M, McGlashan TH. Electrophysiological aberrations in Borderline Personality Disorder: State of the evidence. *J Neuropsychiatry Clin Neurosci*. 2003;15:145–154.
18. Riley T, Neidermeyer E. Rage attacks and episodic violent behavior: Electroencephalographic findings and general considerations. *Clin Electroencephalogr*. 1978;9:131–139.
19. Hughes J, John E. Conventional and quantitative electroencephalography in psychiatry. *J Neuropsychiatry Clin Neurosci*. 1999;11:190–208.
20. Levy AB, Drake ME, Shy KE. EEG evidence of epileptiform paroxysms in rapid cycling bipolar patients. *J Clin Psychiatry*. 1988;49:232–234.
21. Bruns DE. The STARD initiative and the reporting of studies of diagnostic accuracy. *Clin Chemistry*. 2003;49:19–20.
22. Bussuyt PM, Reitsma JB, Bruns DE. Towards complete and accurate reporting of studies of diagnostic accuracy: The STARD initiative. *Clin Chemistry*. 2003;49:1–6.

Index

Note: Page numbers followed by f indicate figures; those followed by t indicate tables.